Praise for Ramel Rones . . .

"A wonderful and practical approach to Tai Chi & Chi Kung, that can correct stress-related illnesses. By a highly respected Master Teacher."

> Herbert Benson, M.D. Harvard Medical School,
> Benson-Henry Institute for Mind Body Medicine.
> Author of the *The Relaxation Response*

"Ramel Rones has long been at the forefront in integrating the powerful health benefits of Tai Chi and Qigong into Western medicine. *Sunset Tai Chi* makes an essential contribution to that effort. In his dedication to nurturing the mind, body and spirit of people everywhere, Ramel honors the true Tai Chi tradition and serves as a valuable bridge between East and West."

> Yang Yang, Ph.D.
> Author of Taijiquan: *The Art of Nurturing,*
> *The Science of Power*

"This book is a gift to anyone interested in maximizing his or her health. Practicing Chi Kung or Tai Chi with Ramel Rones is an energizing and enlightening experience. His guidance empowers people to take control of their lives, develop their resiliency, increase their zest, and improve their physical and emotional well-being. He is also great fun.

Recent research has demonstrated the importance of mind/body techniques, like Ramel's Sunrise and Sunset Tai Chi, for people with challenging conditions such as fibromyalgia and osteoarthritis. My cancer patients, who attend his classes, report increased stamina and improved sleep and mood. I am recommending this book to everyone."

> Ann Webster, Ph.D.
> Director, Mind Body Program for Cancer, and Staff
> Psychologist at the Benson-Henry Institute
> for Mind Body Medicine, Massachusetts General
> Hospital

"Ramel Rones is a pioneer in the development of mind/body/Tai Chi interventions for patients with chronic illness. His work is a cornerstone of our integrative oncology mission and allows us to offer our patients the best supportive care available today. Hundreds of our patients and staff have benefited from his expert instruction and now by reading *Sunset Tai Chi,* everyone can learn the practical exercises, meditations, and visualizations that he teaches. I strongly believe that no integrative therapies library would be complete without the important works of Ramel Rones."

Anne Doherty-Gilman, MPH
Associate Director
Dana-Farber Cancer Institute

SUNSET TAI CHI

SUNSET TAI CHI

SIMPLIFIED TAI CHI FOR RELAXATION AND LONGEVITY

Ramel Rones

with
David Silver

YMAA Publication Center
Wolfeboro, N.H., USA

YMAA Publication Center
 Main Office: PO Box 480
 Wolfeboro, NH 03894
 1-800-669-8892 • www.ymaa.com • info@ymaa.com

ISBN-13: 978-1-59439-212-2
ISBN-10: 1-59439-212-9

Cover design by Axie Breen
Edited by Susan Bullowa

Illustrations by Ilana Rosenberg-Rones

10 9 8 7 6 5 4 3 2 1

Publisher's Cataloging in Publication

Rones, Ramel.

Sunset tai chi : simplified tai chi for relaxation and longevity / Ramel
Rones with David Silver ; forewords by Irwin H. Rosenberg, Yang,
Jwing-Ming. -- Wolfeboro, N.H. : YMAA Publication Center, c2011.

p. ; cm.

ISBN: 13-digit: 978-1-59439-212-2 ; 10-digit: 1-59439-212-9
"Relax and rejuvenate your mind, body, and spirit"--Cover.
Companion publication to the author's "Sunrise tai chi" (2007).
Includes bibliographical references and index.

1. Tai chi. 2. Chronic diseases--Exercise therapy. 3. Relaxation.
4. Stress management. 5. Breathing exercises. 6. Physical fitness.
7. Mind and body. 8. Health. 9. Longevity. I. Silver, David. II. Title.

GV504 .R662 2011   2011925485
613.7/148--dc22   1101

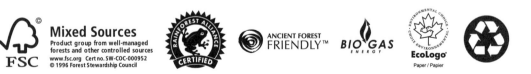

Printed in Canada

Contents

Romanization of Chinese Terms

This book uses a mixture of both the Pinyin and Wade-Giles methods of Romanizing Chinese words. Usage is based on the mainstream popularity of each term, but the authors also aim to educate the reader by offering both Wade-Giles and Pinyin for many terms. Most terms in this glossary are presented only in Pinyin. Similarly, in some cases, the more popular spelling of a word may be used for clarity.

Some common conversions:

Pinyin	Also Spelled As	Pronunciation
Qi	Chi	chē
Qigong	Chi Kung	chē göng
Qin Na	Chin Na	chǐn nǎ
Jin	Jing	jǐn
Gongfu	Kung Fu	göng foo
Taijiquan	Tai Chi Chuan	tī jē chüén

The authors and publisher have taken the liberty of not italicizing words of foreign origin in this text. The decision was made to make the text easier to read. Please see the glossaries for definitions of Chinese words.

Foreword
by Dr. Irwin H. Rosenberg, M.D.

With the release of *Sunset Tai Chi* as a sequel to his bestselling *Sunrise Tai Chi*, Mind/Body Master Teacher Ramel Rones closes with the setting sun on this self-empowering series. This pair of brilliantly explained and illustrated books (with matching DVDs) makes essential reading and use for all those interested in learning to take control of their own centers—physical and spiritual.

As we as individuals, as a nation, and as a population interested in fitness over 40, accept our responsibility to practice a life style which assures health for decades to come, we must accept the fact that physical activity is an essential component of that healthy life style for longevity. We need a greater understanding and adoption of practices such as regular exercise but *principally* the kind of activity that will ensure flexibility, balance of body and mind, and physical resilience for decades. No activity is more important than preservation of flexibility and balance than the stretching and balance postures that are embedded in the Tai Chi/Chi Kung/Yoga approaches of the Eastern arts as described in this book by Master Ramel Rones. No other guide will be more important for the practitioner of active, sportive life.

Ramel's teaching empowers individuals to take control of their lives and evokes faith and belief in times of health, especially when encountering illness. This knowledge of Chi Kung and Tai Chi is one of the ways to achieve better quality of life but most importantly can be used as a preventive approach to better health and higher mental and physical performance. The balanced approach that is presented in this book allows individuals to use this knowledge to improve their bodies, minds, energy, and spirit.

Recent reports in peer-reviewed medical journals confirm the importance of mind-body approaches like Ramel's Sunrise and Sunset Tai Chi programs to disease management as well as health maintenance. When well applied, these techniques can add greatly to our capacity to treat even very challenging conditions like osteoarthritis, fibromyalgia, aging, and even cancer.

This ancient knowledge of using the setting sun to dissolve and cleanse the body from physical and mental stress is rarely taught and is unique to the Eastern arts as well as to this book.

Irwin H. Rosenberg, M.D.
Distinguished University Professor of Medicine and Nutrition, Tufts University
Formerly Director of the USDA Human Nutrition Research Center on Aging at
Tufts University and Dean of the Friedman School of Nutrition

Foreword
by Dr. Yang, Jwing-Ming, Ph.D.

This foreword is written on behalf of Mr. Ramel Rones, one of my senior students, who, as my disciple, is authorized to carry on my teachings. Ramel has been my student for over 20 years. He had moved to the United States from Israel in 1983 to pursue training at my YMAA academy in Boston. It is at the academy and in my in-depth training seminars conducted at academy affiliates nationally and internationally that his main learning took place. Many of my teachings come from my intensive training with my own teachers in Taiwan. These teachings have been reinforced and supplemented through my reading and translation of previously unknown (to the Western society) ancient Chinese texts on meditation, martial arts, and on qigong (the science of human energy) as filtered through my academic training in physics and mechanical engineering (in which I hold a Ph.D. from Purdue University). Ramel's training at the YMAA academy has been deeply ingrained with knowledge of ancient, traditional practices including Chi Kung (Qigong), Tai Chi (Taijiquan), Long Fist, White Crane, Chin Na (Qin Na), meditation, and various weapons, with the focus of analyzing these arts from a Western scientific perspective.

I accepted Ramel as one of my disciples in 1995. Ramel has traveled to YMAA branches in Poland, France, and elsewhere where he has led successful, intensive workshops and summer sessions, and administered tests of skill in taijiquan and kung fu (gongfu). I personally witnessed Ramel winning numerous gold medals, and national and international competitions in North America and in China in both internal and external martial arts. The owner of YMAA Publications, Mr. David Ripianzi has been so impressed with his teaching that he has filmed a series of instructional health and martial arts DVDs created by and featuring Ramel. The first DVD *Sunrise Tai Chi* was published in the spring of 2005 and since then has been published as a best-selling book on Amazon.com within the tai chi category.

Ramel's dedication and focus are notable: I have witnessed his growth from a young martial artist to an accomplished martial arts teacher, healer, and researcher who is able to translate the Eastern healing arts into terms that are accessible and understandable by Western patients of cancer, arthritis, and fibromyalgia as well as physicians and investigators. As a healer, he has worked with numerous students of mine who have been challenged with life-threatening diseases. In speaking with these students, I have been impressed with the way he has been able to take Eastern teachings and apply them specifically to the needs of each student. I am also impressed with the way his instruction has strengthened my students' confidence, optimism, and quality of life.

Ramel Rones is a certified qigong and tai chi instructor and a Tai Chi Master, obtaining his final certifications as a full instructor in 2009 from the YMAA/YMAA CA Retreat Center. He received his qigong certificate instructorship on April 11, 2009, and his certification as a Tai Chi Master on December 20, 2008, as a result of his extensive training and capabilities.

I am very pleased to write this foreword for Ramel. I am confident that he, as well as his books, will bring the same diligence and passion for the healing traditions of the Eastern arts to his work with the various diseases as well as with cancer patients in hospital settings as I have witnessed during his studies with me. I also believe that the bridge he is building linking Eastern practices with Western clinical science is of critical importance and will benefit patients, as well as all complementary and holistic practitioners and researchers. It is without any reservation whatsoever that I enthusiastically give Ramel my highest recommendation.

Dr. Yang, Jwing-Ming
President, YMAA International

Dedication

This book is dedicated to my funny, smart, good-hearted late father, Arie Rones, and my wise, open-minded, balanced, loving mother, Zicria Zakay Rones.

My sincere and full acknowledgements conclude this book on page 417.

Introduction

The things we hear most frequently from new students coming to qigong and tai chi classes are: "I can't relax," "I can't sleep," "I'm too tense," "I have a hard time changing pace," or "I cannot wind down." The pace of activity in modern life is accelerating rapidly. We are inundated with stimuli and information constantly on television, on the Internet, and during our daily interactions. For our jobs, our brains need, more than ever, to stay for long periods of time in a highly-concentrated state—a must for success in the competitive world in which we live. An unfortunate side effect is the toll this level of performance takes on our health and quality of life. Our employers benefit and so does production, but the price we pay may not be worth it in the long run. I am a strong believer in modernization. I love the new-age gadgets, as well as the developments in both medicine and technology, but I am also a strong believer in recognizing what we lose and in trying to incorporate the important principles for better health and improved physical and mental performance. Cars, for example, are a wonderful convenience, but as a result, we do not walk enough. It is important to find time to walk or we will have to deal with muscle and bone loss. Recognizing what we lose when we use modern conveniences will help us find effective ways to address that loss and will allow us the best of both worlds.

The racing mind at the end of the day is part of the game. If you keep thinking and concentrating on your problems for hours, you will experience difficulty in cooling down when you are finished working. Pure instinct tells us to cool down and take a break so we will be ready for the next day. In reality, this break does not always happen. Some people cannot change their working and racing minds into calm, recuperative minds until eleven at night, even when they finish work at six or seven in the evening. Some can only let go by using various substances such as alcohol or other legal and illegal drugs. Some people sit and vegetate in front of the television. These are some of the common ways to change the brain waves from the alpha state with its very active focus to the theta state that is between awake and asleep, the relaxed, healing, and rejuvenating state of mind. There are other methods that are a little more healthful and give you more than just a change in your brain waves. These also give you other benefits, e.g., reading a good book, or exercising, going for a walk or other sports, or just pure joy, such as playing with the kids and maybe your wife.

But even knowing and performing all those techniques and various methods, many still have a difficult time changing pace, falling asleep, and getting a good night's rest. That is the motivation behind this book. This book offers you mind/body exercises and a tai chi program, which together with the powerful pulling energy of the setting sun can facilitate the body and the mind to change more easily between the various brain wave states. This change will not happen overnight. You need to determine the time and the place to practice. The optimal length of time for this practice should be between 15 to 45 minutes and the place you practice should be quiet and peaceful, not too warm or cold, and definitely have no distractions, such as cell phones, Blackberries, or annoying sounds or people.

There are many ways to achieve this skill of fluctuating with control between the various mood stages or brain waves. The best method, the one I like the most, is sunset meditation that coordinates the energy of the setting of the sun and the power of the brain, both dissolving and melting. One encourages the other. On the days you do not use the setting sun, use the mind/body program as well as the tai chi routines in this book. On the days you are very busy, some of the visualizations or just doing work on your breathing will go a long way. Over time and through practice, you will be able to change between the brain wave states more quickly and easily, and learn to relax deeply. This change will translate to a much more relaxed evening, a better night's sleep, and enhanced performance, both physically and mentally, the next day.

How to Use This Book

In order to obtain the full benefits of this book, first read through it thoughoughly and completely so that you understand the theory. Become familiar with what I call the 'mind/body prescriptions.' If you have read the *Sunrise Tai Chi* book or watched the DVD, some of the basic preparation exercises and visualizations will be a repeat for you. In *Sunset Tai Chi*, another layer has been added to keep you stimulated and interested. These skills cannot be excluded for they are the basis for understanding the new techniques. For example, the mind/body prescription Zen mind is as essential a practice before any work is done with raising your energy system as it is for the visualizations evoking spirituality, and the relaxation techniques on which this program focuses. You will find that both programs work together and can provide you with a complete and effective mind/body practice for the entire day. They are an outline for your own effective daily practice. Approach the techniques as if it is the first time. These are fundamental skills that ultimately we all should be constantly mindful of, not only during our scheduled tai chi practice. Remember that the goal is to make both the physical and the mental skills you will learn in both books a regular daily behavior. As a result, at the end of the day you will BE it, instead of only practicing it.

Within the Sunrise and Sunset Tai Chi, you are also learning 16 of the movements common to most tai chi forms. The traditional long Yang-style Tai Chi Chuan (Taijiquan) form is comprised of 37 postures for a total of 108 movements. Although Sunset Tai Chi is a short form, the movements are derived from authentic Yang-style Tai Chi Chuan that will give you a correct foundation. By learning both the Sunrise and Sunset Tai Chi forms you are about halfway to learning the traditional long forms. If your goal is to relax, improve your health, learn to manage your energy, and feel good, then either of the Sunrise or Sunset programs will provide you with the more than enough skills needed.

When you first begin training, practice the physical skills separately from the mental visualizations. Work on the mental exercises, and even if you do not *feel* it, continue the practice. Try moving away from 'feeling' it to more of 'sensing' it. Over time, the internal skills taught in this program will reveal themselves to you. The more you tune in to yourself, the more you will begin to notice small details in your practice. Train the various physical and mental skills individually until you sense that it is time to put them together.

Develop your skill in the 'art of using 80% of your effort.' Do not stretch so far that it inhibits your breathing. Do not breathe so deeply that it inhibits your movement. Inhale deeply and fill your lungs to 80%. Learn to recognize when you are stretching too far or too little. Learn to know how many repetitions are too many and when you are not doing enough, and learn to know how long you should spend doing an exercise. Learn to let go and not to be too hard on yourself. All of the above recommendations pertain to learning to train at your 80% effort. There is a lot more to this concept than you might think. I challenge you to think about it and develop your ability to use this skill. Progress slowly and naturally. Do not strain or make yourself uncomfortable.

Being able to visualize three or four visualizations at once is not easy. It is a process that takes time. Do not overload your brain. Give yourself time to learn this skill. For beginners, it is natural, when you are trying to put your mind in the energy centers, for other thoughts to steal your mind away from staying focused on the visualization. When you realize a thought has taken your attention, visualize looping your attention, first into the breath, because the breath is 'nothing.' Follow the breath in and out. Stay on top of it the same way you stay on a surfboard, and then get back to the visualization. Move your mind in through the third eye, straight through the spiritual valley and down into the pituitary gland area; connect into the baton in the center of your body, and then lead your mind down into the lower energy center two inches below your belly button or what I call the center of gravity energy center. This trick of using your breath to empty your mind from any thoughts I refer to as 'surfing the breath.'

Remember that using the influence of the setting sun is the main concept of this book, but often your practice will happen during other hours. It is still beneficial to practice whenever you have the time. The more you practice, the more benefits you will derive when you have the opportunity to use the setting sun. Once you develop these internal skills of 'listening' inside the body, i.e., feeling your energy and a strong sensation of your energy centers, you can gradually mix these skills with stretches, stances, tai chi drills, and the Sunset Tai Chi form.

Study the theory and as you continue to practice, refer often to the detailed instructions until you have a strong understanding of the various exercises, the separate tai chi movements, and the tai chi form. Be careful especially at the start to build good habits. Practice the tai chi drills and the form to the left and right equally to develop the symmetry of your mind and body.

One of the main objectives of this program is to free your skeleton from being a prisoner of the soft tissue by stretching and loosening your physical body while using the knowledge in the book as well as the power of the setting sun. If you cannot perform certain physical skills, it is often because the muscles and tendons are restricted from lack of use or insufficient stretching that will in turn restrict the full range of motion of your skeleton. After you have developed strength and flexibility in the muscles and tendons, and regain a healthier range of motion and correct alignment, the quality of your life will change tremendously.

Evoke your spirit in each exercise while maintaining a meditative state, which means to relax deeply so that your brain waves shift to the meditative state between being awake and asleep, and then bring in a sense of spirituality. I like to visualize the spirit of nature, the earth spirit, a sensation of the earth beneath me, the mountains, trees, and oceans around me, and heaven above me. If you are interested in evoking spirituality using your personal religious visualizations, you are more than welcome to do so. One of my students visualizes the three angels, Gabriel, Daniel, and Samuel, coming down and holding their wings around her. Another student, who is a priest, told me that he visualizes the internal energetic baton as the light or the rod of God. Who am I to argue with this concept? I sincerely thanked him, and told him that he had brought me to a deeper sensation with this visualization.

Sunrise Tai Chi emphasized drawing the morning energy of the sun inward and charging every cell of your body with clean, natural energy. It is a special routine for the morning that supports having an enjoyable, healthy, and productive day. As the title indicates, the Sunset Tai Chi program involves connecting to the sun's energy as it sets, or at any time after 2 P.M. Later in the day, the natural energy outside is waning, and you can gradually allow this setting energy to dissolve stress, tension, or any problem or trauma that is stored in the physical or energetic body. I refer to all of it as impurities. The force of the setting sun reinforces your mind power to draw out and release the impurities from your body. Together with the mind/body program and the tai chi form, you will have the perfect mind/body prescriptions to finish the day and start the evening so you are fresh and ready for the next day. This ancient practice of connecting with the forces of nature, especially the sun, and utilizing those forces for health and prevention, is a powerful and effective meditation skill, which every individual should learn, practice, and enjoy.

Sitting Tai Chi. Tai chi and the mind/body prescriptions can be done sitting as well as standing. Sit using correct alignment: lengthen the spine, drop your shoulders, relax your face as well as your groin, breathe deeply, and relax. Sitting tai chi is good for those who are unable to stand or for those interested in refining the training by first isolating the upper part of the body. Training on the edge of a chair offers many benefits for beginners and for more advanced students because doing so restricts movement and causes the practitioner to focus on fine-tuning certain aspects that are needed in the body, breath, mind, energy, and spirit. These five building blocks are discussed in detail, beginning at the end of Chapter 1. (The *Sunset Tai Chi* DVD presents a complete sitting workout that you may follow. Try practicing the cool-down exercises and the tai chi drills and form both ways, standing and sitting, to experience the value of this training.)

Tai Chi—Grand Ultimate

WHAT IS TAI CHI?

About the Internal Arts

For centuries, tai chi chuan (taijiquan) has been a practice acknowledged to promote deep relaxation and excellent health, to prevent injuries and illness, and sometimes to reach higher levels of skill in martial arts. This gentle, moving meditation helps you balance strength and flexibility, offers a low-impact workout, and engages all of the various soft tissues in your body: muscles, tendons, ligaments, fasciae, and skin. When practicing the low stances, you maintain or increase your range of motion through your joints, as well as build bone density.

Commonly known by its abbreviated name, tai chi (taiji) practice improves the circulation of blood and qi (energy) that enhances the body's natural healing capabilities. In addition to learning fundamental tai chi stances and postures, these body-conditioning exercises also help you to increase muscle mass, while the gentle movements continually massage your internal organs, leading to increased flow of blood and oxygen through every cell in your body. Tai chi is an excellent way to improve your quality of life and daily physical performance. You learn to optimize your internal energy use and to allow the natural energy from your surroundings to rejuvenate your body. Relaxation is an essential key to successful practice and should be the primary goal of students new to tai chi. Wherever there is tension in your body, your energetic circulation is stagnant or blocked. Therefore, the primary aspect of studying any internal art is relaxing the entire body, first and foremost.

So many books focus on only one aspect of tai chi, the form. This approach can sometimes give the reader an incomplete understanding. It is important that you have a basic overview of the true meaning of the ancient art of tai chi chuan. Many people believe that tai chi is a kind of 'New Age' exercise for health, but in fact, tai chi is a Chinese philosophy that dates back at least 5,000 years. Some recent archaeological findings suggest that the yin-yang concept of balance and harmony, which is the root of this philosophy, may be over 10,000 years old. This concept predates the moving art of tai chi chuan by many thousands of years.

The yin-yang theory of tai chi philosophy is based on the idea that everything in the universe is created, developed, and constantly changing due to the interaction, balance, and imbalance of yin and yang, which can be described as any two opposing forces, such as light/dark, cold/hot, or force/yielding. This concept of constant change and yin-yang balance is an approach to understanding the laws of nature, and the universe itself.

Tai chi chuan is often shortened to tai chi, but the practitioner should be clear about the distinction between the martial art of tai chi chuan and the more ancient tai chi philosophy. Tai chi, which translates as grand ultimate, is the creative force that lies between wuji, the state of no extremity, and yin-yang, the state of discrimination. In tai chi chuan, this creative force is the mind, the origin of all movement and therefore the origin of all yin-yang in the body. The tai chi philosophy was later blended with several ancient physical exercises and martial arts forms to create a new martial art style known as tai chi chuan, or grand ultimate fist.

Lao Tzu, an older contemporary of Confucius, wrote and taught Taoist (Daoist) philosophy in the province of Hunan in the sixth century B.C. The classic collection of ancient writings attributed to him, the *Tao Te Ching* (*Dao De Jing*), or *The Way of Virtue*, offers insightful discussions of the Taoist philosophies that lie in the heart of tai chi chuan, such as yin/yang, two opposite extremes, and wuji, a place of no extremities.

The essential principles of tai chi chuan can be traced back thousands of years to ancient Chinese health exercises and to classical yoga in India. As early as the fourth century B.C., Life-Nourishing Techniques (Yangsheng) were being practiced. These techniques included bending, expanding, condensing, and extending movements; breathing techniques; and qi circulation methods similar to the later internal aspects of tai chi.

These ancient exercises and breathing techniques, known as Dao Yin and Tu Na, were created to adjust the imbalance of qi energy in the body, to build more energy, and to increase adaptability to the natural changes in the environment. Dao Yin is the art of guiding the energy in the pathways of the body to achieve harmony, and of stretching the body to "massage" the qi pathways in order to reduce qi energy stagnation and to attain flexibility. Tu Na is the art of breathing that was taught and studied in the Buddhist Shaolin and Wudang monasteries.

Many people ask in class, "What's the difference between qigong and tai chi?" There is a simple answer: tai chi is qigong, but qigong is not necessarily tai chi. Qigong is the cultivation of your qi energy in the body. Tai chi is a form of qigong, but its movements may also be applied at full speed as a martial art. Tai chi is martial gong. It is a form of qigong that is designed for both health and martial arts. Both medical qigong and tai chi emphasize the power of the mind and the importance of cultivating energy and evoking our spirituality. Many of the internal skills are acquired through meditation.

Qigong is the study (gong) of human energy (qi). It embodies a total system of physical, mental, and spiritual exercises that deal with different aspects of our being. Many popular qigong exercises were developed as long as 2,500 years ago.

Qigong was developed in China and has evolved into four major schools of thought:

1. Scholar Qigong or Confucius Qigong: Ethical development, refinement of personal temperament, and self-cultivation

2. Martial Qigong: Enhancement and development of the strength, endurance, and spirit of the warrior

3. Medical Qigong: Improvement of quality of life. Complements Western treatments. Relieves symptoms of illness

4. Religious Qigong: Divided into two schools—Taoist and Buddhist

   Taoist: Cultivation of physical body and spirit, merging with nature to achieve longevity and immortality

   Buddhist: Spiritual cultivation as a way to reach enlightenment, freedom from the cycle of life and death

Tai chi is a martial qigong. It is a form of qigong that is designed for both health and martial arts. Both medical qigong and tai chi emphasize the power of the mind and the importance of cultivating energy and evoking our spirituality. Many of the internal skills are acquired through sitting, standing, or moving meditation.

Often, people memorize a tai chi or qigong sequence of movements without learning the internal skills, which are the essence of the art. However, it is through these skills that deeper benefits arise. Your health will improve, your balance will improve, your energy will increase, and your mind and spirit will become more focused and clear. The goal is to make these subtle internal skills as easy as possible for you to understand so you may enjoy these benefits in your daily life, rather than focus on the external forms and becoming frustrated by trying to memorize dozens of intricate tai chi movements. First and foremost, you must learn to relax, and then through practice, you will master the internal skills, after which you can learn external moves and various forms.

My Journey in the Healing Arts

My Involvement in Tai Chi and Complementary Medicine

Since I wrote a detailed history of Tai Chi in *Sunrise Tai Chi,* I decided to write a different history for this book, which describes my personal journey thoughts, and some important principles as I developed through the martial arts world and into the growing world of complementary medicine and its recognition and acceptance by health care providers and patients.

In my work with the Dana Farber Cancer Institute and the Harvard and Tufts medical school research departments, I have seen tremendous changes in relation to the methods, techniques, and goals of health care. There is a growing awareness within health institutes and by individuals of the effectiveness of alternative or complementary medicine. The unique wisdom developed through thousands of years of experience of the Eastern healing arts and the modern profound knowledge of Western medicine are coming together to offer us the best of the two worlds. When weaving the two approaches into one tailored health care, we are not only increasing our chances of success in defeating disease, we are also adding a preventative element to our concept of health. This combination will not only improve health care, it will save millions of dollars for everyone involved. It is empowering individuals to become positive and to take an active role in their journey toward better health. This effort will tremendously improve the physical and mental performance of everyone involved, and soon health, nutrition, mind/body, and spirit will be covered by one comprehensive holistic health care system.

Practice, Practice, and More Practice

I came to Boston in 1983 with a suitcase and $1,200. My goal was to study martial arts with a Chinese master whose book I had read. At the time, I was serving in the Israeli Army. Before the army, I had practiced Chinese martial arts with an American from the New York area who taught both Zen and the internal and external Chinese martial arts. His name was "Tzvi" Harold Weisberg, and he had studied in New York in a Zen monastery. We three or four Israeli friends would train a few times a week for three to four hours. After four years of training, Tzvi told me that if I was interested in furthering my study in the martial arts, I should find an authentic Chinese master who would be able to teach me the entire philosophy. I was fortunate to have studied with Zen master, Tzvi. He is very unique: he has the ability of an enlightened individual to first recognize the truth without being selfish and second, to let go.

So there I was, knocking on Master Yang, Jwing-Ming's door after an 19-hour flight from Israel. When he opened the door, he could not believe that I was on his doorstep. Our only prior contact was a letter I had sent a month before. He never thought that I would come to study with him, especially because he was halfway across the world.

I started training every day from 8 A.M. to noon and took a break for four hours so I could go to work to make money and pay the bills so I could keep training. I would come back at 4 P.M. and keep practicing until 9 P.M. On Saturdays, we would practice from 8 A.M. to noon, take a two-hour break, and then get back in the studio from 2 to 5 P.M. I loved Saturdays because there were always special training and special individuals to meet, like visiting masters of other martial art styles.

Within a few years, I realized that I did not have time to work because the training took so much out of me. In order to dedicate myself entirely to the Chinese arts, I started to offer massage and help to individuals who were looking to improve their martial arts. Very quickly, I realized that there is little money to be made in the martial arts world, and before I knew it, I was utilizing my knowledge of the mind and body to help individuals outside of the martial arts world heal an injury or deal with health problems that were not responding to the Western approach, which promotes pills and more pills or pharmaceutical solutions, and then some surgery.

It is not easy to go against the pharmaceutical industry and its pills. One of my dear family members who has reached a very high-level position in the pharmaceutical world told me, "Rami, we do not want you to succeed." Also, because I was doing qigong and working with energy, many individuals thought that this energy work was some kind of miracle. I guess the mysteries of the unknown led certain individuals to believe that I could help their dying family members and friends.

The Early 1980s

I would receive phone calls from individuals explaining that their loved ones were at their last days of life—especially people with cancer. The individuals who called me expected miracles. Of course, I would tell them that I could not reverse the situation, but I could make the last stretch more comfortable and help the patients die feeling empowered. I would be straightforward and talk honestly to those patients about their feelings. Were they afraid to die? Did they have any pain from symptoms or being bed-ridden? We would talk about their death and their pain. When we talked about death, they felt better. We even came up with ideas such as recording messages to be played on their children's birthdays after they had passed away. It empowered their spirit to have something positive to do with their death. On the physical level, some stretching helped the lower back and neck, which becomes stiff from being in bed for so many hours. Some deep breathing helped quiet the mind and gave them a small break from constant fear and negative thoughts. Evoking spirituality with various visualizations put them in a different place and gave them some strength for a short time.

I remember wishing to have more time with those individuals because I saw that even in the short time we spent together that symptoms abated. In the five or six years of working with this population, some of the individuals who were supposed to die would come around and improve, which was considered by their doctors and families to be a miracle. I just saw it as the power of the mind. Because time was of the essence and I could not reverse a health problem that had taken a long time to form in only a short time, only a few survived. Most of them died, but through their practice, spiritually and physically, they had a better death, if one can understand that concept.

THE HUNGER FOR COMPLEMENTARY MEDICINE

More and more people are now using alternative medicine. or what is accepted as complementary medicine to treat problems for which Western doctors have no clear solution, and as complementary medicine to various Western treatments. Methods such as acupuncture, herbs, massage, qigong, tai chi, and yoga are growing in popularity. Some find different ways to evoke their spirituality. It was not that long ago, however, that many Western doctors did not even know that their patients were tapping into all these alternative/complementary methods. A large number of patients thought their doctors would not approve or understand alternative approaches, so they did not tell them. Mostly, doctors did not think that anything other than proven Western approaches would work. I am not telling you how and why alternative or complementary methods work, but I can tell you that a negative attitude and lack of belief from doctors does not allow even a small chance for activating the placebo effect, which could be one explanation for some of the success of the alternative or complementary approaches. Like my mother keeps telling me, "If it does not hurt you, try it."

In the 1970s, the U.S. Senate was approached by a large group of lobbyists who represented alternative approaches. Afterward, the Senate asked doctors to consider research on other ways of treatment. The doctors came back and told the National Institute of Health (NIH) that all positive outcomes were the result of the placebo effect and there was no legitimacy to any other method besides the Western approach. Five or ten years went by and more and more people tried alternative approaches. Life and history sways from side to side. The point was reached where some individuals would not use Western approaches at all and would use only alternative medicine, thereby creating a dangerous situation. For example, certain individuals would not be vaccinated against specific diseases, putting all of us at risk. However, the ongoing pressure from individuals who were using alternative methods eventually forced the Senate to recognize that there is more to better health than only the Western approach.

In the early 1990s, the Senate ordered the NIH to research and investigate alternative methods, and validate or prove which approaches worked and which did not. In 1998, a new division opened at the NIH called the National Center for Alternative and Complementary Medicine (NCCAM). (The common usage today has changed from 'alternative' to 'complementary.' A major reason for this change was that alternative symbolizes a different approach, which may scare away certain patients and may put the Western doctors in a difficult position.)

At first, entire methodologies were put together: acupuncture with herbs and the mind/body exercise, but after a short time, researchers realized that the methodologies should be separated into different parts in order to understand the whole. Acupuncture was separated from mind/body approaches, and the herbs got their own division. In the year 2000, 13 billion dollars were spent on out-of-pocket expenses for complementary approaches. In 2008, 34 billion dollars were spent.

Now, many doctors prescribe complementary approaches for their patients and probably the same number of patients has tried complementary approaches at one point or another. Many institutes are offering complementary approaches in their facilities. Places like the Dana Farber Cancer Institute have their own complementary divisions; at Dana Farber it is called the Zakim Center. Massachusetts General Hospital has the Benson–Henry Mind/Body Institute, and the same is happening at John Hopkins Cancer Institute. The NCCAM Funding History from 1992 to 2008 shows that in 1992, two million dollars was spent on research with complementary approaches, while in 2008 it was almost 13 billion dollars.

If you go to the NIH website and search for tai chi grants, out of the 11 grants, two are grants that I am involved with. I designed and implemented the intervention under the supervision of my principal investigator Doctor Chenchen Wang from Tufts University School of Medicine.

If you are interested in reading how we go about bringing the Eastern and Western healing methods together, go to my website, http://www.ramelrones.com for a complete list of our research.

My Role

From the beginning, I divided the practice into two main categories: passive complementary and active complementary therapy. When you are on a table and being treated by someone else, you are experiencing passive complementary therapy. When you are doing the action yourself, you are practicing active complementary health. Both are needed for success. In ancient China, if you were sick you would go to the tai chi master, often far away in the mountain, who was also an acupuncturist and an herbalist. He would ask you to come a little earlier than the rest of the students, would stick some needles in you, then have you practice mind/body exercises, and finally he would ask you to stay after class so he could make you an herbal mix to take at home.

The treatment in those days was complete: like a good cake, the mind/body exercise is the plain cake, acupuncture is the frosting, and the herbs are the cherries. When you put them all together, you have a delicious cake. When you use only one part, you are missing an important component and you are taking a chance of not succeeding. If you get only acupuncture and do not include an active component, you might feel you have tried complementary healing. In reality, you tried only a passive method and your health issue might require a bit more than that.

Over the years, I noticed that when people were tapping into the various complementary approaches to improve a medical condition, they would usually choose a passive complementary discipline like acupuncture or massage. Passive complementary treatments are an important contribution to your health, but you also need to incorporate some active approaches to bringing balance to your body. Complementary medicine is most effective when both active and passive approaches are practiced together.

In the old days, students would study with a teacher for twenty to thirty years. They would live in their master's house and learn the complete art, which included mind/body exercise, acupuncture, massage, and the use of herbs. They would apprentice for another ten years under the eyes of their guidance and only then would they have been considered a master.

Often present day practitioners are not ready to commit to more than six to ten years. In fact, some people call themselves a 'Master' after a weekend seminar! Be careful about your selection of a practitioner. Ask questions. Do not be afraid to change practitioners if you feel you should.

Also, today people tend to specialize. That means you need to find two or sometimes three people to achieve your goal—a mind/body expert, an acupuncturist, an herbalist, and a good massage therapist. Sometimes, you can still find an acupuncturist who is also an herbalist and may be an M.D. as well. In this way, you can remove one person from your team of complementary helpers, but you would still need an extra person for a good massage.

Complementary Approaches Gain Acceptance

Because there was money to tap into with specific guidelines from the NIH, many institutes created complementary task forces that held meetings regularly to decide how to approach this new field and how to become approved through well-written grants for the money set aside by the NIH. I was and still am part of the group at Dana Farber Cancer Institute that brought some recognition and some awareness to the Western world about the complementary methods. At first, we met in the basement of the institute. There were twelve of us—eight outsiders who were practicing complementary medicine and four from the institute. It was a meeting of both worlds. We tried to see with whom we were dealing, if we could get recognition, and if perhaps we could get some work at Harvard. I remember one of the top oncologists explaining that it is not known how complementary methods work, or even whether they work at all. For the next two years, because Dana Farber was interested in collaborating experts of one of the complementary approaches, every Wednesday, a complementary practitioner would present his or her approach for two hours.

Because I was there in that first meeting, I was able to present my method within a few weeks. There were healers who used their hands to emit energy, there were people who used chanting and loud voices for healing, and there were individuals like me who empowered the patients with basic stretching and strengthening techniques as well as encouraging deep breathing and visualization to help the mind to quiet the negative thoughts that often coincide with cancer.

I remember purposely not introducing the whole 'energy' side of my approach because I felt there were enough beneficial aspects of my method without delving into the less understood facets of energy. My plan was to introduce it later on. Two years later, I received the news that Dana Farber had chosen my approach to be taught and researched at the institute.

At this point, our group was honored with a gift from Lenny Zakim. He had cancer and had experienced massage and other complementary approaches. Lenny had decided to help with the goal of making complementary health available to every individual who steps through the doors of any institute, especially Dana Farber. Thanks to Lenny and a few other generous visionaries, Dana Farber now has a complementary branch called the Zakim Center with four acupuncturists who are herbalists, and medical doctors as well.

The Zakim Center runs qigong and tai chi classes twice a week. It also has a half dozen tables for massage and nutritionists, and offers meditation, music, Reiki, and art classes on a regular basis. Eastern medical studies utilize both mind/body and acupuncture to learn exactly how and why they work. The road is still long, but times have changed. Twenty years ago, I would receive telephone calls from family members of people who were dying soon. Now I receive calls from individuals themselves who are sick, within the first few weeks of their diagnosis. I even receive occasional calls from doctors interested in referring patients to me. Dana Farber has ongoing evening classes in Sunset Tai Chi and morning classes in Sunrise Tai Chi. Classes are available to patients, their families, and the staff.

What is Complementary Healing?

Complementary Healing: Passive Versus Active

Over the years, I noticed that when people were having medical problems and were tapping into the various complementary approaches, they would usually undergo acupuncture or massage treatments and would tell me, "I am doing complementary." My answer to them was that they were doing passive complementary and were missing a big part of what I consider complementary. When doing partial complementary, it is easy to be led into not giving the complementary the best chance to work. This practice leads to the second problem; you could lose your belief altogether in the complementary approach without giving it a fair chance.

If we ask what is complementary healing, we should ask first from where these disciplines derive. The answer is that most of them, especially the ones that are introduced in hospitals and cancer centers, come from the East: China, India, Japan, and other Asian countries. The Eastern view of the body is different from ours. They see the human body as being comprised of five building blocks: the body, breath, mind, energy, and spirit. Once we accept that each block is essential, we will realize that the treatment should include all building blocks and not just some of them. Eastern science works from the view that we have twelve internal organs and not ten as viewed in the West. The difference in the numbers comes from a different view of what is considered an organ. For instance, in Eastern medicine, the pericardium, which is the sac that wraps around the heart, is considered as a separate organ from the heart.

When you are lying on a table and being treated with acupuncture, you are working mostly with the energy building block. Sitting on a chair and breathing deeply works mostly with the breath building block. Going to a psychologist would be dealing mostly with the mind building block. Going to church or temple is fine-tuning the spirit building block. You need to balance each one of the building blocks first, and then harmonize among them. Once harmonized, you can then work toward harmonizing with 'the three forces': heaven, human, and earth.

To achieve internal harmonization, you first need to follow a mind/body approach that gives you tools and empowers you to maintain a routine that can be incorporated into your entire day. Then you need to work on the breath block throughout the day, as well as use meditation and other visualizations to quiet the mind block and strengthen the energetic system. You should evoke spirituality again and again throughout the day. You might choose to be treated by an acupuncturist, who may also prescribe herbs. Also, a good massage every day would be the optimal situation, but once a week will do as well.

This mind/body approach to optimal health, as opposed to a system that fights illness only when symptoms strongly manifest, will create lasting changes from the inside, and external stimulation such as massage, needles, and herbs will strengthen your system from the outside. They are both important for success—the passive and the active techniques are essential for the best results. One activates the other, while at the same time, one helps to maintain the other. The two are the ingredients to achieving a positive chain reaction versus a negative one. They are the yin and the yang, which, when put together, makes the whole.

Finding the Right Complementary Care Giver

In my opinion, it is not easy to find a good tai chi person or an expert in qigong. First, the teachers who can teach the entire art are numbered, and second, the students who are willing to spend twenty years studying are rare. If you are lucky and you do find one in the Western world, consider it not as luck, but as destiny.

If you are seriously interested in learning the Eastern arts, especially qigong, tai chi, or yoga, and you want to find the right teacher, here are some concepts you should be introduced to in your first few years of practice: a teacher who will teach you to free your body from being a prisoner of the soft tissues and, at the same time, will work with you on building strength. Balance between the two is one goal in your journey. Your second goal is to isolate your joints and create a gentle movement in them to stimulate the entire energetic system. You need to learn correct alignment when standing, sitting, walking, and moving slowly. Also important are techniques for deep breathing throughout every mind/body prescription, as well as throughout the day. In addition, various techniques of meditations are crucial: standing, sitting, as well as meditating while moving slowly, i.e., tai chi.

It is very important to work with your energetic system. An expert should know qigong massage because that demonstrates hands-on experience. I, for example, massaged my teacher for ten years for the purpose of learning various aspects of our bodies (usually for two hours at a time).

The teacher you are looking for most probably has training in the external as well as the internal arts. The two arts give your teacher an array of mind/body tools that can be used in different situations. A strong background with various traditional martial arts weapons gives a teacher more insights into understanding the energy field beyond the body.

A good teacher leads you to evoke spirituality and eventually harmonize the three forces: heaven, human, and earth. Your teacher may utilize techniques using some of the forces of nature, or by doing movements or meditations to the various directions: South, North, East, and West. Look for a teacher who has a sense of humor and has faced or dealt with death, a teacher who has an open mind and still keeps learning, a teacher who is open to the contribution of other disciplines toward understanding the art. These attributes are worth searching for as you seek out your teacher and your healthcare provider.

Yoga schools, especially the schools of B.K.S. Iyengar Yoga, are very good for many goals. The schools require teachers to invest time in learning and earn a license that ensures the quality of teaching is very high. Of course, you always have to deal with the individual's personality, which has nothing to do with his or her knowledge. Remember, those are two totally different things. Many times students 'fall in love' with their teachers, but they do not really love the teacher but actually the methodology itself. It is just that at the beginning we have a difficult time separating the methodology from the individual. Remember, learn the art—separate the teaching from the person. Good luck with that one! It is part of developing your tai chi skills.

Finally, if you are interested in learning martial arts, your teacher should have ten years of experience working in martial arts, teaching the form, pushing hands, weapons, and knowledge of the theory of the style. If you are looking for a teacher who will help you regain health, look for someone with at least ten years of experience working with cancer, arthritis, or other debilitating diseases. Of course, if your teacher is involved in research, you can tell that he or she is, first, knowledgeable enough to be chosen by those institutes, and second, that your teacher is curious and interested in really understanding the methodology, which will only benefit you. Remember, most probably, being involved in research means your teacher is sacrificing time and energy for knowledge rather than for money. If your teacher has a good relationship with his or her partner, husband, wife, and children, it is a good sign that he or she embodies the philosophy and styles and is not just teaching them. Remember, you can find a coach or you can find a master; the coach can teach but not necessarily practice. The master can perform the internal arts but not necessarily be a good teacher. There is a saying that I believe to be very true: "It can take you ten years to become a master but it can take you twenty years to find a good one." You may find yourself going to a few teachers. Keep searching. Keep learning.

Tai Chi for Relaxation: Dealing with Stress

We are faced with many kinds of stress every single day. Modern life is fast-paced. The images we see in advertising and on TV are flashy and rapid-fire. The media and Internet blast millions of images before our eyes and minds every day. Prime-time television is cynical and obsessed with action, murder, and mayhem. The war, work, family, friends, healthcare … there is always a source of stress in our lives. How you choose to react to stress and how you choose to internalize it affects your health and the health of those around you. Realize that when you are stressed, even at a very low level, you are hurting yourself physically. The moment you are stressed even slightly, your blood chemistry changes for the worse and your breathing becomes shallow. You are moving to negative hormone production, such as overproduction of adrenaline and away from positive hormone production, such as the production of endorphins, serotonin, and endostatin.

Your reaction to stress is a choice that you make daily, perhaps without realizing it. Awareness is the key. You can choose not to internalize any stress you encounter, not let your emotional mind race, not raise your heart rate and blood pressure, and not constrict your breathing. Strive to maintain equilibrium under all conditions. Breathe slowly and deeply when you encounter stress.

We are shallow breathers. Most of us need to make a conscious decision to breathe more deeply until over time we develop a healthier habit of breathing deeply all day, every day. Breathing deeply is not just good for you; it is the single most important aspect of your practice of tai chi for health as well for relaxation. Shallow breathing will make you sick, reduce your energy, hamper your productivity, and shorten your life span. When you breathe deeply, every one of your internal organs functions better, and you feel better. Every minute, millions of cells die in our bodies. With a healthy diet, the respiratory system should be responsible for eliminating 70% of your metabolic waste. The remainder is eliminated through perspiration (19%), urination (8%), and defecation (3%). If you do not breathe deeply or sweat regularly, waste elimination is slower, or worse, it stays in your body and your circulation slows to a halt. We need to exhale deeply to get rid of dead cells and carbon dioxide, and inhale deeply to provide optimal oxygen levels to make the cell replacement process as efficient as possible. When your elimination is as efficient as possible, your physical aging slows down, and you may even appear to reverse the aging process.

Do we have shallow breath because we are under stress, or are we stressed because we have shallow breath? Both. Certain typical breathing patterns trigger physiological and psychological stress and anxiety reactions. Many of these unhealthy breathing patterns are just bad habits, and they can be re-trained. Do not take this recommendation lightly. Find some time each day to practice deep breathing and build some healthy breathing habits, and an improved quality of life will be your reward.

Stress is sometimes confused as being only on either a physical or mental level. But actually stress is often both mental and physical. We have different ways to stress ourselves physically. For example, bad posture, improper alignment will create stress on the joints and the vertebrae. A collapsed spine can create stress on the individual vertebrae and on the internal organs. Our body is not designed for leaning or collapsing into the joints. It is designed to use the muscles to support the bones. When we lean into the joint, we put stress on the ligament. Over a certain period of time, this stress can take a toll on the ligaments, leading to swelling, shortness, and atrophy of muscles, as well as arthritis. If you do not use certain muscles, you lose them, they turn to fat, and that creates stress on other groups of muscles as well as your bones and joints.

Three Levels of Relaxation

There are three levels of relaxation. The *first level* is that you appear to be relaxed, but you are not relaxed either physically or mentally. You give an impression outwardly of a relaxed person, but you are unstable mentally. You may even have physical backache and neck ache, but you look relaxed. Looking relaxed comes from an outward perception.

The *second level of relaxation* is that you feel relaxed, but physically you are slightly stressed because you are not maintaining proper alignment; you are leaning into the joints and collapsing into the organs. That is not the most relaxed posture; it is a little bit of relaxing but much collapsing. There is a tendency for some to be confused about the difference between being relaxed and collapsing. Collapsed does not necessarily mean relaxed even though there is some relaxation within collapsing. Feeling relaxed, but still being unaware of the stress caused by your alignment, is not true relaxation.

Sensing relaxation is the *third level*, the deepest level of relaxation. It includes both the physical and the mental aspects. In sensing relaxation, you are relaxed mentally and physically, and you are correctly aligned so the stress on the skeleton, the joints, is reduced. Organs can be stressed from misalignment as can the vertebrae in the spine. Slouching and collapsing the thoracic spine, which is a posture that most of us carry when we sit at the computer, or at dinner, or with friends, is one of our worst enemies. Collapsing the thoracic spine compresses against the internal organs as well as the lungs, and slows down the movement in the digestive system, which reduces the oxygen intake. When your thoracic spine is aligned and straight, the lungs are open and you can breathe fully. When the thoracic spine is collapsed, it compresses the lungs and could decrease your oxygen intake by half. In sensing relaxation, you are mentally and physically alert and aware, aligned, and calm.

There are a few keys to reduce or prevent mental and physical stress. On a physical level, the method of prevention and healing is through learning healthy alignment, finding balance between your strength and flexibility, increasing your lung capacity, and understanding the alignment within the spine and within the various stretches and resistance training. Once your alignment and balance between strength and flexibility are achieved, learning the correct use of the *body* alignment in the various motions and actions is the next step. You learn how to utilize the body in ways that reduce stress on the various groups of muscles and train your strength using optimal movement. An example is shoveling snow. Once you learn to lift snow using your legs rather than using your lower back, tremendous stress is removed from your lower back and shoulders. Also, using the leg muscles and using the waist to turn to dump the snow reduces stress on the knees and the lower back. Correct action or movement is an important behavior to reduce stress on the joints and skeleton. Increasing your oxygen intake brings more oxygen into the bloodstream, which upgrades every cell in your body, leading to a better ability in dealing with stress.

An excellent tool for dealing with stress is your *breath*. The breath is the way to quiet the frantic emotional monkey mind—the breath is the banana that will quiet the monkey mind. That is why it is very important to have correct posture especially in the thoracic spine, not pushed in and up like military posture and not collapsed down when we slouch, as well as in the shoulders in order to create the optimal space for the lungs. That is why it is very important to train the lungs with the various breath work from my two books, *Sunrise Tai Chi* and this book, *Sunset Tai Chi*: trapezius breathing, three-chamber breathing, seesaw breathing, etc. The training allows you to develop your lungs and have longer oxygen intake and longer exhalation, or carbon output. Slow deep breathing is a strong tool for quieting the monkey mind when it is bothering you and creating stress within. Try it the next time you are much stressed. Put your attention on your breathing and surf the breath. Follow the air in and out for a few minutes. Some days when the monkey is very strong, you will need to use fire breath breathing. In fire breath breathing, you inhale with a sound through your nostrils and when exhaling whispering "ha" sound from your mouth. Fire breath breathing is useful in intense situations. It will help you move your thoughts away from the stressful situation and release tension. Of course, sometimes you may need to take a few deep breaths and simply relax. Once you do that, you can then deal with the mental stress. First, use fire breath and eventually use a quiet water breath. You have options in different situations: a breath with a sound like "ha" or "oy-gevalt," or a quiet, deep, long, peaceful breath.

The *mind* is the next building block or tool you need to develop to prevent or reduce mental stress. The ancient Chinese describe us as having two minds: the monkey mind, which is the emotions, and the horse mind, which is your wisdom. The monkey mind is the wild and scattered emotional mind. The monkey mind is also the mind that allows us to have passion, excitement, and other beneficial emotions as well. We cannot and do not want to get rid of the monkey or the horse.

The Chinese have a saying, "seize the monkey and train the horse." Most of us train the horse over a lifetime, from our life experiences and by having individuals who we believe in and hold up their personality as an example for our behavior and path in life. Until we reach our mid-twenties, the part of the brain that commands our logic and rational thinking is still being constructed, and our emotional mind is in charge. The emotions are much stronger when we are children, and as we mature we learn to control them. Wisdom is acquired and eventually we develop deeper wisdom as we age if we tame our emotional minds.

In order to learn how to deal with stress, we need to keep emphasizing training the horse and seizing the monkey throughout our lives. For example, the horse decides, "Tomorrow morning I am going to get up at 6:00 and train." But that night you go to sleep at the same time that you always do, so you are not really prepared for waking up early. At six o'clock when the alarm rings, your monkey mind says, "Oh, not today, let us do it tomorrow," and then you push the snooze button and go back to sleep. This scenario is an example of how the monkey mind is controlling the horse mind and not the horse controlling the monkey. Each time you choose to listen to the horse mind and get up and train, you strengthen the horse mind.

The amount of *energy* that you can manifest is directly related to your breathing and to all of the building blocks. You will gain control over your body's energy levels as you continue on the path of tai chi. The energy building block is one that slowly becomes easier to understand with regular, repeated practice. You will feel the difference in how you handle negative stress, and how much more energized you feel as you master the skills of deep relaxation. The energetic block is a very important part of your physical body that is often overlooked. By fine-tuning the body, breath, mind, and spirit, your energy will follow, will be stronger and abundant, and will flow smoothly. But also by focusing on the energetic circulatory system itself, building up the various energy centers, and opening the energy paths throughout your body will help you deal with stress. The energy that flows through the soft tissue will allow stress to dissolve away. Stronger energy is a better tool for dissolving stress, and stronger energy is also a better tool for the mind to dissolve the impurities within the body. When you have more abundant energy, the mind has a stronger tool to work with.

When we have a high *spirit*, stress is not as noticeable, either physically or mentally. Raising and maintaining a positive mental attitude can be one of the most powerful tools for your health and quality of life. When we have a broken, low spirit, stress is more noticeable and will get to us more easily. After all, mental stress often originates from your perception and awareness. You can choose to control it.

Refine your skills until fine-tuning is not needed within each one of the blocks we mentioned—body, breath, mind, energy, and spirit. Perfecting this skill will contribute tremendously to reducing stress on both a physical and mental level.

THEORY OF THE FIVE BUILDING BLOCKS

Fine-tuning until fine-tuning is not needed.

The ancient art of qigong, which means 'energy cultivation,' has been passed down for over 4,000 years. The five basic elements or pillars of practice from the philosophies and styles of both qigong and tai chi that I would like you to focus on are the five building blocks of our being: body, breath, mind, energy, and spirit. You must apply the five building blocks in each movement or mind/body prescriptions from both books. Each block needs to be fine-tuned until fine-tuning is not needed. In other words, within each block there are a number of skills that need to be acquired.

Body: When you first focus on the body, emphasize the alignment of the skeleton, softness in the soft tissues, empty/full moon breathing, stretching and releasing of the bows, dropping the sacrum, suspending the head as if by a thread, dropping the shoulders, relaxing the face, and a gentle pulsing within the joints. Strive to attain your maximum physical potential to create the best environment for all systems to function to their fullest.

Breath: Inhale with a slow, deep, quiet, continuous, peaceful breath, through the nose. Exhale the same way, through the nose, and soften the muscles around the lungs. Move the air to different parts of the lungs using the various postures that stretch the ribs and spine. The postures can be enhanced by moving the limbs and bending the torso. Pause briefly in the space at the end of your exhalation. Do not hold your breath, but breathe as slowly as possible. If you get only as far as mastering the body and breath, you are doing very well. Breathing deeply and taking in more oxygen is the key to wellness. Once the breath is regulated, you will rarely or never get sick, and you will live longer. In the internal arts, breathing is of utmost importance. The amount of air you take in is directly proportional to the amount of qi you can manifest. Learn to use both the fire and the water breath as needed.

Mind: Here is where the training can become more difficult to understand and master. If you persevere through the earlier stages, these will come in due time. Recognize the two minds: the emotional (monkey) mind and the wisdom (horse) mind. Do not allow the emotional mind to control your thoughts and actions. Gradually develop a meditative mind in the mental state between awake and asleep. Warning: you must be entirely truthful inside and out before you can progress within this stage.

Energy: Spend time practicing only your internal visualizations, such as your two main energy centers, the upper and lower energy centers or the energetic baton (Figure 1). You can visualize this center as an energy ball in the center of your belly (your center of gravity energy center) (Figure 2), that is energetically connected to the upper energy ball in the center of your head (your pituitary gland energy center). Practice visualizing the energetic bubble surrounding the body. This bubble is also known as your guardian energy (wei qi) (Figure 3). Finally, work on leading the mind and energy to the four gates at your extremities, both palms and both soles of your feet, and then beyond, and then back to your lower energy center, center of gravity energy center, coordinating with your breath. Remember, the yi (wisdom mind) leads the qi (energy). Energy follows consciousness. Wherever you hold your attention within your body, your energy will gather there.

Spirit: The mind is the general, qi is the soldiers, and spirit is their morale. Develop a strong spirit and powerful intention. Say what you mean, and follow through with

THE ENERGETIC BATON

THE CENTER OF GRAVITY ENERGY CENTER

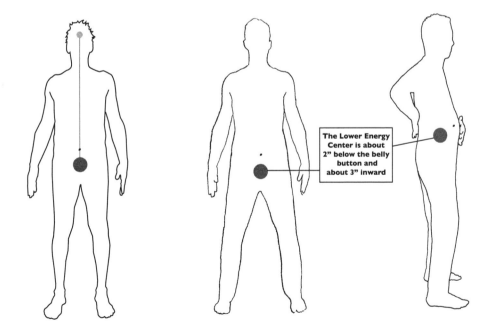

The Lower Energy Center is about 2" below the belly button and about 3" inward

Figure 1. The energetic baton.

Figure 2. Center of gravity energy center.

BUBBLE VISUALIZATION

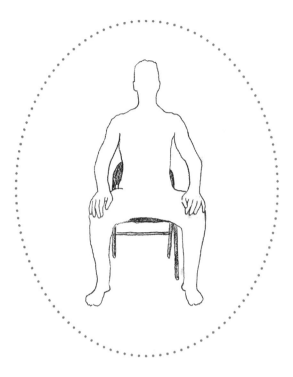

Figure 3. Guardian energy (wei qi).

your plans. Exercise your spirit as you would any other part of yourself. The ability to utilize a strong spirit will help you achieve any objective, and it can make the difference between life and death in a healing crisis.

———————————

The entire cool-down set of exercises, stretches, visualizations, and meditations is meant to prepare you for the tai chi form. Just learning a tai chi form is not enough. Memorizing movements and following along can be a good way to start, but if you are seeking deep relaxation and the full benefits of tai chi practice, then you must go deeper. These skills, which we have been discussing thus far, are the essence of the internal arts. The perpetual refinement of your breath, your alignment, your qi, and your spirit, are the essential skills that we learn through the practice of tai chi. As balancing and developing these skills becomes a habit throughout your day, every aspect of your life is transformed for the better. Without awareness of all these things, the five building blocks, the energy centers, and the relationship between yourself and nature, your practice cannot be called tai chi.

CHAPTER 2
Qi is Real–Understanding Human Energy

Qi is energy. All things in the universe are comprised of energy at their fundamental level. Most often, when qi is discussed as it relates to health as well as internal arts practice, the energy being referred to is that which circulates throughout your body, through energetic pathways: the twelve meridians and the eight extraordinary vessels. It is your vital life force. The ancient Chinese described the living energy within our bodies as qi. The experience of qi and its circulation is well documented in ancient China and India.

Over the centuries, millions of people have tried to connect to their energetic system, build it up, remove stagnation, and improve circulation. They did it through various techniques, such as sitting meditation, tai chi, or qigong. Some philosophies and styles do not always talk or practice them, but instead they emphasize body, mind, and spirit with the belief that if you fine-tune and cultivate each of these elements, your energy will be strong and abundant. This technique results in not only good health but in a superior quality of life, as well as longevity. Those who sit in meditation or practice yoga, tai chi, or qigong have experienced this subtle flow of energy within their bodies. It is believed in the Eastern philosophies and practices that every one of the trillions of cells that our bodies are comprised of contains energy, which is transmitted from air to blood to tissue to bone marrow and back out to the energetic bubble surrounding our bodies.

Practitioners of tai chi, qigong, and other internal arts practice many energetic visualizations for the sole purpose of upgrading this energetic system. It is the same system that the acupuncturists and Chinese herbalists use to help their patients. This belief that we have an energetic system in our bodies is not proven yet by Western science. Many individuals in the West do not believe that this energetic system exists, but some may be convinced that this system represents the power of the mind and maybe in order to tap into this power, we first need to practice with the mind moving through the body in specific paths that over time strengthens the mind and its abilities both on the inside of the body and beyond.

To understand our body's energy system, we need to learn the theory behind it and practice the mental visualizations and the physical movements that lead to a stronger, abundant system. The first step that we are trying to take is to develop our awareness, learn and sense the locations of the energy centers, the channels and the meridians, and lead our minds through the eight extraordinary vessels. Typically, the first task in a beginner's journey, when being introduced to the energetic system, is first to reside in one of the major energy centers. Usually we reside in the lower one, or as I refer to it in my books as the 'center of gravity energy center.' Some traditional masters will have you reside at this center for a year, twice a day for 40 minutes until you can move to the next level, which is residing in the upper energy center, or what I call the pituitary energy center.

Learn to recognize the energy centers in your body. Once you 'know' your energy centers, tune into the movement of energy through the limbs, into the fingers, and down into the toes. Try to feel or sense the energy paths, the channels and vessels. When you become comfortable with the energy centers and the flow through the limbs, you can move to the next visualization and move the mind beyond the body and sense the energetic field around us. Sense the energy around your body, which extends to about the distance of a fist. Move through the different stages with patience and make sure you master each one of them.

The next level is building up the different energy centers in order to upgrade your source of energy. The energy centers are like batteries. They are sources of energy. Putting the mind in those centers while balancing the entire system will upgrade and strengthen each energy center. Strengthening the centers will lead to a stronger, smoother flow of energy throughout the system. The system naturally tends to be stagnant and the batteries tend to deplete. They do not remain constantly powerful and strong for different reasons: aging, lifestyle, soft tissue tension around the skeleton, diet, emotions, and environment. Your energy changes with the day and night, the seasons, and your nutrition. All these reasons and more affect the energetic system and can lead to stagnation or lack of circulation or a weak flow in certain channels, which affects, eventually, our internal organs, our daily performance and quality of life, and our immune system. As you can see, a large part of dealing with the energetic system is mental multitasking that will take time and practice.

ACTION OF THE FIVE BUILDING BLOCKS

In order to achieve a strong energetic system, we fine-tune each of the five building blocks until fine-tuning is not necessary. Starting with the body building block, we balance between strength and flexibility, which is one of the first steps on a physical level to help the energetic system. By finding balance between your strength and flexibility, stagnation will be removed and the system will be one step closer to its full potential performance. The lack of balance between strength and flexibility creates stress on the energy channels and does not allow the mind to flow smoothly through the body, leading to an unbalanced situation within the system.

One other step is massaging the internal organs through movement or through self-massage. By massaging the internal organs, you remove and circulate energy that is stagnant in the organ area; you lead it into the channels and out throughout the extremities. Also, working with the joints allows the energy to move smoothly between the bones and the muscles, and between the inside and the outside. Maintaining flexibility in the joints, tendons, muscles, and ligaments is very important.

Through developing the second building block, the breath, we increase and improve the function of the lungs, allowing more energy to move in. We are supplying every cell in our body with more oxygen, allowing those cells to function and perform better. Moving more oxygen in and more carbon out is a process that also helps you attain a more balanced energetic system. By developing the lungs, you not only take in more oxygen, but also train the mindfulness of your breathing that in turn develops the skill of using the banana to capture the monkey.

The third building block is the mind. The mind is probably the most important aspect of balancing the energetic system. Emotions can create excitement or depression, which leads to lack of balance in the energetic system. If it were only up to the emotional mind, we would not have a balanced system. We are able, however, to monitor ourselves and calm the emotional mind using breathing or other methods. The Taoists refer to this process as "seize the monkey and strengthen the horse." When the monkey is quiet, it will allow the energy to be strong and balanced, which can eventually allow you to connect and harmonize with the energy of the three forces: heaven, human, and earth.

The fourth building block is our energetic system. There are two major schools of thought: the first believes that through fine-tuning until fine-tuning is not needed, each of the other blocks will fall into place naturally. The second believes that all five building blocks need to be fine-tuned, especially the energetic one. The second school of thought is more Taoist than Buddhist. You can find a world of energetic visualizations in Taoist thought that you will not find anywhere else. My personal experience is that both schools have excellent tools so I use the best from both worlds. Some individuals can work and practice every block except the energetic one and will get excellent results, and others will not get results, in which case, focusing on the energetic block sometimes achieves results. That is the reason I keep my mind open and I first try to sense which block will be the most appropriate for each individual to clear.

Through developing the fifth building block, the spirit, we boost our energetic system to places that words cannot describe. Learning to evoke (yang) the spirit and cool (yin) the spirit can lead to abundant energy and great spiritual achievement.

The energetic system consists of two elements, fire and water. The theory is that the system is fiery to start with because of the food we eat and the air we breathe. Because we are more fire than water, we need to constantly cool or calm down the system for the simple goal of achieving balance. One of the methods of cooling the fire is through strengthening and draining the internal energetic baton within the core of the body.

After we strengthen the energy centers, we connect the upper and the lower energy center. This connection creates a baton of energy: two balls of energy in the head and the abdomen and the line connecting them. This baton of energy can become stronger and stronger. The baton is in charge of managing the functions and the operation of the inner body including the immune system. The stronger your baton is, the stronger your immune system is. The Chinese refer to this part of the energetic system as managing qi (energy).

Surrounding the body is a *bubble* or the energy that is about a fist away from our skin, all around us. It is the energy mechanism that deals with forces around us. This energetic bubble behaves as a shield and also as a filter. The stronger your system is, the more efficient this filter is and the better its ability to strain and filter negative forces, as well as deal with positive forces. An efficient filter will allow positive constructive energies to move in and allow negative energies to leave the body. This efficient process is another key element to having a better-balanced system, healthier life, and a stronger performance on a daily basis.

As you can see, once we fine-tune the system, remove the stagnation, build up the center, create a stronger flow, and upgrade the shield and filters, we are one step ahead in promoting better health. We are now in a state of prevention. Cultivating longevity, and not just health, involves prevention, which requires spending time and energy even when you are not sick and even when you are in your best shape, in order to achieve more success as you age.

Striving for and achieving this balance is a journey that needs to be enjoyed. If you do not enjoy and make the most of this journey, you are defeating its purpose. Building up the system and upgrading it eventually allows you to connect to the other forces around us, the heaven and the earth, or what is considered in Chinese qigong the three forces: heaven, human, and earth. Once your energetic system is strong, regulated, fine-tuned, and balanced, you will be able to fully connect to the other forces. We can all connect to the other forces at certain times in our lives, but by strengthening our own systems, it allows us to experience and sense the other forces at all times, not only when we are deciding to bring our minds into it. A good example of this mind being in two places, or actually one, is your martial artist mind; it has a strong sense of the lower energy center throughout the day and should have that strong sensation even as you fight and deal with strong forces from the outside. When you can hold the mind in the lower energy center even when you fight, you will be able to have it there throughout the day. If you strengthen and upgrade your energetic system, you will connect to the other forces, experience them, and be one with them at all times.

GOALS OF THE MIND/BODY APPROACH

When we talk about a mind/body journey, we are not just talking theoretically or in general about philosophical ideas. In order to succeed and advance, we need specific targets and goals that we strive to sometimes just understand and many other times try to actually reach. Some of the benefits as well as goals that you may encounter once you embark on a mind/body journey using the principles of the various Eastern arts are

- Complement Western treatment
- Develop sensitivity and awareness
- Journey into the self
- Tap into the power of the mind
- Deal with and prevent illnesses and their symptoms
- Prevent disability and increase physical performance
- Empower individuals, families, physicians to play an active role in health care
- Improve martial skills
- Utilize and tap into the powerful energy of the rising and setting sun

Find a teacher. Without a teacher, you may practice for ten years and learn very little. Your practice will improve much more efficiently with the guidance of a skillful and qualified teacher. If you cannot find a teacher, continue searching for the correct path with books and DVDs. Ask any tai chi teacher a few questions before you sign up to study with him or her: What lineage or family style is it? Where did the teacher study? Does the training incorporate Yi Chuan, i.e., standing meditation? Will it progress from the form to other aspects of tai chi, such as qigong, pushing hands, silk reeling, martial applications, weapons, etc? Does the practice include internal visualization to develop your energetic system visualizations, such as lower and upper energy center, four gates, or bubble breathing? If you understand more than the teacher about internal energy work for both health and martial arts, keep searching.

I have said it before and will say it again: whether or not you have a teacher, practice, practice, practice. Only through repetition of the movements will some of the finer points reveal themselves to you. Only when you have mastered one aspect of the training will your mind, body, or both be prepared to assimilate the next piece.

BETWEEN AWAKE AND ASLEEP

The mental and energetic elements of practice must be discussed here again as they are an essential aspect of the internal arts that is often ignored. You may have learned some of these fundamental skills in *Sunrise Tai Chi*. I have expanded the teaching in this section with more detailed content so you may step deeper into your practice.

Most Eastern arts seek ways for the practitioner to spend more time with a meditative mind. This deep level of meditation is an essential step for achievement in all Eastern disciplines: seeking enlightenment (meditation), better performance (kung fu), improved quality of life (Taoism), and better health (qigong). Through centuries of accumulated experience, the Eastern arts discovered that the mind is usually in an active state, even during sleep. This theory has been scientifically researched and verified. A common realization is that in order to achieve a deep level of relaxation and high skill in internal arts, one must develop a concentrated and meditative mind, which can be difficult to reach for any person. In fact, achieving this skill of reaching and maintaining this state for long periods of time is an art in itself. It has been explored by many disciplines, if not all, such as Buddhism, yoga, martial arts, Zen meditation, dance, and various sports. Even the ability to be a sniper requires achieving this skill. If you have ever experienced being 'in the zone' during a favorite activity, you may better understand this concept.

Over the years, individuals have renamed the concept of meditation to appeal to a wider audience. These new names describe both the intended actions and the results of performing this ancient practice. For example, Dr. Herbert Benson calls meditation the 'relaxation response.' Twenty years of research into the practice of being and staying in this specific state of brain wave activity, i.e., the relaxation response, has proven that the relaxation response, or meditation, has many benefits for both healthy and sick individuals.

In the West, we also found ways to express our ability to stay in a specific meditative brainwave state. For example, when we perform at our highest level in sports or sex, we call it being in the zone. When runners reach a point that they can just keep running without feeling any pain and feel a total physical transparency, it is called 'runners' high.' When a baseball pitcher or a batter achieves extraordinary performances, we consider him a 'high focus' individual.

With cutting edge brain science, such as CAT scans and MRIs, exploring the brain bucket that is occurring at various universities and institutes, I decided to rename the concept of meditation to 'reaching the brain waves between awake and asleep.' I would have called it the skill of reaching and staying at will within the brain waves between awake and asleep whenever one desires, but this name is much too long. I hope that the shorter name will still give individuals clear instructions as well as a goal to achieve this concept of relaxation response, meditation, or residing between awake and asleep (Figure 4).

You enter this state when the brainwave activity slows from the usual beta and alpha brainwaves of daily activity toward the borderline near-sleep state, which is theta brain waves. Staying in this state of mind and keeping the mind relaxed and calm is not only difficult but is rarely achieved. It is hard to find opportunities in our normal daily routines to spend time in this state, except during the few seconds right before we fall asleep. It is that sweet sensation a few seconds right before we fall asleep when you can still hear the outside but your body is transparent and then, you are 'gone.' The next thing you know, you wake up. In the Eastern arts, this state of mind is considered very important. Techniques were created for reaching this state, staying there, and not falling asleep during exercises practiced lying down, sitting, standing, and even moving slowly.

The light physical tension in sitting meditation that holds the spine upright prevents us from sleeping, but allows the mind to reach and stay between awake and asleep. The same goes for Yi Chuan (standing meditations) and moving slowly (i.e., tai chi chuan). The minimum physical tension allows individuals to keep the body standing or moving while practicing and maintaining the state between awake and asleep and staying or in meditation. The untrained mind tends to stray toward activity and daydreaming or deeper into the delta sleep state. Do not be discouraged. Through knowledge and practice, this skill can be acquired.

THE BRAIN WAVES

BETA brain waves (13 to 22 cycles)	ALPHA brain waves (4 to 7 cycles)	THETA brain waves (8 to 12 cycles)

BETA - Normal waking state
ALPHA - Calm, peaceful state of mind with many physical benefits
THETA - State between awake and asleep: deeply relaxed, meditative mind

Figure 4. EEG Brain scans.

Even before this skill is fully realized, moving toward this mental state is a profound experience. Once you have had the experience of staying between awake and asleep, you may refer to it often. It can become an essential tool for relieving stress and maintaining balance under duress.

A basic technique you can use to get into this state is to observe your breath as it moves in and out, slowly, deeply, silently, and continuously. Relax physical tension. Pay no attention to random thoughts. Keep your spirit alert and engaged in observing the breath. Spend several minutes observing your breath. We will walk you through this technique at the start of the Sunset Tai Chi program, along with the first few cool-down exercises.

Knowing how to utilize the breath is a vital skill in reaching this deep level of relaxation. This meditative mind creates the correct environment for greater success in the martial arts and is one of the key secrets of awakening the self-healing mechanisms within ourselves.

FUNDAMENTAL ENERGETIC VISUALIZATIONS

Here again we must emphasize the importance of understanding both sides—the yang physical body and the yin mental, or energetic, body. Both bodies are one and cannot be separated, but at times they can be trained separately for better results.

The various internal visualization skills presented below will be utilized during the preparation exercises, during your tai chi practice, and hopefully during all your daily activities. These visualizations are tools we will use throughout the program. The visualizations are a fundamental aspect of the training that needs to be explored deeply before you move on to the tai chi form.

If you do not feel comfortable with more than two visualizations at the same time, your mind is not ready, and you have advanced through each stage of your training too quickly. The length of training for each stage is different for each individual. Take your time and enjoy each stage. Some days are better than others. As I mentioned earlier, do not be too hard on yourself. Take each day of your training in stride. One day, you will find that your awareness of yourself, your surroundings, and the meaningfulness of your life have expanded greatly.

First Steps in the Journey of Internal Visualization

The first step that will help you begin to become aware of your physical and mental body is to sit cross-legged on the floor or on an edge of a chair with proper alignment

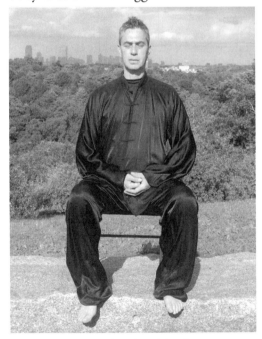

Sitting on the edge of the chair.

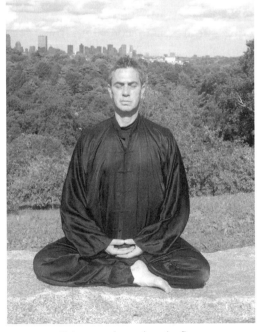

Sitting cross-legged on the floor.

and to experience the various basic energy centers, channels, and vessels that run through our bodies and distribute energy (qi). Sitting this way allows you to focus on experiencing your torso. Once you are able to sense the movement of this qi (energy), you can move on to more advanced stages of internal visualizations with standing and moving postures that include other energy concepts and work with channels in the limbs and the forces surrounding us.

Step 1: Physical Journey

Establish a good sitting foundation. The legs should be crossed comfortably if possible. You may sit in a half-lotus posture, or if you are able, sit in a more advanced full lotus posture, with the right foot on the left thigh and the left foot on the right thigh. Sit up straight on the edge of a cushion so gravity does not pull on your lower back and distract your mind. Slouching even slightly will cause a sore back very quickly. The edge of the knees should rest completely on the floor to create a strong, triangular base between the sitting bones in the rear and the outside of the knees. This posture will slow down the flow of energy in the legs, so you may begin to experience the energy in the torso, circulating in what is called the microcosmic orbit, or small circulation. Your energy naturally circulates down the front of your body from your navel, underneath, between the legs, and then up the center of the back and neck, over the top of the head, down the center of the face, and then down the front of the body to the navel again. Your tongue should touch the roof of your mouth, right behind the front teeth, to complete this circuit.

Step 2: Mental Journey

Follow the breath with your mind to calm the thoughts and reach a basic level of physical relaxation and awareness. Your complete attention should be continuously held on the breath as it moves in and out. This awareness is the first requirement for training, as taught in Zen meditation, which is known as 'Chan' in Chinese.

Physical and Mental Breath Work

When you inhale, feel your abdomen expanding to draw a breath. Feel the breath entering the nose, moving the nose hairs, then moving to the back of the throat to the bronchial tubes, and then filling the different sections of the lungs. Pay special attention to the feelings and sensations of the interactions between the air moving in and out, and the body cells it is touching. Put your mind into each part of your body, experiencing each sensation. Experience the end of inhalation and then linger for a moment before exhaling. This experience is considered the quietest time in our body. By training this skill of putting your mind into your body, you will develop a stronger mind/body connection that will enable you to be aware of your health and other aspects of your life on a much more sensitive level.

During the exhalation, feel how the air leaves the different areas of the lungs, out of the bronchial tubes, through the throat, past the nose hairs, and out the nose. Pay special attention to those feelings or sensations. Experience the end of exhalation. Linger again for a moment on this part of your breathing and try to sense other movement in your body while you are in this quiet, still place. This sensation is called 'looking for the motion in the stillness.'

When you focus your concentrated awareness and intention (the wisdom mind, or 'yi' in Chinese) entirely on the breath, you will help to create a state of 'no thoughts.' When random thoughts arise, simply observe them with a neutral emotional state, and then turn your attention back to observing the breath. The Chinese call this state 'the horse mind seizing the monkey mind.' The breath should be long, quiet, peaceful, slender, continuous, and soft. Inhalation and exhalation should be balanced and equal in length, unless the student is in the more advanced stages of training in which we use the breath differently to balance the kan (water) and li (fire) in the body.

Step 3: Relaxing the Physical Body

While sitting in the emperor or empress posture, use the minimum physical muscular force to lengthen the spine upward in comfortable correct physical alignment. Let go of unnecessary tension in the entire body. Remember, where there is tension, your qi circulation is inhibited. One by one, relax your face, your shoulders, your arms, your torso, your belly, your hips, your legs, and your feet. Become aware of the up and down forces in the body during sitting meditation; the bones and muscles are lifting and holding you up, while the shoulders and the soft tissue, including the face, are 'melting' downward as gravity pulls on you. Do not slouch! Do not collapse the front of the body and compress the organs (Figure 5).

Physical and Mental Breath Work Combined

The torso of the body can be equated to three spheres resting on top of each other. Balancing these three spheres on top of a strong foundation is the first step toward experiencing physical transparency, which will help the mind 'forget' the body and focus on reaching the required brainwave or the meditative state. Of course, in reality the body and mind cannot be separated.

Each sphere has an upward and downward force that occurs simultaneously. The upward lifting feeling is usually associated with inhalation. The downward sinking/ relaxing feeling is usually associated with exhalation. Once this pattern occurs naturally, you should try switching the combination of forces and breathe to increase your internal control. When inhaling, emphasize the downward forces while monitoring and maintaining the upward forces, and when exhaling emphasize the upward forces while monitoring and maintaining the downward forces (Figure 6).

EMPEROR/EMPRESS POSTURE

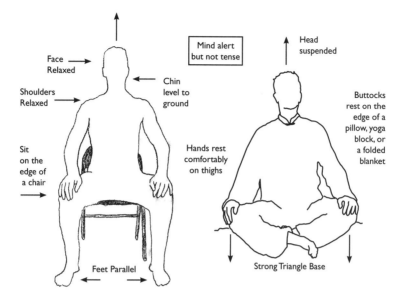

Face Relaxed

Shoulders Relaxed

Sit on the edge of a chair

Feet Parallel

Mind alert but not tense

Chin level to ground

Hands rest comfortably on thighs

Head suspended

Buttocks rest on the edge of a pillow, yoga block, or a folded blanket

Strong Triangle Base

Figure 5. Use minimum physical effort to lengthen the spine upward.

THE UP AND DOWN FORCES
IN EMPEROR/EMPRESS POSTURE

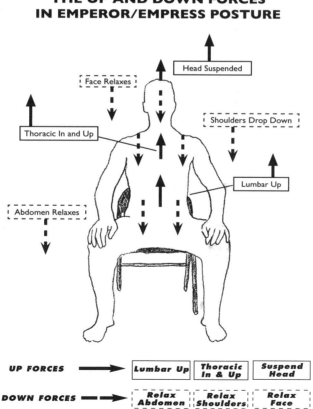

Head Suspended

Face Relaxes

Shoulders Drop Down

Thoracic In and Up

Lumbar Up

Abdomen Relaxes

UP FORCES →	Lumbar Up	Thoracic In & Up	Suspend Head
DOWN FORCES ⇢	Relax Abdomen	Relax Shoulders	Relax Face

Figure 6. Push up through bones;
dissolve down through shoulders and soft tissues.

THREE SPHERES

The three spheres divide your trunk as follows: the biggest sphere goes from the pubic bone to a little bit above the belly button, which is the first sphere. Then from above the belly button to above the sternum, i.e., the solar plexus, is the second sphere. The last sphere is the smallest, and it goes from the solar plexus to the top of the head. As you can see, the bottom sphere is the biggest, the middle one is a little smaller, and the top one is the smallest. The shape of the three spheres reminds those of us who live in the cold countries of a snowman or woman.

The three spheres each have one power that moves upward and a balancing power that moves downward. They are the major forces that should be emphasized within each sphere for a beginner or as a first step.

The three spheres correspond to the following body parts.

Sphere 1: The Lumbar Spine and Abdominal Muscles

The upward force: Push into the sitting bones of the pelvis to allow the lumbar spine to open and start to lift upward. Do not push too much in the direction of the stomach. Notice that in order to lift the spine you may tense your groin. Once you achieve the lengthening through the lumbar area in the lower back, relax the legs and the groin area.

The downward force: Relax the abdominal muscles and the organs and start to feel a downward force. Concentrate on properly positioning this sphere before working on the next spheres. The legs should remain crossed, and may go numb. Periodically uncross your legs and allow them to recuperate as your legs slowly become conditioned (Figure 7).

First Sphere: Typical Body Behavior

There is a tendency to collapse the lower back, the lumbar. This collapsed posture creates much compression through our internal organs. The main idea of the up forces in the lower sphere is to open up the lumbar, that is, the main force that is moving up in the lower sphere. But at the same time when you try opening up and and lengthening the lumbar, you will find there is a tendency to achieve this movement to tense the abdominal muscles in order to lift up the lumbar. There is no need for tensing the abdominal muscles that are also the next down forces within the bottom sphere. Let go of the abdominal muscles. As your lower back lifts or lengthens, the abdominal muscles relax. You have two forces: the up force in the back and the down force through the front.

Sphere 2: The Thoracic Spine Up, Shoulders/Upper Back/Upper Chest Down

From behind the sternum, lift up the thoracic spine to create a rising upward force. You also want to sink the chest slightly and arc the back into a 'turtle back' so as not to have a militarily straight posture.

THE THREE SPHERES

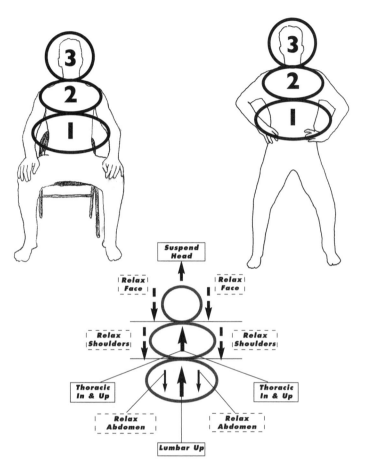

Figure 7. Each sphere has a power that moves upward and a balancing power that moves downward.

The downward force: Relax the shoulders by pulling them horizontally outward and simultaneously downward at a 45-degree angle. Some individuals will also need to draw the shoulders gently backward. At first, check your alignment in a mirror until you can recognize the sensation of good posture.

Second Sphere: Typical Body Behavior

In the second sphere, there is a tendency to collapse the thoracic spine between the shoulders. Most people do not sit or stand with an erect spine or lengthening through the spine. Many of us just collapse that part of the spine, especially when working on computers, watching TV, or sitting in the car. Many aspects of the modern lifestyle do not encourage the thoracic spine to open up. Actually our lifestyle encourages doing the opposite, collapsing that section of our spine. In fact, it is a large section that has 12 vertebrae. When this section collapses, there is much pressure on the lungs, stomach, intestines, and other internal organs. When the thoracic spine is collapsed, we utilize just a third of our lungs, not to mention the pressure on the discs and the spine itself as the shoulder blades and the neck are pulled forward, thereby pulling them out of alignment and creating a whole chain reaction of physical problems leading eventually to mental-emotional issues.

Lengthening and keeping the thoracic spine upright is very important in promoting smooth circulation and better health. When you lift the thoracic spine up and hold the spine straight, the next issue that may happen within this sphere is that the shoulders rise up with this lengthening of the thoracic spine. The next step is dropping the shoulders and relaxing them while lifting through the thoracic spine. As you can see again, you have two actions in the second sphere: the thoracic spine lengthens upward and the shoulders drop down.

When we talk about the shoulders, we can have three common misalignments. The first one is floating shoulders. Many times it is the opposite shoulder to your dominant side. If you are right handed, it would be the left shoulder that will slightly float up. Some individuals can have both shoulders floating up toward the ears. As you can see, dropping the shoulder down toward the ribs prevents it from floating. If you put your mind underneath the armpits and push the shoulders down toward the ribs, you will feel the muscles under your armpits connect the muscles around the ribs. This down action is experienced as a 'slide' of one muscle into another or movement of muscles by each other. Experiencing this down drop through the shoulders will also allow more opening upward of the spine. Remember yin, shoulders down, creates yang, spine up.

The second common mistake or misalignment with the shoulders is that they have a tendency to roll forward. First, they rise up and then secondly, some people have them rolling forward. In this case, the shoulders need to be pushed back and then down.

The third common mistake or physical misalignment that happens in the shoulder is that the left shoulder, or the one that we do not use, the one opposite the dominant side, tends to shrink in toward the neck laterally. That is why there is a need for keeping an emphasis, throughout the day, on opening through the shoulders so they are out and away from the neck. As you can see, there are three directions or motions that you want to emphasize with your shoulders in order to find correct alignment—down, back, and away.

Sphere 3: The Cervical Spine. Top of the Head, Up/Face Muscles, Down

The **upward force:** Imagine a string gently pulling the top of the head, slightly lifting the cervical spine and skull.

The **downward force:** Relax and allow the muscles of the face to relax with a downward melting sensation.

Third Sphere: Typical Body Behavior

The upper sphere is the neck and head. The up force is through the top of the head while the head is suspended. There is a tendency to collapse the head and have it not aligned; the tendency is also to keep the chin a little bit too low. The chin should be parallel to the floor, slightly lifted. That position, in the beginning, may give you a weird sensation, almost as if you are looking up into the sky, but that is the correct alignment of the head and over time, your eyes will adjust.

This upward energy movement through the spine may lead to excitement of the soft tissue in the face. The next thing is to balance this up-force with working on deep relaxation of the various layers of muscles in your face. Because the face is very important to relax and not many methods are offered, I developed the face meditation: visualize your face melting, starting with the skin; then move to the areas in the face that are tighter or closer to the skull, like the corners of the eye, corners of your nose, corners of your mouth, and the temple area. Allow those areas to melt or dissolve downward, layer by layer. A good metaphor for this experience, or exercise, is dividing the face into many thin layers, like an onion.

While in meditation, I work on suspending the top of the head, lengthening through the lumbar and thoracic spine, dropping the abdominal muscles and the shoulders. Next, I work on cooling down and calming the excited soft tissue in the face, melting layer by layer, and moving, mentally, inward very slowly. I spend about 20 minutes until I dissolve each layer. Every now and then, I have a sensation of just being a skull: no identity, no me. At first, it was a scary experience but over time I became used to it and now when it happens, it is a special, unique experience. It does not happen that often but when it does, I know that I reached a very deep level of dissolving and letting go.

Please note: there are also the minor up and down forces to become aware of in the body, such as the up force of gently lifting, or lengthening, through the spine, and the down force of relaxing the groin area. Another example of these minor forces is the up force of the air moving up the nostrils as we breathe in, while the down force of the relaxation of the nose, throat, and lungs takes place on a cellular level.

Training the Up and Down Forces within the Three Spheres

Training and working on the up and down forces within the spheres is a day-to-day challenge. If you can mix the up and down forces into your daily routine, you will increase the benefit of the exercises and develop deeper body awareness. You can practice this skill throughout your day in all your physical actions, but you can also sit or stand, and meditate and emphasize the up and down forces during this time of meditation. When sitting, you can work on the up and down forces in a few ways: First, you can lengthen from the lumbar, upward to the thoracic spine, and then continue the sensation to the top of the head. Once you monitor these three up-forces within the three spheres, you also become mindful of the down forces. Emphasize letting go of the abdominal muscles. Next, work a little bit on dropping the shoulders. Then, spend time melting the face. Some days you can work on the up and down forces, in what I call zigzag: lengthen up through the lumbar, and drop down through the abdominal; lengthen through the thoracic spine, and then drop the shoulders, suspend the head, and relax the face. During some of your sitting meditation, keep the spine upright and for 20 minutes emphasize the down-forces. As I mentioned before, some days I will spend the entire 20 minutes only on dissolving the face, or I may spend a minute or two just lengthening the spine and dropping the shoulders, but then the rest of the time I will spend on dissolving my face, layer by layer.

Other Experiences with the Up and Down Forces

There is also a tendency when working within the three spheres to overemphasize the movement of the up or the down forces. For example, when I first learned the up and down forces, I was told I needed to move the lumbar in. Over the next three weeks, I moved the lumbar too much in and pushed it toward the stomach; that gave me back pain. Of course, balance is a keyword. You do not want to let the lumbar collapse, but you also do not want to push it in too far. The same with the thoracic spine, which should be lengthened but should not be stiffened military style. That is too tense and creates tension in other soft tissue around the trunk. Dropping the shoulders over time will become easier and easier because once you drop them and emphasize relaxation, the soft tissue will lengthen and you will be able to move the shoulders farther. Dissolving the face is done more on a mental level, but definitely there is a connection when you put your mind on the face and dissolve it. You are also releasing stress and tension from the soft tissue. A good facial massage is recommended, at least one time, to help you understand the sensation of dissolving and relaxing your face.

Combining the Three Spheres and the Up and Down Forces

When achieving the fine-tuning of these skills, emphasizing the up and down forces, you will discover that your whole trunk may feel transparent, your lungs have as much space as possible, and your organs are not compressed. Your movement will no longer be stagnant and this correct alignment allows the function of the various systems within your trunk to be optimal.

This alignment through the trunk will allow a more open space and a better functioning of the various systems within the trunk. Remember, stress is not just on a mental level—stress can also occur on a physical level. A collapsed spine or lack of alignment through the three spheres equals stress. These up and down forces will also reduce stress on the spine or the disks between the vertebrae, and that will contribute to having stronger energy throughout the day. Of course, while emphasizing the up and down forces, do not hold your breath. Keep breathing with deep, quiet, long, peaceful inhalation. Utilize the sigh sound to help the muscles relax around the lungs. Sometimes you can linger at the end of exhalation and inhalation to maximize your oxygen intake and elimination of carbon dioxide.

LOWER (CENTER OF GRAVITY) ENERGY CENTER

One of the main energy centers of the body's energetic circulatory system is located two inches below the belly button and about three inches inward from that same spot, in the center of your abdomen. In the West, we refer to this spot as the center of gravity.

In qigong, this area is known as the lower dan tian, which translates as field of elixir, and is believed to be the main area of the body where qi energy is stored and from where it is circulated. The first skill that is needed for both martial arts and health is the ability to reside mentally in your physical center of gravity, the lower energy center (Figure 8), while physically moving the abdomen and back muscles in and out with each breath. I refer to this controlled expansion and contraction of the abdomen and back muscles as empty moon and full moon breathing (Figure 9).

CENTER OF GRAVITY ENERGY CENTER

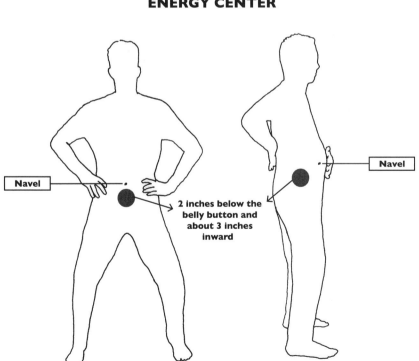

Figure 8. Visualize the Lower Energy Center.

EMPTY—FULL MOON BREATHING

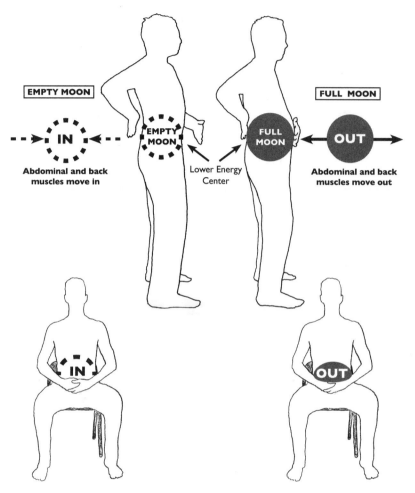

Figure 9. Move the abdominal muscles in and out with each breath.

This skill is the secret to storing qi (energy) and upgrading the battery in the center of our human electromagnetic field. The practice of residing in the lower energy center should not be only an exercise. It should eventually be practiced throughout all your daily activities. There are many benefits that this skill will give you for martial and health training. In this section, we will focus on the training and not the theory. It is best not to fill the mind with too many concepts and thoughts because we are trying to develop a more sensitive internal awareness.

Lower Energy Center—Obstacles

What will typically happen is that you will put your mind at the lower energy center, and then the thoughts will steal your mind from the visualization of concentrating on the lower energy center. The solution is to loop the thought that stole your focus from the lower energy center back into the lower energy center. Because we have so many thoughts, 18 thoughts per second, it is very difficult, at first, to keep the mind on the visualization. Accept the fact that other thoughts will come in and will steal your original thought of the energy ball in your abdomen. Instead of being upset that there are *more* undesired thoughts, just loop those thoughts back to the visualization of the energy ball at the lower energy center. Repeatedly return your attention back to the visualization every time that you realize your mind has wandered. The more cool and relaxed you can stay the better. The more you hold your attention in your lower energy center, the stronger this main battery will become. The stronger this main energy center is, the greater your quality of life, health, and martial skills will become.

After some practice, you will be able to maintain your focus for longer periods of time within the energy center. One day your mind will be able to sense the center even while you are fighting negative forces and impurities from within or outside. Later in this book, you will also learn that the more we quiet the brain, the eye energy, and the upper energy center, the easier it is to reside in the lower energy center.

Alignment/Space is an Essential Part of Creating the Lower Energy Center

Alignment throughout the spine and the pelvis floor is essential in order to create the right space within the torso and a better sensation of the mind. Think of your pelvis area with the bottom trunk as a container. When alignment is correct, this container would have the most space possible and the least tension to distract the mind from staying at your lower energy center. That is why before starting your visualization of your lower energy center on a physical level, drop the tailbone down, move the lumbar slightly out, and lift the thoracic spines. For energetic purposes, slightly bend forward and arc your upper back into what is called in the tai chi world as turtle back. Creating this alignment through the spine and the pelvis will feel like you have more space and less tension from the soft tissue, which will lead to an easier and stronger visualization. If you push the lumbar inward too much, it creates tightness in the muscles and that prevents you from attaining deep relaxation and having an easy visualization. If you tighten the abdominal muscles, again, you create stress and tension that will prevent a better visualization of the lower energy center. If you drop your head, you will have a hard time 'holding' the visualization.

Holding your mind in the lower energy center can be done when you are sitting, standing, or moving slowly and practicing tai chi. Practicing when lying down is not as effective because the mind is not centered and it is too easy to fall asleep. Lying down is more of a relaxation, letting go, or a way to fall asleep than a meditation. The sitting or standing postures, or moving slowly is strongly recommended for practicing the lower energy center visualization. When sitting, you can use a chair, sitting on the edge, or just sit on the floor. Over time, when sitting on the floor, the lower back will pull you backward and will distract your concentration on the visualization. It is recommended you sit on a block or a pillow to just lift the tailbone off the ground while tilting forward toward the knees two to three inches. This tilt allows the lower back to be more relaxed over longer periods of time, which is needed for the visualizations to become strong.

When standing and putting your mind in the lower energy center, you will find that when the eyes are open, it is a little harder to visualize the lower energy center than when your eyes are closed. Over time, close your eyes and focus on the lower energy center, and then open them and try to maintain that visualization. If that has become difficult, you can practice an in-between stage and half-close your eyes, and go from closed to half-closed, and then eventually to holding the visualization with your eyes open. After you have trained this way for a while, you will be able to create the same strength visualization when the eyes are closed or open. One day, when you are looking at people in front of you, your mind can think about them, but at the same time your mind will also be focused on the lower energy center. At this point, the question is are these two places, your lower energy center and the person in front of you, or is it ONE? Is your mind in two places or is your mind in one place? When you are relaxed and focused deeply, you will find that it is in one place.

One of your tasks, eventually, will be to hold the mind in both the upper and lower energy centers and sense the common elements, as well as the different characteristics in each of the energy centers.

Some Reminders about the Lower Energy Center

Remember, when training your lower energy center, divide the training into two parts—physical and mental. On the mental level, visualize a ball of energy in your abdomen and go over the process of the stages described above. On the physical level, move the abdominal and back muscles in and out, coordinating with your breath, while you hold the visualization of the energy ball. Remember that you have two ways to move the abdominal and back muscles with coordination of the breath, the Buddhist and the Taoist. Over time you may find words that characterize the personality or behavior of your lower energy center, like 'slow movement,' 'molten lava,' or associate it with certain colors like green, purple, white, red, or orange. Different people see and feel different colors, which symbolize the different energy situations throughout the body.

EMPTY AND FULL MOON BREATHING

For this exercise, we will focus on the physical muscles surrounding the lower energy center area. This skill, coordinating the movement of the abdominal and back muscles with the movement of the lungs and diaphragm, should be practiced and emphasized on its own. This exercise is one of those pillar principles that should eventually be incorporated into every mind/body prescription throughout the Sunset Tai Chi program. It is ultimately used with every breath you take. Physically, this exercise will allow you to regain control over the abdominal and back muscles. Many of us have lost the firmness and control over those muscles. If you do not use it, you lose it. Starting to move them with the help of your hands, one on the back and one on the abdomen is the first step.

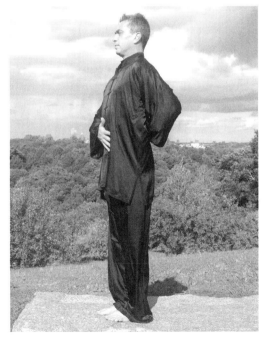

Move muscles with the help of your hands (standing).

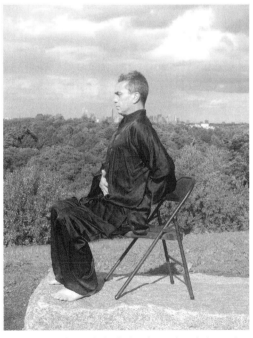

Move muscles with the help of your hands (sitting).

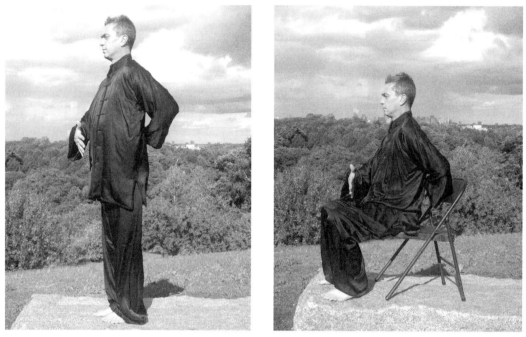

Full moon (standing).   Full moon (sitting).

Once you experiment with the movement of your back and abdominal muscles, you will realize that you can choose to move the muscles in or out during inhalation or exhalation. When the muscles move out, it is full moon and when they move inward, it is empty moon. At first, just breathe naturally and deeply with your lungs, and then with the help of your hands move the back and abdominal muscles in and out with only 80% effort. If you move and inhale to 100% it will create tightness in the muscles, which inhibits your circulation. You may initially experience little movement and control over the back and abdominal muscles, especially the back, which moves significantly less. The movement at this stage of training can be compared to the pulsing of the skin of a drum, just moving in and out without much control. As you progress, you will be able to move the muscles while counting 30 levels or stages between full moon and empty moon, meaning that you have developed excellent control over those muscles and can imitate the actual cycle of the moon.

The final idea is not to move quickly from empty to full moon positions but to create as many stages in the movement as possible. Once you are able to create all the different stages of the moon from empty to full, you have very good control over the abdominal and the back muscles. Next, try moving only one side of the abdominal muscles.

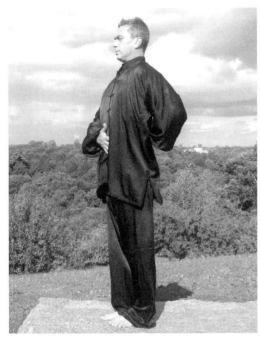

Empty moon (standing).

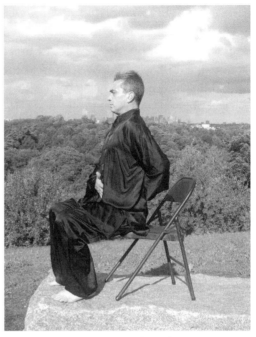

Empty moon (sitting).

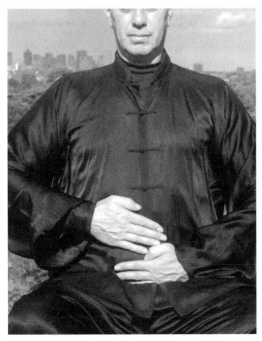

Use 80% effort.

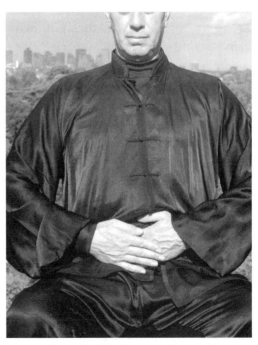

Move abdominal and back muscles through 30 stages.

Get Started with Empty and Full Moon

At first, you may want to use your hand to help the movement of the abdominal muscles either in Buddhist or Taoist breathing. Use your hand to shape the muscles and help you gain back control of those muscles. Many people lose the ability to move the abdominal and back muscles especially around the pubic area and the solar plexus. The back muscles are sometimes particularly difficult to control and move. Over time, by using your palms or your fists, or a partner's, you will gain more and more control over this group of muscles and you will not need the help of your hands.

When moving the abdominal muscles in and out, you will discover that the front abdominal muscles move a lot more than the back muscles. That is because the front muscles have a few more layers of soft tissue than the back ones. The back muscles are very thin and close to the spine. You can easily feel the spine within the soft tissue of the back, but you will have a harder time feeling anything through the front. The front has many more layers than the back.

Even though the front is bigger and has more layers, when you move the back and the front muscles they should both reach empty and full moon at the same time. As the abdominal and the back muscles move in or out, even though the back muscles have a shorter distance to cover, it is your job to make sure that they reach out or in at the same time. If you cannot do this stance, train the movements separately. Train the front muscles and then train the back muscles. Once you are able to isolate and move each group separately, you can then put them together. You will be amazed how quickly you achieve control over those muscles, especially with the help of the hands. Within a few weeks, you may find that you can move the abdominal muscles all the way down from the pubic bone to the solar plexus, emphasizing the movement of front and back at the same time.

Once you have more control over the muscles, you will notice that you can move them in a wave instead of just in and out like the skin of a drum. The more control you have, the easier it is to move them as a ripple or wave. It will also be much easier to move slowly from full moon to empty moon. As you can see, achieving a higher quality with the physical skill of empty and full moon comes down to controlling the front and back muscles in coordination with the breath. This control will lead to our main goals of this skill—strengthening the abdominal and the back muscles while massaging the internal organs, and constantly strengthening the energetic system, especially the lower energy center, or, as it is referred to in this book as well as in *Sunrise Tai Chi*, the center of gravity energy center. This skill will strengthen and upgrade your energetic system, remove stagnation, and increase circulation throughout your entire system. This constant abdominal and back muscle movement will also strengthen what is today popularly referred to as your core.

Slow, Fast, Small, Large Muscle Movements

On some days in your training, you will want to emphasize three to five minutes of intense movement of the abdominal and back muscles. When practicing this way, you are building tension. In order to make efficient progress in regaining control of those muscles, tensing techniques are occasionally needed. The nice part is that when you go back and perform the empty and full moon with only 80% effort, you will find that doing so becomes much easier. You will also experience a larger and better movement throughout the abdominal and the back muscles after these three to five minute intense sessions. Every now and then, just take a few minutes and emphasize vigorous physical empty-full moon breathing.

Buddhist Breathing and Taoist Breathing

When performing the empty-full moon exercise, we can coordinate the breathing with two methods of movement. In Buddhist breathing, we inhale, expand the lungs, and the moon expands at the same time, and when we exhale, the moon and lungs contract. The moon and lungs expand and contract at the same time. Inhale slowly into your lungs through the nostrils and, with control, expand through the abdominal and the back muscles. Keep visualizing the lower energy center. Notice how the walls of the abdominal and back muscles move outward away from the visualization of the energy ball at your center of gravity energy center. Eventually, see if you can mentally reside within the energy ball and then 'see' the walls of the front and back muscles moving away from you or where your mind resides.

If you are interested in achieving this skill, you need to take it slow and easy. Work on one side, the abdominal or the back muscles—isolate the side you chose for a while, as you did for empty full moon. Regain control over the movement of the front and back muscles. Once you are comfortable, move from this skill and emphasize, for a month or two, the visualization of the energy ball at your center of gravity energy center. Once you are comfortable with doing each one separately—the physical skill as well as the mental one—put them together. Your mind still may move from the ball visualization when expanding the abdominal and back muscles, but after some time you will be able to maintain the energy ball visualization while sensing or seeing the walls of the moon (abdominal and back muscles) moving away from you.

Taoist breathing is the opposite. When inhaling, the lungs expand and at the same time draw the abdominal muscles and the back muscles inward. The lungs expand while the moon contracts and the lungs contract while the moon expands. The diaphragm is in the middle between the two forces. You may feel more tension in the diaphragm area because you have opposite motions within the trunk. That is why, in qigong and tai chi, we hold the thoracic spine slightly forward in a posture referred to in tai chi as turtle back, whereas in yoga we hold the spine slightly straighter. The curving of the spine in the turtle back posture does not misalign the spine. The thoracic spine just slightly relaxes forward to create space for the diaphragm to move down without pressure from the walls of the back and front muscles.

One of the questions I always ask myself is "What is the healthiest and best position of the spine to reduce stress as well as use minimum effort?" Through years of doing both yoga and tai chi, I realized that there is no single position where we should always hold our spine. We want to develop a healthy zone. For this reason, we need to emphasize stretching the spine or the soft tissue around the spine further away from that zone, to all 360 degrees, in order to create a comfortable environment within that zone. Comfortable means there is a lack of the physical stress that pulls on and changes the alignment of the bones and joints. When inhaling in the Taoist breathing method, the lungs expand, and the abdominal and the back muscles slowly draw in while

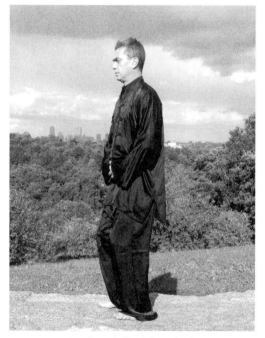

Tai chi turtle back (standing).

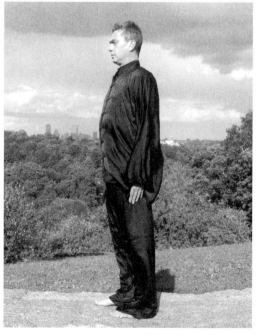

Yoga spine (slightly straight).

maintaining a visualization of the lower energy center. As you exhale, allow the abdominal and the back muscles to open outward with control until you reach full moon.

Buddhist Breathing–Mental Visualization

On a physical level: When inhaling, expand the abdominal and back muscles to full moon, and when exhaling, move the abdominal and back muscles inward to empty moon.

On a mental level: When performing or practicing Buddhist breathing, put your mind in the lower energy center. The mind needs to reside there with the sensation of a point or a ball without being distracted away by your thoughts. At first, when putting the mind in the lower energy center, your thoughts may pull your mind away, and you will find that you are thinking of something else entirely. The trick is not to fight this distraction when it occurs but just to keep looping from that thought back to the visualization of the round sensation in your lower energy center (Figure 10). It is natural that the emotional monkey mind is trying to steal your horse mind away from being focused on your energy center. Allow the thoughts to pass, and return your awareness to the energy center. This gentle looping visualization technique is an important skill.

MIND RESIDES IN
THE CENTER OF GRAVITY ENERGY CENTER

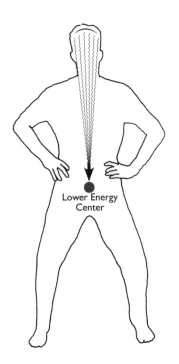

Lower Energy
Center

Figure 10. Keep looping your thoughts back to the Lower Energy Center.

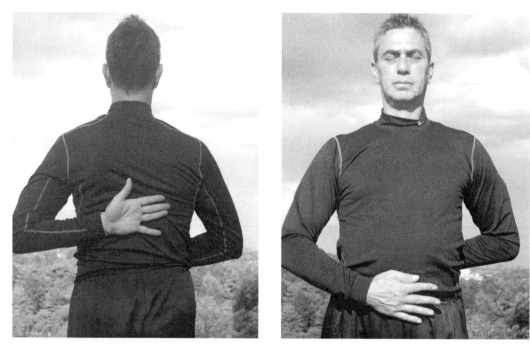

Place your hand on your lower back.   Place your hand on your abdominal muscles.

Another good technique is to place one hand on the abdomen and one on the lower back, and visualize the spot between your two hands until you develop a strong sensation there. Yet another method of achieving this same focused awareness of mentally residing in the center of gravity energy center is to drop an imaginary fishing line down the inside your body from the center of the top of your head, the heavenly gate, until it reaches the lower energy center (Figure 11). There are many different visualizations that can be effectively used to reach the goal of mentally residing in the lower energy center. Find one that works for you, or even make up one.

Taoist Breathing–Mental Visualization

On a physical level: When inhaling, contract the abdominal and back muscles to empty moon, and when exhaling, expand the abdominal and back muscles out to full moon. Taoist breathing is more aggressive than Buddhist breathing and will help you to generate abundant qi (energy) more quickly (Figure 12).

IMAGINE A FISHING LINE DROPPING DOWN

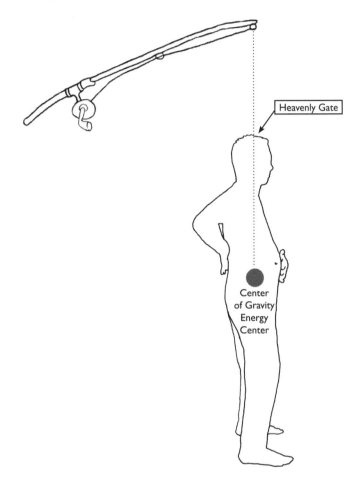

Figure 11. Imaginary Line from the Heavenly Gate
to the Lower Energy Center.

On a mental level: Put your mind in the lower energy center as you did in the Buddhist visualization. Once you are able to reside in this center, start mentally pulsing the sensation of the ball of energy that you have created in your center of gravity (Figure 13). When inhaling, the ball condenses, and when exhaling the energy ball expands. As your center condenses, imagine that it also glows brightly like a ball of light, and when you expand, imagine the sunlight expanding slowly around you, then around your house, then around your city, growing until it expands around the world, as if there is a dimmer switch in your belly and you are slowly turning it on.

TAOIST AND BUDDHIST BREATHING
Physical Skill

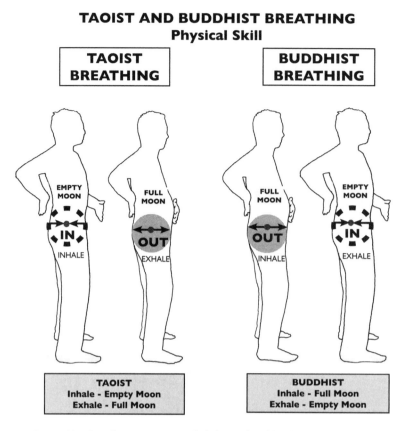

Figure 12. Coordinate movement of abdominal and back muscles with breath.

TAOIST AND BUDDHIST BREATHING
Mental Skill

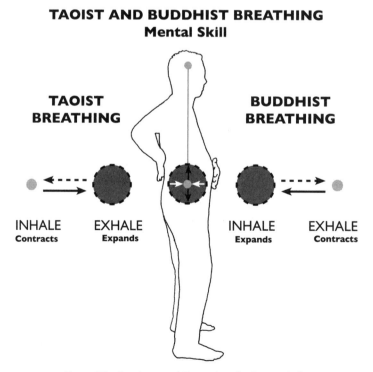

Figure 13. Condensing / Expanding the Energy Ball
Visualization in the Lower Energy Center.

Differences between Buddhist and Taoist Breathing:

The two breathing methods, Buddhist and Taoist, are used for different purposes and different reasons. Many students say that they can learn the Buddhist breathing easily, but not the Taoist. We do, however, use both of these breathing techniques naturally throughout the day for different purposes. I like to challenge my students, and before I tell them the answer I like to ask them to spend about 16 minutes—eight minutes on the Buddhist breathing and eight minutes on the Taoist breathing—and then I ask them to answer three questions: 1) Which one of the breathing techniques creates more tension? 2) Where is that tension? 3) What is the reason that one of them is tenser than the other? Answering these questions brings the students one step closer to understanding and realizing when and how we use the two different breathings throughout the day.

Here are the answers if you did not figure them out already. Taoist breathing creates more tension. The area of tension is in the diaphragm, and the reason is that when your lungs expand, the diaphragm moves down while you contract the abdominal and back muscles. That creates a conflict between the movements of the diaphragm, and those of the abdominal and back muscles. Because of this conflict, tai chi practitioners and yoga practitioners stand slightly differently. The tai chi individuals stand with the thoracic spine gently curved or slightly forward, which is referred to as turtle back. Performing the turtle back posture creates space for the diaphragm to move down with less conflict and tension with the back and abdominal muscles moving inward. Yoga practitioners stand with the thoracic spine slightly straighter. Use of the Buddhist breathing is more conducive to this posture because it does not create conflict between the movements of the back and abdominal muscles and the downward movement of the diaphragm.

PITUITARY GLAND ENERGY CENTER VISUALIZATION

Upper Energy Center

The upper energy center is at the cross section of an imagined straight line from the nose through the middle of the head and a line between your ears. It is located underneath the two lobes of the brain near the brainstem, the central area where the spinal cord connects to the brain. It is also the area where the pituitary gland (the master gland) is located. We will focus our visualization not only on the pituitary gland but also the whole area around it. I call this upper energy center the 'pituitary gland energy center.' It is about three to four inches in diameter. If you cut the skull into four symmetric pieces, this upper energy center would be in the middle. You can also find this energy center by stretching an imaginary line straight from the nose to the soft part of the back of the skull, in the area the Chinese refer to as the jade pillow (Figure 14).

Many people think that the upper energy center is in front of the two lobes in the forehead. This spot is not the upper energy center; it is the third eye energy 'spot' or 'gate.'

THE PITUITARY GLAND ENERGY CENTER

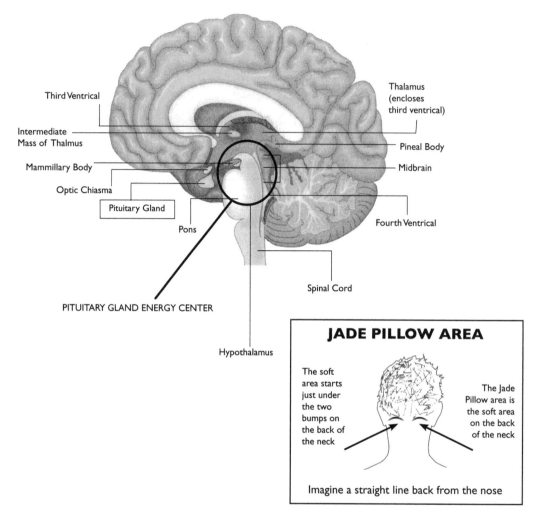

Figure 14. The brain, glands, and the Jade Pillow Area.

The upper energy center is harder to visualize than the third eye gate because it is closer to the brain and the eyes, which are two very active and distracting energetic elements. I found over the years that investing a few minutes in cooling down the eye energy and the brain energy will help tremendously in the task of acquiring the skill of residing in the upper energy center. This preparatory exercise will save time and give you an easier and stronger experience. You need to practice residing in this center while you are sitting, standing, or moving slowly when practicing tai chi.

Upper Energy Center–Progress

The more you practice, the more you develop your ability to concentrate. Eventually you will have the ability to maintain the mind in the center while, simultaneously, your mind is outside, holding attention within the body while being outwardly active at the same time. Most people, when closing their eyes, can put their minds in the upper energy center and sense it, see it, or feel it. But not many people can open their eyes and still have a sensation of that energy center. That takes practice. Of course, there is always the exception; some people are just going to get it faster than others. The trick to achieving this sensation is repetition. Practice while people talk to you, while you are walking, or while you are waiting at a stop light. The ability to maintain the visualization of the pituitary energy center while your eyes are open is a sign of very strong mental and energetic abilities.

For some people, it is harder to start with the upper energy center so I recommend starting with the lower energy center. People who have a difficult time with the lower energy center may have an easier time starting with the upper energy center. The idea is eventually to strengthen both by residing in them as much as possible.

Important Happy Reminder

When working on both upper and lower energy center visualization, there is a tendency to become too serious. Keep a little bit of a happy sensation throughout the chest area and allow it to spread through the body and up to your face—what is referred to by Taoist qigong master Mantak Chia as the 'inner smile.' This sensation is the feeling of joy throughout the trunk and a slight happiness throughout the face. Just remember not to become too serious because seriousness leads to stress. On the other hand, you cannot do this meditation when you are too excited and happy because that will lead to more excitement that will charge the soft tissue and distract you from residing in the upper energy center. Find a balance. A gentle sensation of joy throughout the body will be sufficient. You may find out that this feeling or sensation will result in a slight smile on your face. Over time, when dissolving the face, that smile disappears and just stays within the body and spirit.

External Energetic Baton Visualization

If you connect the upper and the lower energy center with a rod of energy, you will have an energetic baton with two energy balls on each end. First, before we do that internally, emphasize this sensation externally. We can use our fists, a tai chi ball, or any other round object. Placing the round object in front of the energy center that you would like to strengthen will help the mind to transform the feeling of the round object deep into your center. Once you have the round objects in front of your energy centers, work on the visualization of the energetic rod between the two objects you are holding. As you can see, I am a strong believer in breaking the larger visualizations into smaller ones. After you are capable of visualizing them separately, the upper, then the lower, and then the rod between them, when you put them together you will have an easier time.

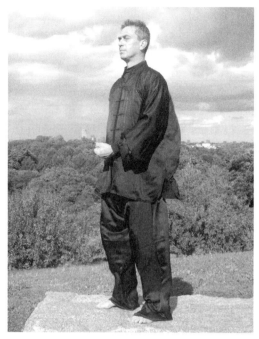

Placing the round object, or your fist, in front of your lower energy center.

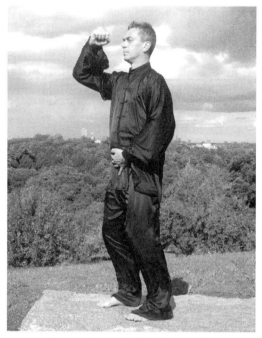

Placing the round object, or your fist, in front of your upper energy center.

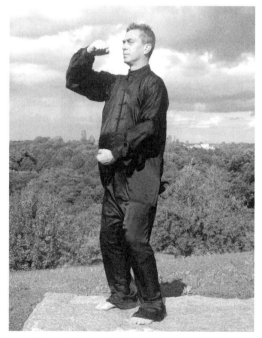

Placing the round object, or your fist, in front of both your energy centers (standing).

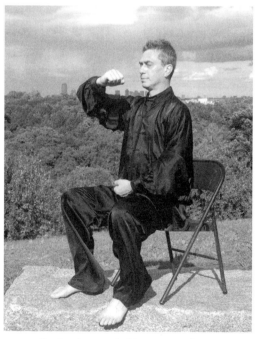

Placing the round object, or your fist, in front of both your energy centers (sitting).

Visualization of the rod between the two external pretend energy centers is just a baby step toward having the real visualization, which is the entire internal energetic baton. See if you can notice the various differences in each ball or in each energy center. You discover that even when you are visualizing energy centers, the upper and the lower, the centers will have totally different characteristics and sensations.

Internal Energetic Baton Visualization

Once you are able to stay focused on both the upper and lower energy centers separately, you should then connect the two with a straight line, or an energetic rod, through the center of the body—not the spine but right in front of it—like a baton (Figure 15). This sensation of an energy line through the center of the body will strengthen over time after you develop a stronger sense of the relationship between the upper and lower energy centers. The pituitary gland energy center is the top head of the

CONNECT THE TWO ENERGY CENTERS

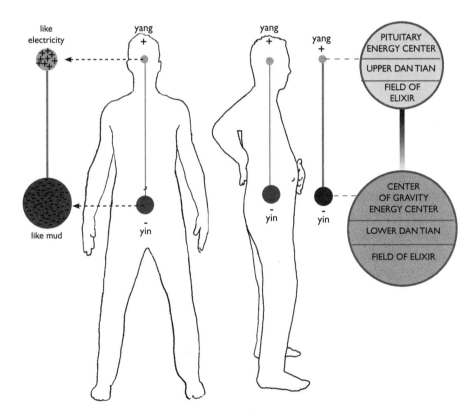

Figure 15. Observe similarities and differences
between the two Energy Centers.

baton and the center of gravity energy center is the lower head of the baton. You can also use a more spiritual visualization like a baton made of light, the light of God, as one of my students taught me. Pay attention to the various sensations of each of the energy centers, i.e., the balls of the baton, and observe the similarities and differences in the sensations that are revealed during quiet observation of each.

Many people mention that by visualizing the two energy centers within the baton, it is easier for them to see each one of the centers, as opposed to visualizing one at a time. This reaction is understandable because the two centers are interconnected. By trying to visualize one center separately, you are actually trying to eliminate the other. It may be that emphasizing the two may be easier for certain people than starting with the bottom, and then adding the top, or vice versa. Because visualization is very different for each individual, I recommend trying both options and seeing which one works best for you.

Moving Energy down the Baton

Once you are able to maintain a strong visualization of the energy baton through the center of your body, try leading the energy from the top head of the baton down to the lower head of the baton energy center (Figure 16). As you progress, one day you may experience the sensation that you are sitting in the lower energy center and looking up the baton toward the upper energy center. You may sense the energy from the upper center dropping gently on top of you like rain falling. Some people experience a feeling like honey dripping down the outside and inside of their body.

Cooling the Upper Energy Center

Because energy naturally moves up, the upper energy center has a tendency to become overly stimulated. To balance this energy, you need to cool the upper energy center. This cooling can be done by putting your mind in the upper energy center and slowly moving your mind down through the energetic rod (baton) into the lower energy center. Slowly move the mind from the upper energy center toward the lower energy center, and your energy will follow. Utilizing the setting sun to help cool the fire energy in the upper energy center will strongly enhance the effect. At the same time that your mind is moving down the energetic baton, face the setting sun and use this powerful drawing energy to cleanse and cool the head and the chest. Gently close your eyes and allow the warmth of the sun to caress your face and chest area. Let the setting sun draw out the energy from these areas. Keep moving the mind down the baton either straight down or, with further training, in a spiral.

When you become experienced with this visualization for cooling the upper energy center, you can *be* at the lower energy center, look up, and draw the energy downward from the upper energy center repeatedly, bringing more down with each pass. Do this visualization a few more times to move the energy you were not able to move down the

Cooling the Upper Energy Center

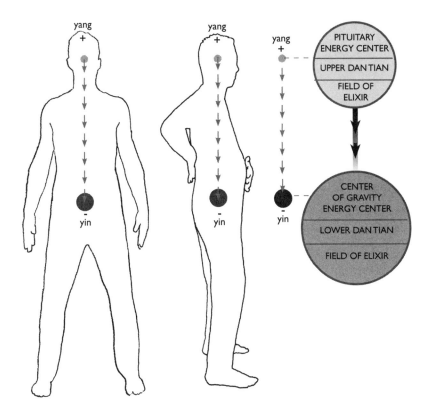

Figure 16. Energy should be led, not pushed.

first time. At this point of the process, you can use the waterfall and the elevator visualizations. Just keep moving the energy down using whatever visualization it takes. Eventually, you will be able to reside down in the lower energy center, look up, and lead the energy from the top into the bottom. At this stage, the fishing line and the bob visualization can be more helpful. The focus of the visualization is on being the bob and looking up. The fishing line is very thin. You do not need a strong visualization at this point, such as the elevator or the waterfall to build the visualization of the downward movement.

Here are some examples that I have used over the years to help strengthen my visualization of this skill: at one point I would visualize the down movements as a waterfall. The smooth and strong visualization of the water moving down kept my mind focused and was consistent with my goal of moving the mind down to the lower energy center while cooling the upper one (Figure 17). Some days when I would need a more 'solid' down movement feeling/sensation, I would visualize being in an elevator. I would get in the elevator through the eyes or the top of the head and just shoot down to the basement where I would stay until my thoughts would steal me away. Instead of thinking at this point, "Wow, I am not there anymore," I would just go back and take the elevator again. No thoughts, I just kept taking this elevator down over and over. On days that my mind was quieter, I used a fishing visualization. While I practiced, I would drop an imaginary fishing line through the center of my body starting from the top of my head and would visualize the bob floating in my center of gravity energy center. The gentle bobbing within the abdomen would help me keep my mind focused down, while the line helped me maintain the visualization of the movement downward.

THE ENERGETIC WATERFALL
Cooling the Upper Energy Center

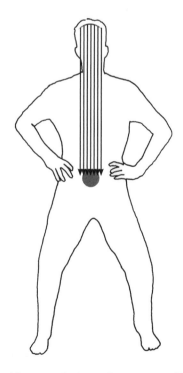

Figure 17. The mind flows into the Lower Energy Center like a waterfall.

Moving in a Spiral

Once you can easily lead energy down from the upper energy center into the lower one, you can try moving the energy down with a spiraling sensation, like water moving down a drain. Move the mind in a spiral, down the energetic rod from the upper energy center into the lower one. Certain people feel more comfortable starting with spiraling down the baton as opposed to moving straight down. I first trained by visualizing the energy moving straight down and then I was introduced to the spiral. This method is the more traditional progression. But during my teaching, I realized that some of my students were able to spiral down better than just moving straight down. For them, a stronger experience was created. I prefer to introduce both methods and allow individuals to experiment and see which visualization works best for them.

Important Reminders about the Baton

It is very important to notice the differences between the two energy centers.

When draining the baton and cooling the upper energy center, first move straight down from the top like a waterfall. Eventually, reside in the lower energy center and watch the energy coming down from the upper one.

Afterward, spiral downward from the pituitary energy center; upper energy center to center of gravity energy center; lower energy center, spiraling down along the visualization of the energetic rod that connects the two energy centers.

Distractions from Having a Strong Energetic Baton–Eyes and Brain

There are two energetic components that interfere with having a strong visualization of the pituitary energy center and with moving the energy from the upper energy center to the lower one. The two components are the 'eye energy' and the 'brain energy.'

The Eyes

We use our eyes all day, causing much energy to continuously flow out of the sockets. Even when we close our eyes, we do get some relief, but that energy continues to be emitted from the eyes. This movement of energy distracts us from focusing on the upper energy center, from cooling the upper energy center, and from moving energy down to the lower center. You must first spend time cooling the eyes, relaxing the area around the eyes, and eventually calming the eyes so they are no longer an energetic distraction.

Cooling the Eyes

While sitting in meditation, gently close your eyes, relax them, and let your eyeballs drop into their sockets. Notice that even though you close your eyes and slow down the movement of energy, there is still energy moving out through them. Now draw your sensation through the closed eyelashes toward the brain. Remember, your sight comes from the brain. The eyes are just lenses. Moving the energetic sensation toward the brain will eventually slow or cool down this constant moving-forward energy that usually moves through the eyes.

When you are practicing while the sun is setting, allow the energy of the setting sun to draw the excess energy from the eye and face. Do not wait only for that time. Do it because so much cooling needs to be done to the eyes that doing it only while the sun is setting is not enough.

After years of practice, one of the visualizations I have found to be effective is to imagine that there is a flashlight in my brain and the light is shining through my eye sockets. I visualize that the flashlight on/off switch is the brain and I can either shoot out the eye energy (on) or cool it down (off). As a beginner, the moving of the mind over and over through the eye tunnels towards the brain was an easier method for me to use to achieve this skill of cooling the eye energy.

The Brain

The second energetic element that interferes with first residing in the upper energy center and then with the process of moving energy down and cooling the upper energy center is the brain energy. The right and left lobes are generating many thoughts and that energy pushes up beyond the skull, beyond your hair, into a field around the head. That energy is strong and distracting.

Cooling the Brain

One of the methods I have found effective for cooling the brain is to sit with your eyes closed and sense the brain: first the brain lobes, from the top, and then the projection of the energy from the lobes. If you close your eyes and notice the sensation around your head, you will sense that the energy your brain generates does not stop at the skull, but is hovering over your head almost a fist away from the skull.

Start by emptying your mind of any thoughts. This step will already cool down the energy significantly but you can take it a step further. Take whatever energy is left over and use the imagery of the morning dew. Let the remaining energy move downward through your hair, which is the grass, down into your skull. If you are bold, just draw the energy down through the skin, which will be like the earth. To move and cool the rest of the distracting energy and to move further down, I use the image of the toilet, which is sometimes a very appropriate metaphor. It flushes the waste from my mind. I imagine that my head (skull) is the toilet and that the brain and whatever is in it will be just flushed down. I start a visualization of a spiral inside my skull and I collect the matter and the energy and just flush them down toward the stem that connects to the base of the brain. Sometimes I sense a total emptiness from both the eyes and the brain and experience just the skull. At first it was scary, but now I look forward to the experience.

Using the setting sun adds a powerful element to cooling the brain. At the same time that you are moving energy down toward the lower energy center, allow the setting sun energy to draw the energy from the skull, especially the forehead, cooling from both the inside, using your mind, as well as the outside. The sunset is an opportunity that only comes once a day and for just about 30 minutes. Enjoy it while it lasts, but do not wait to practice cooling down only at that time. Cooling the brain energy can be done several times a day.

You can use this process every now and then throughout your meditation to cool the eye and brain energies. Your mind will then be able to remain more strongly in the upper energy center and you will be able to drain it in a more efficient way. In my personal practice, if I sit for 45 minutes, I will visit those areas at least three times and cool them down, and then continue with the rest of my visualization. This practice is very important to your progress, this ability to keep checking and monitoring the different skills, the different visualizations, and the different alignments. Eventually you become like a conductor—you monitor the various skills that are like the different musicians, the different instruments, and you make sure that everybody is part of the melody, and that is what makes an orchestra, and that is what makes a holistic or a complete mind/body approach.

BUBBLE VISUALIZATION (GUARDIAN ENERGY)

Visualize a bubble around the physical body, about a fist away from the surface of the skin, like a cocoon. Some of my students feel as if they are within an egg, or some sense a fog or mist around them. Others experience this mist with a color and others with many colors. Whatever visualization it takes to strengthen this sensation and awareness of a bubble surrounding the body is legitimate. In the beginning, when sensing the bubble, you may experience holes or areas that are not as strong in your bubble as other areas. That is normal. Keep patching the weak parts of the bubble with your mind while maintaining and thickening the areas that are already strong. Over time, you will have a thick and vibrant energy bubble around you that can be utilized for both martial and health goals. In Chinese qigong, this bubble is recognized as the 'guardian energy' or the energy that guards us from negative forces from the outside. It is used as both a filter and a shield against negative forces and impurities inside of us as well as outside. I believe it to be an energetic component of our immune system as well as our spirit (Figure 18).

Impurities can be chemicals from our food and air, stagnant energy, toxic emotions, unpleasant encounters with other people, or bad memories we have not yet resolved.

The bubble visualization is an easier one than those previously described because it is easier for the mind to focus outside the body than inside. The bubble visualization will strengthen the external energy that guards us while filtering out negative forces and impurities within us. This energy field is about a fist away from our body, surrounding

BUBBLE VISUALIZATION

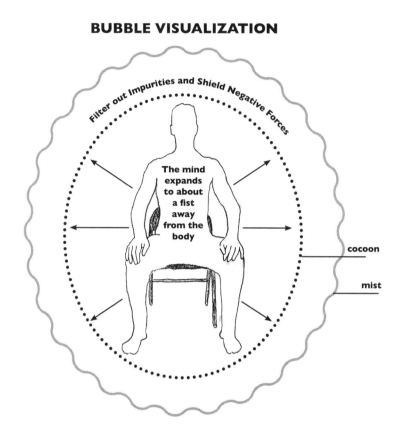

Figure 18. The mind expands out from the body,
enveloping you in a protective bubble.

our entire body. The quality and performance of the filter varies with different people, but everyone can benefit from using this visualization to strengthen our external shield.

This energy can be strengthened by focusing on it specifically, and through the longer and more successful path of fine-tuning all five building blocks: body, breath, mind, energy, and spirit. When it is cold, the bubble moves closer to the skin and when it is warm, the bubble expands further from the skin. When your whole body needs more energy in the core, this bubble energy will shrink and move all the way to the skin and then away from the palms and the feet. Some people experience cold feet and cold palms. That is a manifestation of this bubble shrinking toward the core to protect it. One of the quick ways to strengthen the bubble temporarily is when cooling the upper energy center and residing in the lower one, visualizing deep roots from your feet will strengthen the bubble. The long and more effective and long-term way is through strengthening and developing your energetic system, finding alignment, increasing your breathing, quieting the monkey mind, and evoking your spirituality. Harmonizing these skills will contribute to having a stronger bubble of guardian energy around you.

To develop the bubble, first start with sitting or standing meditation. With your eyes closed, notice the sensation a fist-distance away from the body. Then, visualize a fog or color or energy about a fist away from the body. After a while, you discover that when you monitor the sensation around your body, you find areas that the visualization is stronger and other areas that the visualization is not as strong. Next, spread the areas that are stronger into the areas that are weaker and eventually you will have an even bubble surrounding you that includes the space under your feet.

To strengthen this visualization and to help the mind make it more vivid and real, we can use the sensation of the floor. The floor beneath your feet is the stronger *real* sensation when compared to the sensation of the air surrounding the rest of you. Use the floor sensation and use this physical feedback to help the mind create the same strong sensation around the rest of your body. Awareness of the floor beneath you can help the mind create a stronger visualization around you.

Strengthening the energetic bubble takes time. At first, you patch the areas that are not as strong. After a while, you expand the bubble away from you. Eventually, visualize the bubble and the baton at the same time. Once you can simultaneously visualize the energetic bubble outside your body and the energetic baton inside the body draining downward, you are advanced in your visualizations.

The energetic bubble is a very important skill within the energetic system visualizations because it allows you to control a shield between you and external forces, and gives you a mechanism that filters impurities away from you and blocks negative forces coming into you. Many people are very affected by external forces and their lives are sometimes even controlled by them: fears, sickness, anxiety, annoying people, and on and on. Building the energetic bubble will help you deal with these stresses or negative energy. The energetic bubble is one more line of defense, a transition between you and the forces that come at you.

Remember that the energetic bubble shrinks in the winter and expands in the summer. You need to dress warmly and protect the energetic bubble from spending its force on protecting you from the cold. Dressing warmly allows you to conserve your energy so you can use it to nourish the internal organs and maintain a stronger and more efficient filter. Protecting the five major energetic gates—palms, feet, and head—is important as well, which means wearing gloves, scarf, hat, and warm socks.

On the other hand, in the summer the energetic bubble is naturally stronger and this kind of protection is unnecessary, but you need to be aware of the effects of modern technology, such as air conditioning and motorized travel: air, ground, and sea. You need to take the necessary steps to not abuse the energetic bubble but instead help this energetic element by using correct behavior to deal with the effects of modernization.

For example, even in the summer when I teach at hospitals, I bring a sweatshirt. I find it necessary, especially when we do lying down relaxation techniques, or sitting or standing meditation. The air conditioned air is too cold when I am yin, i.e., less active in one of the postures I just mentioned, and that affects my energetic bubble. Without protective clothing, I would be forced to spend time on strengthening the bubble instead of focusing on more important skills. Flying around the world results in a change of climate as well as time. Sudden changes, such as flying to another time zone, will weaken the strength and the function of the bubble. Sleep and meditation will help to regain strength in the bubble.

Some of my students who have experienced traumatic events in their lives were not able to sit and meditate, and sometimes could not even close their eyes. They were afraid of just closing their eyes, afraid of the dark, and afraid at night of falling asleep. What could they do? How could I teach them the entire practice if they could not close their eyes and meditate? I found that using the visualization of the energetic bubble as a first step definitely decreased their fears and behavior issues, which allowed them to go further into the training.

Traditionally, the first energetic visualization focuses on the center of gravity energy center or lower energy center. Sadly, I have encountered individuals that were ten years into their tai chi training and still had not been introduced to this visualization or any other one. They were just learning the tai chi moves or what is considered the tai chi dance. Remember, without the internal visualization you are not doing tai chi but you are doing an external dance. There are still benefits, but adding the energetic visualizations is a part of traditional tai chi. After all, that is the reason you are doing the form so slowly. The body is performing with the least effort needed while you tap into the power of the mind. Look for the movement in the stillness and look for the stillness in the movement. This ancient saying refers to the body moving slowly while the mind is active with the energetic experience. Eventually, your physical sensation of these subtle aspects of the body will come naturally to you, and you will no longer require visualizations to experience and strengthen them.

BATON/BUBBLE BREATHING VISUALIZATION

Once you have a strong sense of each one of the visualizations separately, it is time to put them together. Having the ability to hold each visualization for at least 10 to 15 minutes without letting the monkey mind steal away your visualization is important.

Bone Marrow-Skin Breathing

While sitting, reside in the energetic baton. See if you can sense all of the energetic baton components: the two heads as well as the energetic rod between them. See if you can sense the differences as well as the similarities between the two energetic heads of the baton. Then challenge yourself and experiment with the visualization while your eyes are open. Once you are able to hold the visualization while sitting with both eyes closed and open, practice while standing with your eyes closed and then practice with your eyes open.

The final visualization, which is the most difficult, is holding the visualization while moving slowly, doing your tai chi form. Again, start with your eyes closed and after you sense the visualization comfortably while shifting from one move to the other, try doing it with your eyes open. If you can do the form with your eyes open and you are able to sense the energetic baton, you can move on to the energetic bubble visualization. Follow the same steps with the bubble—sitting, standing, and moving slowly. Remember, start with your eyes closed and as you improve, try opening them. Once you are comfortable with each energetic visualization, put the two together. When you inhale, move your mind to the baton and when you exhale, move out toward the bubble. When your energetic baton and bubble become clear to you, move to the next level of visualization. Every time you reach the bubble with your mind, keep strengthening and building it. When you reach it with your mind, use mental actions like patching, thickening, spreading, or stocking energy within the bubble mentally. When you reach the energetic baton, move the energy down from the top energetic head to the bottom or from the upper energy center to the lower one first straight down and then in a spiral. When you are able to move your mind from the energetic bubble to the energetic baton on inhalation and back to the bubble on exhalation, you are ready to move to the next step in the energetic system visualizations in the tai chi form.

Sunset and Bone Marrow-Skin Breathing

Because the setting sun is a form of pulling energy when you emphasize moving your mind to the skin, this pulling energetic force will help you. When, however, you move your mind to the energetic baton, the setting sun can be an obstacle unless you have been practicing to the point that your mind is strong enough to lead the energy inward even though there is a pull from the setting sun. In fact, as the bone marrow-skin visualization becomes easier, the setting sun is used to remind the mind when it is at the energetic baton to keep some sensation at the skin. The idea is that when your mind moves to the energetic baton, you also reside a fist away from the skin; and when your mind moves to the skin or the bubble, you remain mindful at the energetic baton. The setting sun will touch your skin and will help you remain mindful of it when you turn your attention inward to the energetic baton. Visualizations become easier through practice. Use the setting sun to help drain the energetic baton and then use the setting sun to draw the energy from the baton out to the skin; and finally, use the sensation of the sun to remain aware of the bubble while your mind is moving inward to the energetic baton.

First Level: Start leading the mind from one visualization to the other. When inhaling, bring the energy of your entire body inward with your mind from the bubble to the baton in the center of your body. When exhaling, use your mind to lead energy from the baton back outward into the bubble, which you can do with either breathing technique, Taoist or Buddhist. Remember that when using the Buddhist breathing technique, as you inhale your mind moves out into the bubble, and when exhaling the mind moves into the baton. When you use the Taoist breathing, as you inhale the mind moves into the baton, and when exhaling the mind moves out to the bubble.

Second Level: Once you have the ability to maintain the baton/bubble visualization, try to develop the skill further. When doing Taoist breathing, be aware of the bubble as you inhale and notice the baton as you exhale. With Buddhist breathing, monitor the bubble on the inhalation and notice the baton on the exhalation. You will need to stay on each component for longer periods of time, until the two are one, but still are two. In reality, they cannot be separated (Figure 19).

A caution: During long periods that you are practicing only the energetic baton and drawing energy inward toward the energetic baton and staying only on the baton, you can 'shrink' your guardian energy or the energetic bubble. This practice can lead to becoming overly yin, which can lower your immune response and make you more susceptible to sickness. Because you are emphasizing your internal energy, your mind is not as strongly focused on the outside of your body. You are less able to deal with such elements as a cold or bacteria. To avoid getting sick during these periods, dress warmly. Protect your kidneys with an extra layer or even wrap a scarf around them, use a blanket and maybe even a hat when you are sitting and meditating. Drink warm tea or miso soup throughout the day. Other warm soups are great as well. My favorite is going to Chinatown and getting a large bowl of chicken noodle soup.

Moving between the Baton and the Bubble

You are at the point that when you close your eyes, you can visualize the upper and the lower energy center as well as the energy rod (baton) that goes between them. As you are visualizing your energetic internal baton while practicing Taoist breathing, on the next exhalation, move your mind from the baton, from both energy centers out to about a fist distance away from your body into your energetic bubble. As you inhale, bring your mind back from the bubble into your energetic baton. Exhale, move your mind from the baton into the bubble.

If you want to succeed with this visualization, you cannot be too hard on yourself. You need to learn to let go and move from the energetic baton to the energetic bubble and vice versa smoothly. Even though your mind may be stolen by your thoughts along the way, you should just continue the path toward the bubble. If you are moving mentally from the baton to the bubble and along the way you lose the visualization, just

BATON-BUBBLE VISUALIZATION

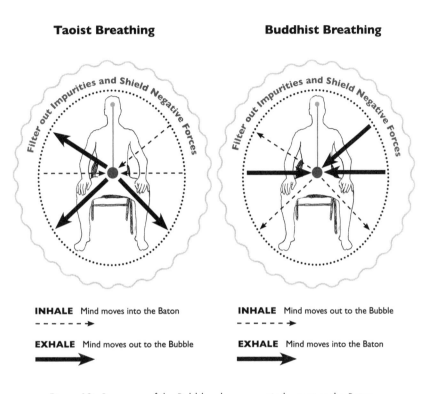

Figure 19. Be aware of the Bubble when your mind moves to the Baton.
Be aware of the Baton when your mind moves to the Bubble.

continue from where you lost it and keep going. Do not try to start again or go back. That means being too hard on yourself. It is like sitting in the car when you are traveling in new surroundings; certain things you see out the window and certain things you miss. But your car is still traveling from point A to point B, and you would not go back and re-start the trip because you missed seeing something. Over time, the more you travel from point A to point B, from the energetic baton to the energetic bubble or from the bubble to the baton, more and more elements will be revealed to you. Over time, you will be able to stay on the path between the two visualizations without allowing thoughts to steal your mind away, and more and more of the internal landscape will be revealed to you.

You may find that in the beginning, it will be easier to visualize the movement from the baton to the bubble with your eyes closed and as you improve, you will be able to achieve this visualization with your eyes open as well. I recommend that you start with your eyes closed and then, instead of going right into open eyes, practice with eyes opened just slightly so the light comes into the eyes. After some practice, you can open them slightly more. There is a stage between closed eyes and open eyes that is like a gentle squint allowing you to be mentally half inside and half outside. Keep using this technique of gradually opening the eyes and eventually you will be able to practice your visualizations with your eyes open. Do not expect to have the same experience when your eyes are opened rather than closed. When the eyes are closed, 98% of the time most people have a stronger and better experience. Every now and then, we have a strong energy experience while our eyes are open. Cherish those experiences and most importantly, when they happen, stay cool and relaxed, or you will lose the experience.

Once you can perform those visualizations altogether, I challenge you to go to the next multitasking visualization, which is to visualize the movement of the energy from the baton to the bubble and vice versa, while at the same time move the energy down through the baton. My personal experience is that the more I settle the energy down through the baton, the stronger my bubble becomes. The movement of the energy in an excited state goes up into the upper energy center as well as to the brain, which takes away and weakens the energetic bubble that is serving as a filter and a shield. When we calm down and cool the upper energy center by mentally moving energy to the lower energy center, the energy that moved down expands and nourishes the bubble, which could translate to our guardian energy expanding.

You can see how strengthening the energetic bubble can be done simply by just moving your energy, using the mind, down the energetic baton and cooling the pituitary energy center or upper energy center and the brain from its natural excitement. Moving the energy down will first build the lower energy center and cool the upper one. It will also strengthen the bubble or the energetic filter around you by making it more efficient in the process of recognizing and dealing with the negative and positive forces from within as well as from the outside. At the same time, moving the energy downward will lead to having a stronger energy shield to prevent sickness and negative forces from reaching you.

FOUR GATES BREATHING

We have five major energy gates in our body and many other small ones. In fact, each of your skin's pores can be considered a gate on a small scale. The five gates are 1) The head, especially the face, ears, and the center of the top of the head (baihui point); 2) The two palms, especially the center of the palms (laogong point); and 3) The two feet, especially the bottom of the soles (yongquan point). In this section, we will work with four of the five gates: the palms and feet (Figure 20).

Moving the Energy to the Four Gates

In order to succeed with the four gates visualization, first practice this visualization in a simple way and then in a more elaborate way. I also divide the mental training into three stages: first stage, practice using only the lower two gates; second, practice the upper energy gates; and finally put them together and practice using all four gates at the same time. Do it with both the simple and the elaborate way.

Four Gates: the Simple Way

The four gates are the two palms and the two soles of the feet. In the first stage of training we only train two gates at a time. I recommend starting with the upper gates, which are the palms. I recommend them because they are the easiest of the four. You can do this visualization sitting on the edge of the chair or standing.

THE FOUR GATES

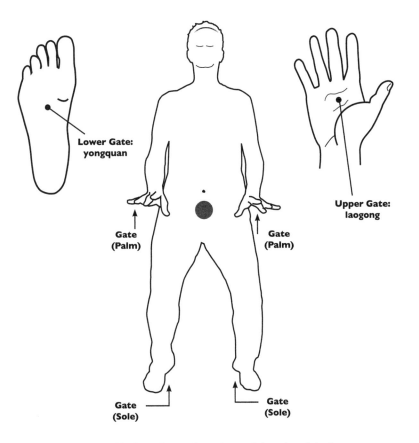

Lower Gate:
yongquan

Upper Gate:
laogong

Gate
(Palm)

Gate
(Palm)

Gate
(Sole)

Gate
(Sole)

Figure 20. The Four Gates—the palms and the soles of the feet.

Upper Two Gates: the Simple Way

Put your hands out, palms facing down about the height of your belly button. Relax your wrists and elbows. Drop your shoulders, lengthen the spine, suspend your head, and relax your face. The tongue should touch the roof of the mouth, and the fingers slightly spread as in the tai chi hand form. On your next exhalation, bring your mind into the palms, about an inch away from the palms. On the inhalation, move your mind back into the lower energy center. On the exhalation, your mind goes to the palms. As you can see, in this case you are not really leading the energy through a specific path. You are just moving your mind from the lower energy center to the center of your palms, and back to the lower energy center (Figure 21).

UPPER GATES BREATHING
The Simple Way

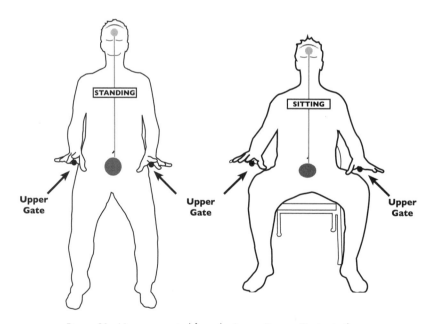

Figure 21. Move your mind from the Lower Energy Center to the
two Gates and then back to the Lower Energy Center.

Lower Two Gates: the Simple Way

After training the two upper gates for a while, place your palms on your center of gravity energy center and practice sending energy to the lower two gates. Inhale with your mind in the lower energy center. As you exhale, put your mind about a few inches below the soles of your feet. Distribute the weight between the ball of the foot and the heel, so your weight is distributed evenly between the two. Inhale, bring your mind into the lower energy center, exhale, put your mind an inch or two beyond the soles of your feet. Continue this process until you feel comfortable with the mind shifting from the lower energy center to the lower two gates, and then back again (Figure 22).

LOWER GATES BREATHING
The Simple Way

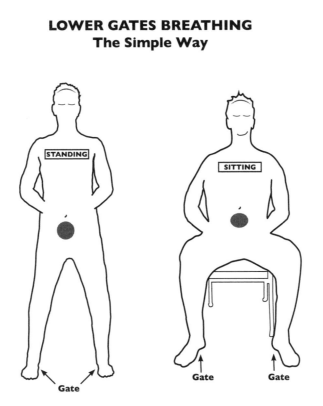

Figure 22. Move your mind from the Lower Energy Center to the two gates and then back to the Lower Energy Center.

All Four Gates: the Simple Way

Once you are comfortable with each of the two gates, it is time for you to put all four gates together. Stand with your feet shoulder-width apart, palms face down in front of your body about two inches below the navel. The elbows are a fist away from the trunk. With the next inhalation, bring your mind from the four gates into the lower energy center and on the next exhalation, shift your mind to the four gates. Make sure that your mind is even at all four gates.

You will notice that two out of the four gates are sometimes stronger than the others. Certain people may sense the bottom two gates more strongly than the upper two gates and others may experience the palms as a stronger sensation than the legs. What needs to be done is to balance the sensation and make it an equal sensation throughout the four gates. If your mind is stronger in the palms, just balance it by moving more of your mind into the soles of the feet and if it is stronger in the soles of feet, do the same by moving the mind more strongly into the palms. Eventually you will find the correct mental balance between all four gates with 25% of the mind in each gate (Figure 23).

Once you feel comfortable with the four gates, go to the next level of visualization, which goes from the gates to the lower energy center through a more specific path.

FOUR GATES BREATHING
The Simple Way

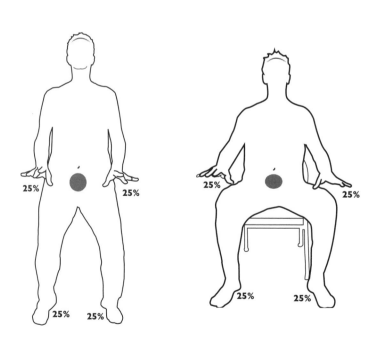

Figure 23. Make sure your mind reaches all four gates at the same time
and returns to the Lower Energy Center at the same time.

Upper Two Gates: The Elaborate Way

Start by standing with your knees slightly bent, and your feet shoulder-width apart. When inhaling, the ball of energy at the center of our lower energy center squeezes into a brighter, focused ball, but at the same time, the energy from that ball rises up in the back through the governing vessel. The governing vessel is an energy path on the back of the torso that runs upward between the spine and the skin on our back (Figure 24). The mind performs two mental tasks: the first, while inhaling, focus in the lower energy center and second, on the same inhalation, the mind raises to the shoulder blades area within the governing vessel; then during the exhalation, the

THE GOVERNING VESSEL

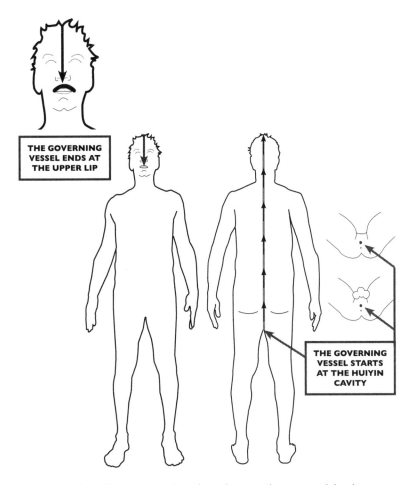

THE GOVERNING VESSEL ENDS AT THE UPPER LIP

THE GOVERNING VESSEL STARTS AT THE HUIYIN CAVITY

Figure 24. The Governing Vessel runs between the spine and the skin.

UPPER TWO GATES (TAOIST)
The Elaborate Way

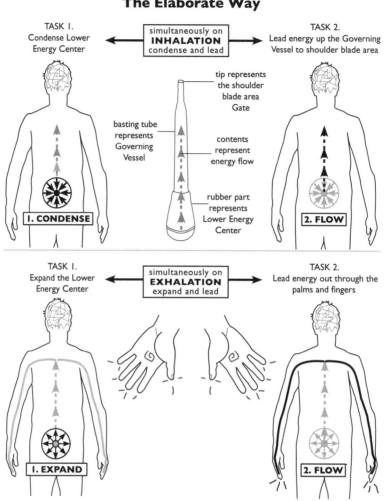

TASK 1.
Condense Lower
Energy Center

simultaneously on
INHALATION
condense and lead

TASK 2.
Lead energy up the Governing
Vessel to shoulder blade area

tip represents
the shoulder
blade area
Gate

basting tube
represents
Governing
Vessel

contents
represent
energy flow

rubber part
represents
Lower Energy
Center

1. CONDENSE

2. FLOW

TASK 1.
Expand the Lower
Energy Center

simultaneously on
EXHALATION
expand and lead

TASK 2.
Lead energy out through the
palms and fingers

1. EXPAND

2. FLOW

Figure 25. On inhalation and exhalation,
the mind performs two mental tasks simultaneously.

mind leads the energy out from the shoulder blade area, through the center of the arms, and out through the fingers and the center of the palms (Figure 25). At the same time, on the same exhalation, the mind leads the energy from the focused energy ball in your center of gravity energy center down through the legs, and out through the toes and the soles of your feet (Figure 26).

LOWER TWO GATES
The Elaborate Way

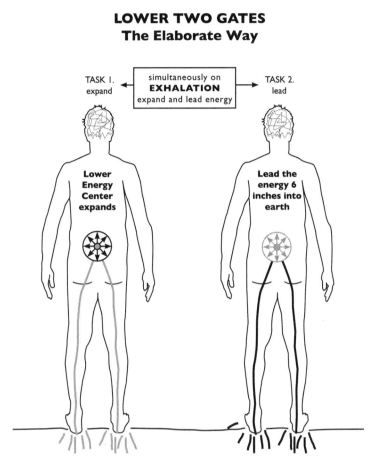

Figure 26.   The mind performs two mental tasks simultaneously.

You may notice that the visualization through the lower gates is simpler. The mind just focuses on leading the energy from the energy ball at the lower energy center down and out of the feet during the exhale, and back up again during the inhale. The visualization through the upper gates is more complex. The mind needs to use one inhalation to reach the shoulder blade area and the following exhale to lead the energy out through the palms and fingers.

Once you are comfortable with this path of visualization, add the last piece of the four gates breathing. When inhaling, also lead energy inward through the palms up through the inner arm and down the front of the body back to the lower energy center. Your mind is required to handle more than one visualization simultaneously. This sequence is called multi-visualizing. Practice leading the energy in through the arms until it becomes a natural, effortless sensation. As you lead energy through these pathways of the body, the pathways will gradually widen, and your ability to have a stronger sensation of what is happening in these energy channels, meridians, and vessels will become clearer, more enjoyable and rewarding.

This practice is the stage of 'regulating until regulating is not needed,' or 'fine-tuning until fine-tuning is not needed,' at which time you can again simply focus your awareness on maintaining a neutral state of mind, and mentally reach 'the thought of no thought.' Four gates breathing is the basic breathing technique that should be used throughout all of your tai chi practice. As you can see, it can take a long time to achieve a high level of proficiency.

Some Lower Gates Practice

On inhalation, your mind is in the lower energy center, and as you exhale lead the energy down again to three to four inches below the soles of your feet as if you were growing roots. Inhale and draw the mind through the center of the legs up into the lower energy center; use the empty/full moon breathing exercise, as well as your mind. Wherever your mind travels, your energy follows.

Pretend your legs are like two straws. Beneath the soles of your feet, pretend you have two cups with your favorite drink in them. I even allow my students to visualize beer, or wine, whiskey, cognac, or anything they want. Now pretend that your lower energy center is a mouth. On the next inhalation using both skills, the mental and the physical, visualize the lower energy center sucking the liquid from the two cups through the two straws, which are the legs. The drink beneath the soles of the feet moves up into the lower energy center. Now you are leading energy because your mind is at the mouth, the lower energy center, drawing the energy from beneath the soles of the feet and through the center of the legs. On the next exhalation, put your mind at the cups beneath the soles of the feet and just wait for the energy to arrive from the lower energy center through the straws, and fill the cups. If you can maintain your mind at the cups or the area beneath the soles of the feet and just 'look' up toward the lower energy center, you would lead the energy from the lower energy center instead of pushing it.

Once you feel comfortable with leading energy from beneath the soles of the feet into your center of gravity energy center or lower energy center and leading it back down beneath your feet, move to practice the upper two gates.

More Upper Gates Practice

When practicing the upper two gates, my experience is that sitting on the edge of a chair is the strongest, fastest way of achieving this visualization. Sit on the edge of a chair, lengthen the spine, and drop the shoulders. Palms are again facing down two inches below the navel with the elbows a fist away from the floating ribs. The wrists are relaxed, shoulders are dropped, and head is suspended. On the next inhalation, move your mind from the center of gravity energy center down and around the huiyin cavity, the area between the groin and the anus, up along the governing vessel in the back until you reach the area between the shoulder blades. This important acupuncture point, or cavity, huiyin, means 'yin meeting place.' The perineum is the most yin part of the body. Now exhale and lead your mind from the shoulder blades through the center of the arms all the way to three inches in front of your palms. First, when you lead the energy from the lower energy center to the shoulder blade area, close your eyes and when leading to two to three inches beyond the palms, open them. Then change and open your eyes when leading your mind up to the shoulder blades and close them when leading the mind and energy out through the palms. Make sure you use both the physical and the mental skills to help with this visualization.

Finally Four Gates Together

Once you feel comfortable with each of the two gates, it is time to put them together. Start by putting your mind in your lower center of gravity energy center for a few minutes. On the next inhalation, the moon moves to empty (Taoist breathing). Do two things: first, condense the energy ball in the lower energy center and second, move the mind from the energy center up the governing vessel to the area between the shoulder blades. On your next exhalation, again do two things: first, move your mind from the shoulder blades to the center of your palm or even better three inches away from them and second, move the mind from the condensed energy in the lower energy center down through the center of the legs three inches below your feet.

There is another path that can be incorporated in four gates breathing. Add this path only after you have been training for several years using other visualizations. For this path, on the inhalation, your mind brings energy into the lower energy center from the inner legs and inner arms. As you inhale, lead your mind/energy from the inner legs as well as the inner arms all the way to the lower energy center.

THIRD EYE PULSING OR SPIRITUAL BREATHING

The third eye is located behind the forehead, between the skull and the brain, in front of what is also called the spiritual valley or the crack between the two hemispheres of the brain (Figure 27). Your first task is to put your mind in that area without tensing the eyes or the face. With your head suspended, totally relax the face and try to just reside in the third eye area. Try to reside in a tiny spot. Imagine a dot, nail head, thumbtack, or maybe a raisin. See if you can maintain your visualization without thoughts stealing your mind away. With practice, you will be able to maintain the visualization while your eyes are open. Once you feel comfortable with having the mind in the third eye, you may start to pulse this visualization. Just enlarge it from a raisin to a grape and back to a raisin. Inhale, shrink it to a raisin; exhale, expand it to a grape. *Remember to monitor the tension of the face at the same time,* continually relaxing the face layer by layer while pulsing the third eye visualization. Remember, the third eye energy center is not

THE THIRD EYE

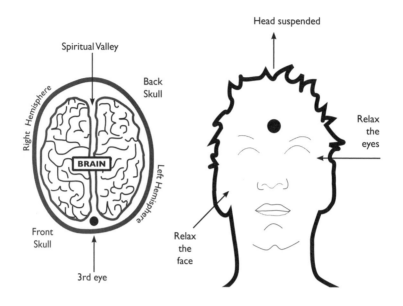

Figure 27. Reside in a tiny spot between the front of the skull and the brain.

the pituitary energy center or the upper energy center in our energetic baton. The upper energy center is located below the brain lobes where the spinal cord connects to the two lobes. The third eye energy center is right behind the forehead in front of the two lobes or in front of what we refer to as the spiritual valley.

The mind resides in a fixed point in this third eye area while cooling the energy of the eyes and brain. When you cool the energy of the eyes and brain, the third eye or spiritual breathing is stronger and clearer. This gate is also the spot through which we lead the sun energy into our body, to nourish our entire being and to boost our energetic system. If you have an uncomfortable sensation of pressure in this area, just stop and massage in clockwise circles and continue another time.

A common mistake is lifting up the eyeballs toward the third eye while visualizing the third eye. Instead, drop and relax the eyeballs into their sockets and then maintain the visualization of the third eye. At the same time, lengthen the neck upward through the top of the head and lengthen through the spine. Breathe deeply, dissolve the face, and relax the neck, shoulders, and the abdominal muscles.

'Dropping the eyes' is part of the minor up and down forces. Imitate the setting sun movement with your eyeballs and allow your eyes to drop and relax. Keeping the spine extended and the head suspended are up forces. Meanwhile, the face relaxing, shoulders dropping, abdominal muscles relaxing are the down forces. These up and down forces are endless in the body. Over time, you will discover and understand more of them. They are essential to smooth circulation and free connection between the three forces, heaven, human, and earth, as well as creating a strong flow throughout the body and stronger guardian energy surrounding your body.

As one of my teachers told me, do not be too quick to attempt to reopen the third eye. Relaxing the face is essential to the success of third eye visualization. Spending a few minutes before this meditation to remove tension from the face will contribute tremendously to the clearness and awareness of the third eye. Opening the third eye should happen naturally, and it will happen only after many years of diligent training of both the physical body and the development of a neutral and peaceful state of mind. People often speak of opening the third eye in terms of attaining enlightenment, but in fact, these experiences are not only metaphysical events—they are physiological processes that take many years to develop and are quite difficult, even for a mighty sage of ancient times.

Pulsing the third eye is the preparation for learning how to cool and raise the spirit. The spirit can be cooled and the spirit can be fired up. When you are in a dangerous situation, when somebody threatens you, you may look at him or her with an intense feeling. That is the sensation of your spirit being raised. When you are in a safe place, you can relax and cool your spirit while maintaining a strong awareness of it. Your spirit is still strong but it is cooled down.

There is one more stage of training the spirit and that is what we think of when we think of having no spirit. It is the sensation associated with being sad, depressed, upset, or discouraged. It occurs when your spirit is low, weak, in the moment of giving up, in the moment of despair. Studies have shown that in this state, your immune response is equally down. The good news is that you can always move from one stage to the other with the power of the mind. You can use reasoning, or the strength of the spirit, or hope, or maybe combinations of positive mindfulness.

Practice moving from a cool spirit to an intense spirit. The eyes are a useful tool in helping this visualization. To have an intense spirit, you want to have 'fury eyes' like a tiger, or the cat, right before it leaps on its prey. Take a mirror and see if you can create those eyes, the fury eyes. If you make the eyes too tense, they are not fury, they are just tense. On an inhalation, withdraw from this intense look and become a relaxed, quiet being, almost as if you are in your favorite spot on the beach lying down just closing your eyes and enjoying the warm sun on your face. That will be more of a calm spirit, relaxed yet vibrant, strong, and alive.

When you are in a low, defeated spirit, it is hard to come out of it on your own. That is when you need guidance and help, sometimes even professional help. At the same time, you can complement your situation by starting first with the body and breath building blocks, and then when you feel stronger, add the mind and energy blocks. Persist and do not stop. The emotional monkey mind will try hard to distract you and it is already strong at this low spiritual moment. Some days you just need to go through the motions and keep working. Sometimes, you can work your way through a bad mood, or depressed state, by practicing these energetic exercises or your tai chi form. Even if you really do not feel like practicing, you will usually feel much better when you are done. Practice the program and continue refining your mind/body skills that were passed down by the masters of the various Eastern arts.

After some time, you will come out of your depression and you will be able to practice raising and cooling the spirit. But when you are healthy, practice, practice, and practice some more, and you will be able to build a positive attitude and maintain a feeling of evoking your spirituality. Remember that while cooling your spirit, it will still be strong and vibrant. It is easier to experience the raised and energized spirit, and harder to experience the cooler one. Try to find the strength of the spirit within the cooling. Spirit does not lose its strength just because it is calm and relaxed. Think of soldiers when they are back home, or police officers on a break from their shift. Their spirits are in the cool position, but they remain alert and strong. When raising the spirit and expressing this energy with your fury eyes, make sure you balance this response with a sense of caution, awareness, maturity, freedom, and above all, compassion.

BATON/BUBBLE AND FOUR GATES SPIRITUAL BREATHING

When you feel comfortable practicing each visualization separately, you may then practice them combined into a whole. This practice can only be done once the visualizations have been trained, regulated, and fine-tuned to a degree where constant mental monitoring is no longer necessary. It is the same as having your third or fourth child. By then, you can monitor all of them and you have become more efficient with all four than you were when you had only one. When combining, you may find it mentally difficult to have all the visualizations happening at the same time. Expect to act like the conductor of an orchestra. Your mind is aware of all visualizations, and it moves naturally between them, while monitoring and staying in a deep and relaxed state.

I often talk about Dr. Herbert Benson and his great contribution to the mind/body world. The relaxed state he talks about is an essential part in becoming a 'Taoist visualization conductor' but remember, it is just a doorway to a palace full of rooms. What you can do once you are in the zone is unlimited and rewarding to each of the five building blocks. Yes, it is true you need to reach the relaxation response state first. This mental state corresponds more with the path of the Buddhist school of thought that emphasizes deep relaxation or 'reaching the emptiness' as the way to reach a natural healthy place. But as a warrior, that is, a type A personality, I personally enjoy and have benefited tremendously from the Taoist energy visualizations, which are on a more aggressive, warrior path. Once you are relaxed, you utilize the power of the mind to remove stagnations and take control over building your energetic system as well as connect to the three forces, heaven, human, and earth. Over the years as I have aged and as I have worked with more and more students, I have become a firm believer in utilizing both schools of thoughts, the Buddhist and the Taoist, according to each individual personality as well as situation.

All Visualizations Together: Try It

Inhale and focus on leading the mind inward from your energetic bubble to your energetic baton, while noticing your mind condensing the energy at the lower energy center. Notice and lead the energy up the governing channel. Focus, while sitting or standing, for a minute or two on the empty moon and full moon, and abdominal breathing, while remaining aware, in the back of your mind, of the four gates, your energetic baton, as well as your energetic bubble simultaneously. These skills are what make tai chi an 'internal art.'

Insight Into What Do I Do?

Let me give you an example of how I grow into visualization multitasking. First, if you sit every day, you have many opportunities to practice and experience many new skills as well as emphasizing old ones. I usually sit between 30 to 40 minutes in one session and a few more times throughout the day for five to ten minutes each time when I meditate standing as well as moving when doing my tai chi or qigong. Many times, I will spend the whole 30 to 40 minutes just on fine-tuning one skill like the mind in the lower energy center or cooling the upper energy center. Many times I just surf the breath, the Buddhist way. This is the Zen mind method taught to me by my first teacher. (Thank you, Tzvi Weisberg.)

When sitting for 30 minutes, I like, at various times, to fine-tune my basic skills and give personal attention to each one separately. I start by spending about eight minutes doing the exercises: surfing the breath, the sigh sound and lingering at the end of exhalation, and at least three minutes on emphasizing and encouraging the up and down forces. Then, I put my mind in my center of gravity energy center or the lower energy center for another eight minutes while maintaining the two other skills I just emphasized. I begin the empty full moon meditation and enjoy it. Next, I move to the pituitary energy center or upper energy center and send my mind downward, first straight down and then in a spiral following the rod of the baton for about five minutes. Then I notice my energetic bubble and put my mind there for five minutes. I strengthen the energetic bubble at the areas that are not strong and use the floor sensation to create a stronger sensation of the energetic bubble around me. For the next ten minutes, I will gently and peacefully monitor the various visualizations, giving each visualization just enough attention that I can sense it while doing the other visualizations. Every now and then, I can be in four or five of them at the same time. Then I move my mind from the bubble to the baton as I inhale and move my mind to the bubble as I exhale. I notice the baton as I exhale and move my mind to the bubble; I notice the bubble as I inhale and move toward the baton. I lightly 'light' the third eye and if the sun is setting or rising, I use it to boost all my skills and connect to the three forces.

As you can see, it is like getting dressed in layers. You put on the t-shirt (lower energy center) and then you put your sweatshirt (bubble energy), followed by other layers of visualizations. You put in the visualizations one by one. *Remember that you also spend time and practice each visualization separately* for 20 to 40 minutes to the point that they are strong and that they are real to you in the same way you actually put on a t-shirt. You do not want to be like the emperor in the story who had no clothes. You do not want to think you are doing the visualizations when actually they are weak and not really there. Traditionally, each visualization was trained for one year, twice every day for forty minutes. Once you do that for a year, you will own that visualization and that is when you can start adding the next layers of visualization.

FIVE GATES SPIRITUAL BREATHING

The five gates in our body are in the five extremities of our body. The bottom two gates are the feet. The top of the feet is yang, which means it has a tougher physical structure and slower energy flow than the soles. The soles are yin, which means that they have a softer physical structure but stronger energy flow. The top two gates are the hands. The back of the hand is yang which means it has a tougher structure and slower flow of energy while the front part of the palms are more yin, which means a weaker structure but a stronger energy flow. The fifth gate is the head. The back of the head is yang and again physically tougher than the front of the head, the face, which is weaker but has a stronger flow of energy. The top of the head has a smaller gate, which is the soft opening at the top of the skull. In qigong or tai chi, it is called the heavenly gate. Acupuncturists call it baihui (Gv-20). It is the entire head, however, which is considered as the fifth gate. The face is a special piece of the five gates because we can actually see when energy is moving in and out of it. For example, when we blush, it is a result of the energy rising into the face. When we faint, our faces pale when the blood and energy leave our face. You can see that the fifth gate has energy moving easily and constantly through it, especially if you are tied up in your thinking for productive reasons or distractive ones. Between the emotions and the wisdom, you can see that the five gates tend to be 'on fire,' or excessively yang, which means that they need to be constantly cooled down.

One way of cooling the five gates is through draining the energetic baton, and another way is through moving energy into the four gates and not allowing it to float up into the fifth one. Balancing the circulation into the hands and feet will reduce the energetic stress in your fifth gate, the head.

Let Us Do Some More Visualizations

Start by training four gates breathing while pulsing the third eye, or at least putting your mind at a fixed spot at the third eye. Start with moving your mind from the lower energy center to the four gates on the exhalation, and back on the inhalation into the lower energy center. Do not worry about the path for now; just move your mind to the four gates and back to your lower energy center. At the same time, visualize a spiritual eye in the center of your forehead. Visualize it as a tiny point and hold it there. Reside in that visualization. At this point, you have two visualizations: one is moving in and out, i.e., the mind moves from the lower energy center to the four gates, and a still visualization, that is, the mind stays in the third eye, right behind the forehead in front of the two brain lobes.

Once you are comfortable holding these two visualizations at the same time, you can try running the mind through the four gates pathways in coordination with deep breathing. On an inhalation condense the energy ball at your center of gravity energy center, and move your mind from the lower energy center up through the huiyin cavity (Co-1) and up through the governing vessel to the shoulder blade area. See if you can still maintain the third eye visualization.

On an exhalation, move your mind from the shoulder blade area through the center of the arms to the space a few inches in front of your palms, and on the same exhalation, while you experience the condensed feeling at the lower energy center down through the center of your legs to the space a few inches below the soles of the feet, maintain the visualization of the third eye. Once you are comfortable with these visualizations, you are at the last step of these multitasking visualizations. Add the pulsing of the third eye.

ENERGETIC LESSONS AND CONCLUSIONS

Sometimes when spending 40 minutes in sitting or standing meditation, I divide the time and spend about five minutes on each visualization and then maybe I will leave the last 10-15 minutes for trying to visualize all of them at the same time. Some days, I emphasize only one. Because I meditate sitting and standing on a daily basis, I am not worried about missing any of the larger visualizations or the multitasking ones.

Emphasizing one visualization at a time and then at the end of each meditation session putting them together makes the multi-visualizations much more powerful for me. Many of my students report similar results. It is an important principle of the Taoist approach, that is, dividing all things into small sections, breaking them into yin and yang, practicing them separately, and then putting them all together. You will find that it is worth pulling yourself back and holding yourself on the individual visualization rather than trying to achieve all of them at the same time. The more I strengthen each one, the stronger are all of them together.

These two visualizations, four gates and pulsing the third eye, become much stronger when you are able to cool the fifth gate, especially the face. You should first cool the face before performing the third eye visualizations.

> ## Reminder: Every now and then pull yourself
> ## back and train one visualization at a time.

Face Meditation

Sit in a comfortable position on the floor or the edge of a chair. Lengthen the spine and suspend your head, drop your shoulders, and slowly start dissolving the face. Dissolve the face layer by layer and melt all the soft tissue on your face—the skin, the fascia, and the muscles.

First, relax your eyes; then start dissolving and melting the areas that are closest to the skull. Relax the corners of your eyes, and relax the corners of your nose, the corners of your mouth, as well as the temple area. Let go of any tension in your face. Keep your head suspended, dissolving the face using a visualization: solid to liquid, liquid to gas. Your face will relax and dissolve over time. You will discover that it had held lots of tension.

Dissolving Your Image/Persona

When you deal with certain individuals in your life, there are certain faces you make to get you what you want. After a while, each one of us develops five or six major faces to get what we want and to make life smoother with no conflicts. If you want your kids to do something you put on a face of 'authority'; some put on a face of 'asking politely.' If you are interested in getting something from your spouse or partner, you put on a 'sweet' (some use 'authority') face. If you are scared or disappointed, your face changes again. Some people who have had a hard life look like they are sad all the time, even when they are not. Some people look like they are always smiling, even when they are not. The muscles in our face are sophisticated, dense, and intertwined with one another. If you keep making the same faces over and over, you will form a certain look that is your image. This perceived image is what gives you confidence and security. This face is what you and others consider as YOU. Over time, you accept yourself and others accept you and your regular face. Sometimes, you do not have the energy to put on your nice face. You may show a side of yourself others have not seen, and it can draw unwanted attention. We spend a lot of energy maintaining this façade. We sometimes do not feel well and do not have the energy to put on the different social faces that others are used to. Sometimes the best remedy for not feeling well can be interacting with others.

When you practice the face meditation, you melt or dissolve the face layer by layer. You are also dissolving your 'image.' Every now and then when doing the face meditation, you may succeed in becoming just a skull. You will be able to melt the entire face and experience total transparency—no soft tissue, no image. If and when this happens, do not be scared, just play it cool and be nothing, just another skull: no you, no image. It is a liberating experience.

When I sit and do the face meditation, I start with the tighter areas and then pretend that my face is an onion. I dissolve the onion layer by layer from the outside in. After I get halfway through, I move my mind to the skull and then I dissolve from the inside out, again layer by layer. Even if you have just a few minutes, close your eyes and dissolve the face. This practice is especially effective when doing it facing a rising or setting sun. An energetic, enlightening experience is very special and powerful.

If you want to go deeper with the face meditation, use the setting sun to help your mind dissolve and melt the tension and other impurities by allowing the energy of the setting sun to pull and draw the impurities away from you. (Look at the *Sunset Tai Chi* DVD animation to get a clearer understanding of this dissolving and cleansing exercise.) Once you are finished with the face meditation or even if you just emphasized it for a few minutes, move on to other visualizations. Spending even a few minutes on the face meditation before other visualizations will help provide stronger experiences because you are cooling down the face energy distraction. That allows you to have a stronger sense of the other energetic components.

Using the setting sun is a powerful experience but do not wait to cool and cleanse the face fire energy only during this time. Practice it throughout the day, even if it is for only a few minutes.

Once the face is relaxed and dissolved, add the next visualization, the visualization of the third eye. *Remember to reside or hold the visualization in one spot.* When moving energy up and through the governing vessel, make sure the energy that moves up the governing vessel, from the lower energy center, reaches the shoulder blade area, goes to the palms, and does not climb up into the head unless you are doing the small circulation meditation or you have other energetic reasons. Maintain a strong horse mind. Stay in control of creating the path or the shape of the energy flow. Your mind leads the energy and that path becomes the container for the energy to flow through. Whatever path you choose, your mind will shape your container. If you choose to work on the four gates and third eye visualizations, energy should not move up into the face. Some energy will always sneak up but what you are doing with your mind is the same as a train conductor. You are opening gates, removing blocks, and changing tracks.

Be easy on yourself. Slowing down the energy going into the face, while doing four gates and third eye visualization, is challenging. Not succeeding right off the bat is normal. Be patient and keep practicing.

SMALL CIRCULATION-YOUR BODY'S MAIN CIRCUIT

Traditional Chinese theory divides the small circulation path into two parts: the yang side, which is the governing vessel or in Chinese du mai and the yin side, which is the conception vessel or in Chinese ren mai. The energy channels are classified by size and function. Vessels are larger and are considered to be similar to a reservoir, while meridians are smaller, like rivers, streams, and creeks, and are considered to be the path as well as the suppliers of energy to the twelve internal organs, as well as to the other parts of our bodies, such as the bones, skin, and most importantly, our brain.

The governing vessel runs on the back and is a positive or yang vessel, while the conception vessel runs on the front, and is a negative or yin vessel. Ultimately, these two different vessels are experienced as one. Influencing the flow of energy in these vessels is a fundamental skill in both qigong and tai chi. These two vessels are an important part of our energetic system.

The governing vessel runs up the back, from the area between the groin and the anus, (huiyin cavity), up in front of the spine and under the skin, over the middle of the head, and ends at the upper lip or internally at the roof of the mouth (Figure 28).

THE GOVERNING VESSEL
Reservoir—Yang

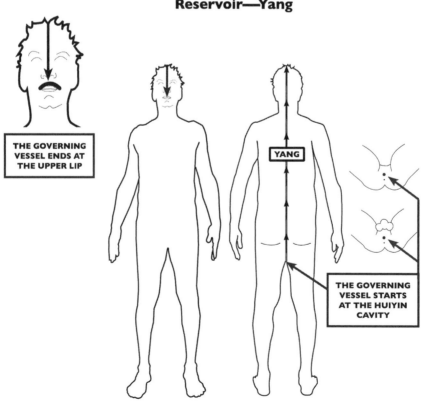

THE GOVERNING VESSEL ENDS AT THE UPPER LIP

YANG

THE GOVERNING VESSEL STARTS AT THE HUIYIN CAVITY

Figure 28.   The Governing Vessel regulates the six yang
internal organs when they are in excess or depleted.

The conception vessel runs down the front, from the bottom lip to where it meets the governing vessel at the area between the anus and the groin (huiyin cavity) (Figure 29).

The tongue is used to connect the two vessels. Putting the tongue on the roof of your mouth closes this energetic circuit. The governing vessel is the reservoir for all of your yang internal organs, while the conception vessel is the reservoir for all of your yin internal organs. Each one is in charge of regulating the needed flow in the channels that lead to the organs. Energy fills the vessels, and then if you have a balanced energetic system, energy will flow efficiently in and out according to the needs of your internal organs.

There are six energy channels that branch out from the governing vessel, and there are six energy channels that branch out from the conception vessel. The six channels that go from the governing vessel to the six positive internal organs or the yang organs are large intestine, gall bladder, urinary bladder, small intestine, stomach, and triple burner. The six channels that go from the conception vessel go to the six negative internal organs or yin internal organs are heart, lungs, kidneys, liver, spleen, and pericardium.

THE CONCEPTION VESSEL
Reservoir—Yin

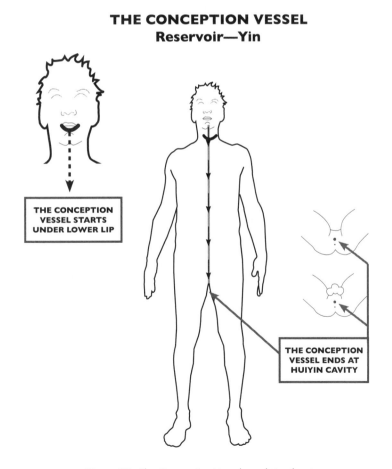

THE CONCEPTION
VESSEL STARTS
UNDER LOWER LIP

THE CONCEPTION
VESSEL ENDS AT
HUIYIN CAVITY

Figure 29. The Conception Vessel regulates the six
yin internal organs when they are in excess or depleted.

Now, if you are a little bit knowledgeable of your anatomy, you may be thinking that there are only ten internal organs. You may wonder if the Chinese have two more internal organs that we do not have. And you are right to ask this question because we really do have only ten organs as defined by Western science. The Chinese, on the other hand, recognize two other parts and functions in our bodies, which they consider to be organs. The first is the pericardium sac that wraps around the heart and the second is the system called the triple burner, which burns and processes essence and converts it into energy. The triple burner is divided into three areas: the upper burner, which converts the air we breathe to energy; the middle burner, which converts the food we eat into energy; and the lower burner, which holds and stores our original essence, or in other words what we have received from our parents, i.e., genetic material. Original essence is believed to be stored in the kidneys, but it is released to the lower energy center. Out of the three parts of the triple burner, the lower burner is the only one that the energy stored in it is considered to have the quality of fresh, cold, and clear water. In Chinese, this quality is called kan. The other two parts of the triple burner are considered as generating fire energy. In Chinese, this quality is called li. The air we breathe, which is not always very clean and the food we eat, which is not as healthy as it could be, generates fire quality qi. According to both practices of qigong and tai chi, at the end of the day you want your condition not to be on fire, or excessively yang. Fresh air and healthful food contribute to a more balanced condition. I do not address the large subject of food in this book. Use the list of recommended books at the end of this book to learn more about this important subject and learn about foods to cool down the body. The bottom line is that we are more fire than water to start with, so in order to balance, we always need to look for the water quality.

In order to connect the governing vessel with the conception vessel, we need to gently place the tongue on the roof of the mouth. When the tongue touches the roof of the mouth in the right spot, you will feel the whole mouth fill with saliva. You do not want to touch the teeth, which will be too forward, and you do not want to have the tongue too far back, which will be too tense. There's a little indention on the palate of the mouth that you can feel with your tongue. Your mouth will fill with saliva when you hit the right spot.

Remember, doing tai chi without this skill means you are not integrating your energetic system into the form; you are doing the tai chi dance and not tai chi (grand ultimate). I have met individuals who have been practicing for ten years and their teacher has never told them about this skill. When I talked to them about this skill, they looked at me with glazed eyes and sometimes tears in their eyes. Just think of all the time they could have been practicing tai chi instead of just the moves and being relaxed. If you are one of those individuals who was taught the tai chi form without the visualizations, either your teacher is very traditional or does not know this part of the art. It is your decision what to do next. I came all the way from Israel to Boston to study with the right teacher for me. Most individuals will tell me that they do not have the time or place but as my first Zen teacher/master kept telling me over and over, "Rami, you are Time." The good news is if you have been practicing a tai chi form for some time and you integrate this skill into your tai chi form, you will have a new and strong energetic experience. You can mix in the other skills in this book as well as the ones in *Sunrise Tai Chi*. Always think positively. Do your best.

Practicing Small Circulation

For the purpose of isolating only the trunk sit, either in the seiza position with the lower part of your legs folded under your thighs, or a modified seiza position, sitting on an elevated yet flat surface or on a block, or you can sit on the edge of a chair, or cross your legs on a folded blanket. Sitting in any of these postures does two important things that are essential for this meditation. It slows down the energy and blood going into the legs, but slows it enough that the legs get slightly numb and you have an experience of 'being' only a trunk. Sometimes to create this illusion, you can use the trick of putting a blanket on your thighs.

Remember that letting the legs fall asleep is a goal of sitting meditation so that you can

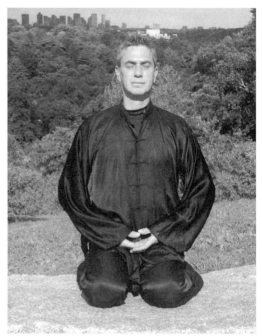

Seiza position with the lower part of your legs folded under your thighs.

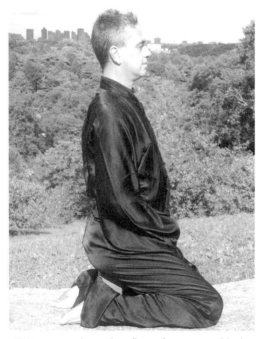

Sitting on an elevated yet flat surface or on a block.

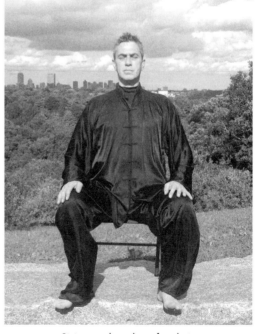

Sitting on the edge of a chair.

experience just the trunk of the body. That is one of the reasons why we sit for at the most 45 minutes, so your legs will get only a little numb. Over time, you will know yourself and the behavior of your legs. My legs usually fall asleep after about 20 minutes. If you move when the legs are asleep, you will reintroduce flow to the legs and at this point you will actually suffer more from the sensation of pins and needles. Your best option is just not to move, and over time your legs become conditioned to this way of sitting. If you do not like this kind of sitting or have any medical issues that contraindicate allowing your legs to become numb, just sit on the edge of a chair. Also you may sit on a block or cushion, or sit with your legs crossed but not in a lotus position, so the legs will still have circulation of blood and energy, which may prevent injury.

Folding the legs decreases the circulation in them, emphasizing the governing vessel and the conception vessel, which when put together make up the small circulation. By folding the legs, we slow down the energy enough from the grand circulation so that we can divert it to the small circle. Sitting in postures that slow down the energy into the legs creates a situation in which the energy in the governing and conception vessels is stronger, and allows you to experience the small circulation more clearly and strongly. The head should be suspended and empty of thoughts. Once you generate the cycle in the small circulation path, the mind becomes empty, or air, or the place of thoughts with no thoughts.

From my personal experience, your arms can be put in one of three positions:
  • If you are cold and want to build up energy and heat, put the palms one on top of the other and place your hands two inches below your navel.

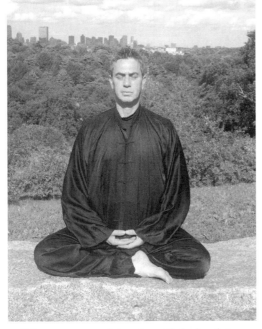

Palms one on top of the other with the hands two inches below your navel (on the ground).

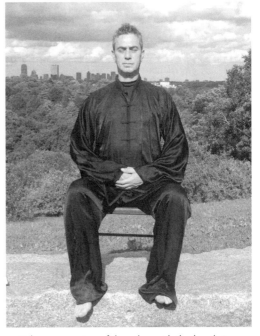

Palms one on top of the other with the hands two inches below your navel (on a chair).

- If you are warm and you want to cool yourself, put your wrists on your knees with the palms facing out.

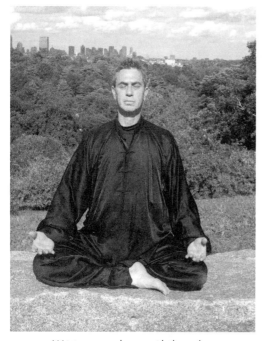

Wrists on your knees with the palms facing out (on the ground).

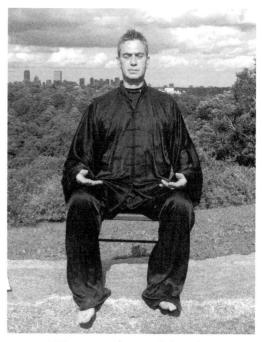

Wrists on your knees with the palms facing out (on a chair).

• If you are neither warm nor cold, put your palms face down on your knees.

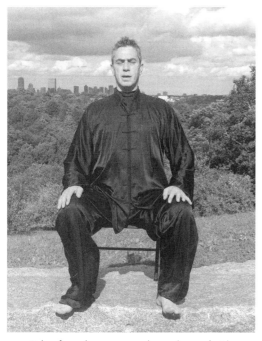 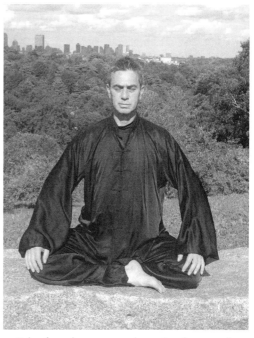

Palms face down on your knees (on a chair).   Palms face down on your knees (on the ground).

Having the hands palms down on the knees helps support the lower back. This is often useful for beginners who need to build up their lower back muscles. Sitting in this posture will be hard at first, especially if you are not flexible through the groin and hip area. If your knees are not flat on the ground within five to ten minutes, your lower back will pull back on you and will not allow you to stay focused on the visualization. Instead, you will be occupied with the posture. I recommend using a yoga block, or books, or a folded blanket. The slight height will create enough of an angle toward the front to prevent pull on the lumbar area.

Once you are comfortable in your sitting position, start circulating your mind along the small circulation path. Start from the

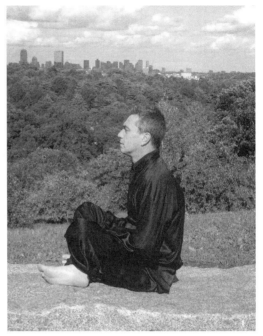

Lower back pulling back.

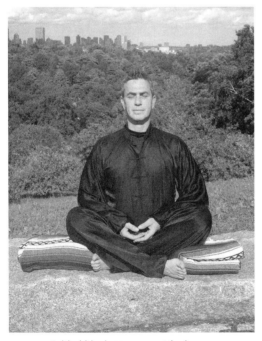

Folded blanket to support the knees.

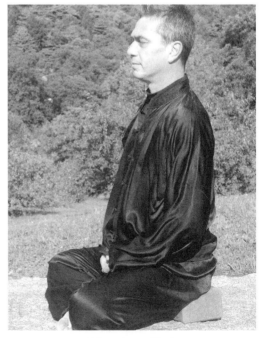

Using a yoga block.

lower energy center, move down from your lower energy center through the area between the groin and the rectum or what the Chinese call the huiyin cavity, up through the back, over the tailbone, between the spine and the skin, all the way around the middle of the skull, down through the front of the face, the trunk, and back through the huiyin cavity to your center of gravity energy center.

When inhaling, move your mind from your lower energy center to the huiyin cavity up along the governing vessel all the way to your upper lip, and when exhaling, move your mind from the upper lip down the front of the trunk into the huiyin cavity and into the lower energy center. You just completed one cycle (Figure 30). Inhale and repeat the action to the upper lip. Exhale and repeat the action, back to your lower energy center. Your mind moves around the trunk and back into the lower energy center.

SMALL CIRCULATION PATH

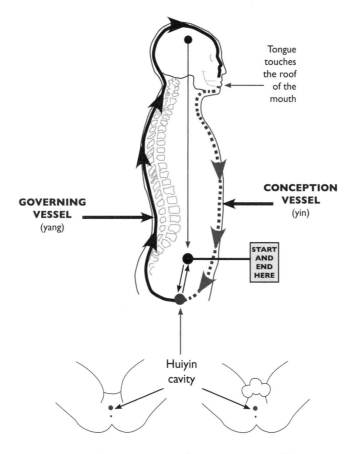

Figure 30.   The Huiyin cavity is between the anus and the groin.

I suggest that beginners use the fingers of the left hand and run it along the path of the visualization. The visualization may be even more vivid if you sit still and allow a friend to trace the path for you. As you exhale, the fingers run from the upper lip all the way to the huiyin cavity. Inhale and from the huiyin cavity, move your finger up along the spine to the shoulder blades and back over the top of the head. Trace the path a few times to make this visualization or path more substantial in your mind. You may notice that when using your finger, your mind did not move back into the lower energy center. At first when you are trying to feel the small circulation path, the mind tends to stay out on the outer surface of the body. That is another possible path for the small circulation; start from the lower energy center and once you leave it, you only come back at the end of your small circulation meditation.

Two Options for the Mind

Let us review the two options:

1. Starting from the center of gravity energy center, up through the governing vessel around the skull and down the conception vessel, then back into the center of gravity energy center or lower energy center.

2. Start from the lower energy center and move up the governing vessel, around the skull and down the conception vessel. At this point, do not move your mind back to the lower energy center. Instead, circle the mind around the huiyin cavity and back up the governing vessel. You are looping from the governing vessel to the conception vessel without passing through the lower energy center.

The Three Paths: Fire, Water, and Wind

There are three paths through which the mind can lead the energy through the small circulation: The fire path, the wind path, and the water path. The fire path as described earlier runs from the huiyin cavity upward along the governing vessel and downward along the conception vessel. The wind path follows the fire path but you lead the energy in the opposite direction, out from the lower energy center through the huiyin cavity. You lead the energy down the governing vessel and up the conception vessel. And last is the water path, which by gently tensing the huiyin cavity, you lead the energy from your lower energy center through the thrusting vessel, which is inside the spine. The three paths, the fire, the water, and the wind, are not known to many qigong or tai chi practitioners but are an essential part of our energetic system and the ability to control fire and water conditions of our bodies. In this book, I will focus only on the fire path, which is the natural way your energy circulates each day. Readers interested in learning more on this subject may do so in advanced qigong books, such as those by my teacher Dr. Yang, Jwing-Ming.

> **Summary of the Paths**
> The Fire Path: Move your mind up the governing vessel and down the conception vessel.
> The Water Path: Gently lift the huiyin cavity to redirect the energy into the thrusting vessel in the
> center of the spine. Lifting the cavity prevents the energy from flowing into the governing vessel.
> The Wind Path: Move the mind in the opposite direction from the natural direction of the flow
> of energy. Lead energy up the conception vessel and down the governing vessel.

Is Practicing the Small Circulation Meditation Dangerous?

All qigong practice should be taken seriously. Proceed slowly and do your home-work, which means to be sure you understand the concept before you train. In my experience, due to the nature of the process the small circulation meditation is a rela-tively safe practice. You should, however, be aware of some of the problems that can occur. Having a teacher or a master who has walked this path of meditation is impor-tant and very useful. Having the luxury of working with another individual who has gone through this path of meditation can make a big difference in how quickly you advance, but is not always necessary.

There are three spots along this path where the skin is very close to the bones and therefore creates a narrower path through which energy must flow. Some masters believe that the mind can get stuck in these areas, and that may lead to energy blockages and to energy problems, which eventually can manifest on a physical or mental level, or both.

The trick to moving through these three areas is to just move forward with the mind and the visualization. Do not let the sensation of the physical tightness block the visu-alization from moving through the small circulation path.

The first problem area is the tailbone. For some, the tight physical sensation in this area blocks their ability to keep circulating the mind through the governing vessel; they just get mentally stuck. The second physical area is the area between the shoulders. The third physical area is the base of the skull where the soft and the hard parts meet. In Chinese, this area is called the jade pillow. As you can see, the areas that are considered by some as problematical are all in the back, the yang side, along the governing vessel.

Another potential problem is allowing the energy that you lead up the governing vessel to get stuck in the head. Sometimes people forget the original task of moving through the circle and they become lost in their thoughts; the energy gets stuck in the brain.

Remember, if your mind is wandering, those brain cells are consuming energy. You can avoid this by moving through the governing vessel to the conception and continu-ing down toward the huiyin cavity.

Another danger could be your personality. If you have too much imagination and you start to put it into the meditation, you can end up with mental issues. You should not get lost in any fantasies. Keep it simple. You are just sitting still, breathing deeply, and circulating your mind softly and easily through the small circulation path. Once you are finished, return with your mind to the lower energy center. Do not hold your breath and do not sit to the point that your legs are numb. Holding your breath, or sitting too long in seiza or lotus position could create circulation problems. Using a belt or rope or other implements to force yourself into different postures for the purposes of achieving various energy goals may result in an injury or even worse.

REFINING YOUR BREATH

In general, the breathing should be associated with these words: smooth, long, peaceful, deep, soft, and natural. Do not hold your breath.

In the *Sunrise Tai Chi* book (pages 49 and 50), you learned three-chamber breathing. In this book as well as in the *Sunset Tai Chi* DVD, you are learning latissimus breathing. Other names for it are wing breathing and trapezius breathing. You will also learn mushroom breathing and seesaw breathing. These breathing techniques help develop healthy and strong lungs that will give you better and deeper breath. Developing the lungs is first the 'banana' to capture the emotional mind or what is referred to as the monkey mind.

Develop the lungs as a separate skill. Isolate the breathing exercises and practice them throughout the day. Later, when you mix the different skills, each skill is diminished a little just because your focus is now on more than one skill at a time. But if you practice the skills separately, just by itself for some time, then when you put a few of those skills together, you still will get just a little more from each one of those skills. This habit will help in giving you a stronger experience as well as more potential for success. This is also the typical behavior of the Taoist school of thought: Break everything into small little pieces, yin and yang, and emphasize each one, fine-tune it until fine-tuning is not needed, and then put it together with the other skills. The yin-yang symbol represents that school of thought.

The breath training described in this book will give you larger lungs and more control over the lungs and the muscles around them. Having larger lungs will allow you to use one breath cycle to accomplish longer mental visualizations instead of disturbing the visualization with the need to change from inhalation to exhalation. For example, if you are working on the small circulation and if you have good lungs with a nice long inhalation, you will be able to circle through the governing vessel very slowly with one inhalation. If your lungs are not well developed, by the time you move your mind halfway through, you will need to exhale and continue the movements up the governing vessel on the second inhalation. You can see how the second option is not as quiet and peaceful as the first. The ability to take long, deep, quiet inhalations allows the mind to travel through the small circulation without the interruption of changing the breath from inhalation to exhalation. Long, deep inhalations allow you to maintain the visualization without distractions from the lungs.

The banana that captures the monkey mind and prevents 'danger.'

Legs: Between Danger and Safety

One more risk comes from impeding the circulation in your legs to a dangerous point. Whether you are sitting with crossed legs or in the seiza position, do not sit more than 45 minutes and do not use belts, or any props, and tools that might further block the flow of blood and energy. The energy is already blocked in the crossed leg or seiza positions. When your legs become numb, you could sit fairly safely for another five to ten minutes before releasing the position. Massage your legs, or tap them to stimulate the circulation, then stand up and walk until the numbness and the sensation of ants running through your leg disappears.

My personal experience is that my legs become numb after 20 to 30 minutes, depending on what I did that week. If I walked the 15 miles per week that I would like to do, then it is 20 minutes, but if I do not walk that week then my legs last almost 10 minutes longer. It is useful to sit through 10 to 15 minutes of numbness in the legs. It helps you have a clearer as well as a more pure experience of the trunk as well as the small circulation. Just play it safe. Do not force yourself to sit too long, and wait until you know your legs, i.e., know how long it takes your legs to become numb.

One- and Two-Breath Cycles in Small Circulation Meditation

When performing the small circulation meditation, one of the goals for optimal practice is to do it in one cycle as slowly as possible with one inhalation; then you run through the governing vessel, moving as slowly as possible, while you exhale. One inhalation should be for moving the mind up the conception vessel, and one inhalation for moving the mind down the governing vessel. Wherever your attention goes, energy flows. Not everyone's lungs are developed enough to follow this specific skill. Until you develop your lungs, there are some options that will make it easier for you and will take some of the physical and mental pressures away.

One-Breath Cycle

Inhalation—Governing Vessel, Exhalation—Conception Vessel.

Two Options:

1. Start in the lower energy center, and then circle your mind from the lower energy center through the governing vessel. Use one inhalation. Once you reach the upper lip, move your mind down the conception vessel back to the lower energy center. Use one exhalation. Keep your mind circling through this loop.

2. Inhale and leave the lower energy center and lead the energy up the governing vessel. Once you reach the upper lip, exhale and move your mind down to the huiyin cavity. Keep your mind in this loop and do not go back to the lower energy center until the end of your meditation period. At the end of your meditation, bring your mind back to the lower energy center.

Two-Breath Cycle

Some people find it is easier to use the two-breath cycle while doing their loop. First, divide the governing vessel as well as the conception vessel into two. On your next inhalation, move the mind from the lower energy center up the governing vessel to the area below the shoulder blades or at the shoulder blades, which is about halfway through the governing vessel. As you exhale, do not move your mind. Use the exhalation to strengthen your mind at the shoulder blade area. Then inhale again and keep moving your mind from the shoulder blade area, go around the middle of the skull, and all the way around to the upper lip. Now exhale and lead the energy down to the solar plexus. Inhale and stay focused on the solar plexus. Exhale and lead your mind down from the solar plexus all the way to the huiyin cavity (Figure 31).

Small Circulation–Conclusions

In the two-breath cycle, on the first inhalation you climb up the governing vessel and pause to exhale, staying focused on the spot at which you paused. While exhaling, you lead your mind halfway down the conception vessel. On the inhalation, you focus the mind in the spot at which you paused and on the next exhalation, you finish the movements of your mind through the conception vessel. You are now at the huiyin and on your way again to the governing vessel.

Once you are comfortable with circling the mind up the governing vessel and down the conception vessel (up on inhalation, down on exhalation), see if you can monitor, at the same time, the up and down forces and the three chambers (*Sunrise Tai Chi*, pages 18, 19, and 20). The more correctly your body is physically aligned, the less physical stress you will have and the more relaxed you will feel. When you are aligned, you are creating a structure with less energy stagnation. Stagnation is a distraction to your visualizations. Learning to maintain correct physical alignment will lead to an easier and stronger visualization of the small circulation path. Having any physical discomfort will detract from your ability to visualize the small circulation.

SMALL CIRCULATION

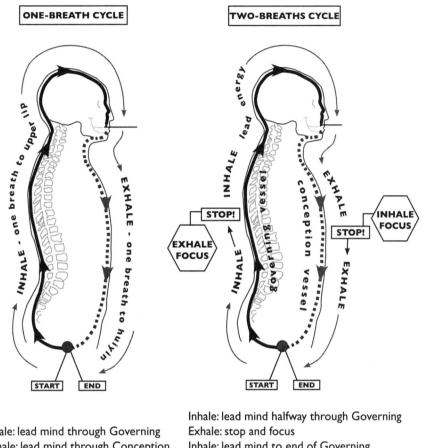

Inhale: lead mind through Governing
Exhale: lead mind through Conception

Inhale: lead mind halfway through Governing
Exhale: stop and focus
Inhale: lead mind to end of Governing
Exhale: lead mind halfway through Conception
Inhale: stop and focus
Exhale: back to start

Figure 31. One-breath and two-breaths cycle.

Notice the different sensations when the mind is moving up the governing vessel and moving down the conception vessel. Many students have expressed that the sensation throughout the back was stronger than the sensation through the front. The energy in the back is more yang than the energy in the front. It is normal to have a clearer sense of the stronger yang energy. Also, the energy in the back moves more slowly than the energy in the front making it easier to notice. Keep spending time and minimum physical effort to practice the small circulation. Your mind will become stronger and stronger, and so will your energetic system. You will open up other energy centers and connect to the three forces, heaven, human, and earth, in new and different ways. You will develop your intuition and awareness, improve your health, and even contribute to your longevity.

When Do I Practice Small Circulation?

The best times to practice the small circulation is during sunrise or during sunset. These two unique times are when earth, human, and heaven energy are changing from yin, night, to yang, day. Each day, the natural energy changes from yang, plants giving oxygen to yin, plants releasing carbon dioxide. As the earth and the universe change, so do we. If we sit during the strongest times that these changes occur, we have an opportunity to experience the change. You can practice the small circulation at any other time of course. It is just a stronger experience to practice when these changes take place. That is the reason I encourage you to practice the small circulation during one of these times.

When practicing during sunset, note the smooth sensation through the conception vessel as well as the stronger and smoother flow of energy in the governing vessel. By using the pulling energy of the setting sun, you could cleanse any stagnant energy in both the physical and energetic body that will lead to a unique and different experience of the small circulation. Sitting on the edge of a chair or on the floor with your spine straight is important because the evening is a time when we are more tired. You need to stay in the state between being awake and asleep, and enjoy the setting sun and the small circulation.

I loved the years that I did Zen meditation. I would get up an hour before sunrise and take a warm shower, dress warmly and stretch for 20 minutes, very passive stretching for the pure purpose of staying in the state between being awake and asleep, then get on my motorcycle and go to a Zen house where twenty to thirty other people would gather. First, we would have some warm miso soup and then sit, in seiza, for 45 minutes. This was a wonderful training experience for me, and years later, I did the same on my own with the small circulation meditation training.

The best times to start sitting is 15 minutes before the sun rises or sets. At the same time, you can experience your energy changing as well as the earth and universe energies changing with you. As you can see, the chances for different experiences is stronger at those times of the day and that is the reason there is no time like when the sun is rising and setting.

If you cannot find time to sit during those two times, just sit whenever you can. Do not practice the small circulation meditation between one o'clock and three o'clock in the afternoon. Our energy moves every two hours along the governing vessel and then the conception vessel. This subject is another book in itself and I will not go deeply into it in this book. During the time between one o'clock and three o'clock, this wave is at the solar plexus area, and the energetic mind/body prescription that is recommended for this time period is to lie down and relax, to cool the middle energy center.

CHAPTER 3

Sunset Tai Chi Mind/Body Program

COOLING DOWN EXERCISES

The following sequence of mental and physical exercises is designed to develop your mind/body connection, and increase and improve your internal skills while bringing you to a deeply relaxed state, especially after a long, draining day at work. If you can, practice while the sun is setting. The energy of the setting sun will aid you in cooling down, plus you will have a stronger experience of the other energetic and spiritual sensations.

Nowadays with the fast-paced lifestyle that we have, more and more individuals are looking for ways to reduce stress as well as enjoy the time they have with their friends and families after a long day at work. Being able to 'let go' is a skill not many possess. Many continue thinking and dealing with the actions of the day and have a hard time transitioning, which does not let them enjoy the few hours of relaxation they have. Some people even have a hard time falling asleep because of this problematic pattern of behavior.

Being able to change from one pace to another without using any pharmaceutical product not only will allow you to enjoy the time you have with your loved ones but will also allow you to enjoy your hobbies and recreational activities. Most importantly, you will have the skill to control the fluctuation of the brainwave state you are in. Learning to slow down and relax will lead to having a better night's sleep, a better experience the following day. Developing the skill of changing from one situation to the other in the most efficient way leads not only to a more productive next day but also to better decision-making.

This ability to change is one of the most important principles of the Tao, which translates as the *Way*. When taking the right path, your life will flow smoothly. Part of this Tao is the ability to change when the situation changes. Learn from the past, live in the present, and enjoy the future. As individuals look for ways to achieve this skill, many end up doing tai chi, qigong, or yoga. In the United States, many people who are practicing tai chi are doing it for health reasons. Tai chi emphasizes the skill of being able to change, rather than studying it as a martial art. Tai chi as well as qigong and yoga are the most effective practices that have many exercises making the best use of your practice time, and help you to transition into a calmer more focused state as soon as you get home from work, or whenever you find the time to train and practice. When stretching, it is best to build up to the point where you can hold each stretch for three minutes to allow the cells of the muscles, tendons, and bones to reach an excited state in which real change can take place.

Turn your attention inward and listen to your body. Try to become aware of the difference between constructive pain and destructive pain, and progress in your training slowly but efficiently. Your physical sensations of pain discomfort, tingling, or muscles burning are your body's way of communicating its needs to your mind. Respect these sensations, and allow the soft tissues the time needed to stretch very gradually. You are re-educating the intellect of the soft tissue. Use your mind to monitor the different muscles you are working with, and pay attention to where you are tight, which side stretches more easily, and how you feel from day to day. Over time, this internal skill will improve. This is the kung fu of internal awareness.

As always, practice each mental and physical skill separately, and once you are comfortable with each, combine them. For instance, practice four gates breathing separately. When you are ready, practice the breathing technique while doing the Sunset Tai Chi form. The key is to perform each mind/body prescription in the program as well as the tai chi drills, and the form, with the five building blocks: body, breath, mind, energy, and spirit. Keep tapping into the setting sun energy whenever you have an opportunity. The setting force is a powerful element in helping dissolve impurities and stress. Remember, when you nourish with the rising sun or when you are cleansing with the setting sun, you can conquer the impurities or you can surrender to them. Try both in the meditations as well as in any of the mind/body prescriptions in the *Sunrise Tai Chi* and *Sunset Tai Chi* books and DVDs. For example, my teacher and master, Dr. Yang Jwing-Ming kept telling me over the years to conquer my hamstrings. Every day, I stretched those hamstrings. I was on a mission to conquer them. Years later, my yoga teacher Patricia Walden saw me stretching my hamstrings with my conquer mentality and she softly told me, "Rami, try surrendering to your hamstrings." It is amazing what one word can do and that is after years of practice. Both approaches are valid, but sometimes we need a new perspective to reach a new level of understanding.

Five to Ten Minutes of Sunset is Better Than Nothing

Although the mind/body prescriptions as well as the tai chi program are designed to help you cool down, change pace for a better sleep during the night, and prepare yourself to perform at a higher quality during the next day; using the powerful energy of the setting sun to support the mind/body goals will make a huge difference. If you are busy during this time, you can always use the drawing force of the moon even when it is empty but especially when it is full or around that time of waxing or waning. The moon is yin as well, and it does pull on our physical and energetic bodies the same way it pulls on the oceans that lead to low and high tides. If you are working or busy during the time of the setting sun and cannot practice any of the programs or the tai chi, just stop what you are doing for five to ten minutes, face the setting sun; outside is best, second best is indoors. Close your eyes and pay attention to the energetic change that is happening through the three forces: earth, human, and heaven. Then with your mind, search and dissolve your impurities and let the powerful energy of the setting sun help you cleanse both your physical and energetic bodies. After you become comfortable with this, you may use the moon to help with further cleansing.

Surfing the Breath

The breath is a tool to achieve our goals and needs. Sometimes we use slow and deep breaths and other times we use fast and shallow ones. We can use the lungs differently according to the different goals we have. Breathing is the method we use to bring oxygen into our blood stream that nourishes every cell in our body, but the breath is also the banana we use to capture the monkey mind. The breathing in qigong is considered one of the tools to affect our ability to be watery or fiery. Fast and hard exhalations lead us to be *fire,* and deep, long, quiet inhalation will lead us to be *water*. If you do too much of either for too long, you will lose balance, and it can have negative effects on a mental or physical level. But if you know how and when to use this principle, you will be able to benefit tremendously from it and achieve balance in both mind and body.

This first breathing exercise is the simple and safe way to start this journey into the science of the breath. It will lead you to the first step of being relaxed or what Dr. Herbert Benson refers to as the relaxation response or what I consider a Buddhist path. But remember, this is just a first step or, as previously mentioned, the relaxation is a doorway to a palace full of other interesting rooms that I consider the Taoist path.

Surfing the breath is the simplest method of achieving deep relaxation. First, close your eyes. Sit in an erect posture with a straight spine. Do not collapse your spine. When the spine is collapsed, surfing the breath will still work on a mental level, but you will not get as much air because the lungs are compressed. Surfing the breath will help you calm the monkey mind. Follow the air through the nostrils down through the windpipe, deep into both lungs, in and out with long, quiet, and peaceful inhalations. Your inhalation and exhalation should be, eventually, equal in length, unless you have other specific goals.

After a few minutes, you will be able to determine which of your nostrils is wider. Our bodies are not symmetrical. One of our nostrils is more open than the other. Move down, with your mind, into the lungs and try to determine which lung is longer and which lung is wider. One lung has three lobes and the other lung has two. I really enjoy the moment when my students tell me they do not know which lung has three lobes and which has two. Not knowing this fact allows them to experience the air moving into the nostrils and the sensation of air moving into the lungs, and then to determine from the sensation, not from looking at an anatomy book, which lung has the three lobes and which lung has the two.

Sometimes the lung that is wider has the two lobes, which makes some people think that it is the longer lung. This 'wide' sensation that the mind experiences throws them off, and they will swear that one is the lung that has the three lobes. But really it is just a stronger sensation in that lung that confuses them and makes them think that one is the longer lung—feel as opposed to real.

As long as you follow the air in and out of your lungs, that is, surf the breath, you will be able to quiet the mind from excess thoughts. Remember we have, on average, eighteen thoughts per second. Relax, reduce the number of thoughts, and bring the mind to the brain activity level between being awake and asleep.

Fire Breath

Some days when it is difficult to quiet the mind, you can use fire breath breathing to surf the breath. Fire breath breathing means that you make a slight sound with the air moving in through the nostrils and a sound when the air is moving out. The breath, the air, and the sound all contribute to helping you to empty the mind. But as soon as you can, go into the water breath—back into the quiet, long, peaceful, deep breathing work.

Eighty Percent Effort and the Power of the Mind

After you have been experimenting and experiencing the various lung skills, you should pay attention to the next very important principle that can also be looked at as 'less is more.' The lungs have a tendency, when putting the mind in them, to become tense. The muscles around the lungs, the smooth muscles, become especially tense when we work the lungs to their 100% air capacity. In this case, this mentality is not always good and it needs to be balanced with the principle of the 80% effort. This principle will help the muscles around the lungs to deeply relax and over time allows for longer inhalations as well as exhalations. As you inhale, notice the air moving into your lungs and the tension in the muscles around them. Use the sensation of the tension in the muscles around the lungs to determine what the 80% effort of your lungs is. The way to find the 80% is by inhaling as deeply as you can while finding your 100%, and then as you exhale, put your mind in the muscles around the lungs and with your mind help them to relax. With the next inhalation, just inhale to 80% of what you just did. Once you have determined the 80% effort of your lungs on every exhalation, use your mind to help those muscles to relax using the metaphor: 'ice to water and water to vapor.' If you become dizzy at any point, stop and take a break. You are trying too hard in holding your breath and tensing the muscles. When helping the muscles relax around the lungs, do not collapse the spine. Keep the head suspended and shoulders relaxed and dropped; relax the face and empty the mind of any other thoughts.

Zen Mind

Stand with your feet shoulder-width apart. Bend your knees and put your palms on your lower energy center, or sit in seiza on your knees with or without a block. Sit comfortably, with correct alignment. Surf your breath. Continue breathing slowly, deeply, and quietly through the nose. Push down through your legs or sitting bones and lengthen your spine up into the heavens. Relax your face, neck, shoulders, and abdominal muscles downward, while lengthening up through your back to the top of your head. Allow your mind to gradually settle into a semi-sleeping state. On the outside, be as still as a mountain. Look, inside, for the motion in this external stillness.

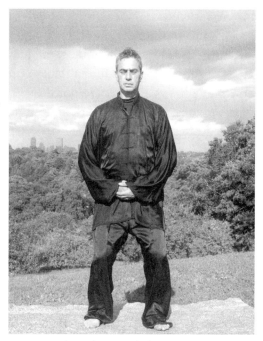

Bend your knees and place your palms on your lower energy center.

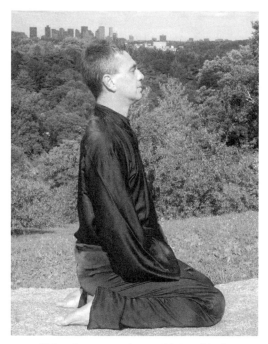

Sit in seiza on your knees without a block.

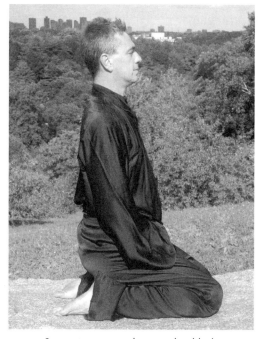

Sit in seiza on your knees with a block.

Remain aware of all your sensations—the sound in your ears, the movement of your breath, and the circulation of fluids and energy inside your body; notice the sensations around you—the air, the sounds, the temperature. Allow your senses of both the inside and the outside to unify into a state of oneness until your body feels light and transparent. Thoughts will come. Do not try to suppress them. Allow your thoughts to rise and pass naturally, using the breath and the stillness, as you settle into deeper relaxation and higher awareness.

This Zen mind exercise is the best beginning to your meditation practice. The idea of the Zen mind is to empty the mind of any thoughts. The mind uses much energy and oxygen. It requires daily rest, but the task of emptying the mind is very difficult for many individuals. Some may isolate themselves and go to monasteries in the mountain and try for years to achieve that one skill—emptying the mind from thoughts. This stage has different names. For example, in the East it is considered as meditation, while in the West, the medical community discusses Dr. Herbert Benson's concept of 'relaxation response.' The idea is that you close your eyes and empty the mind from any thoughts, using different techniques and methods. One way of emptying the mind is using the breath to help you. Surfing the breath is an effective technique to help you reach a place between being awake and asleep—a place of nothingness or emptiness. The thoughts will keep coming in. Your job is not to fight the thoughts and not to become upset. Your job is to loop your thoughts back into the breath or into nothingness.

Sunset and Zen Mind

Try every now and then to work on emptying your mind using the powerful energetic pull of the setting sun. First, use the warmth of the sun to caress and dissolve your face, then allow the warmth to melt any thoughts in your brain, and finally use the energetic pull to draw away any lingering thoughts from your brain. Make sure you maintain the up and down forces. You want to relax but not collapse.

A Small Reminder

It is very important to physically sit still. If someone were to look at you while you were doing your sitting or standing meditation, he or she should not be able to see you move. In my readings, I came across this ancient saying that has stayed with me: "When standing or when sitting still, be as still as the mountain, and then look for the movement in the stillness."

Once you are still externally, it is very important to notice the movements that are happening throughout your body. Notice the many things that are moving internally, excluding your thoughts. The idea is to slowly quiet down the moving elements in the body and allow only the necessary minimal movement that needs to happen in it. Of course, that includes your thoughts. For example, I was sitting and meditating with one of my students when he said, "I am sitting and I am starting to feel relaxed. I'm moving to being between awake and asleep, my number of thoughts is reducing. I am surfing my breath, and then I hear the sounds around me, such as the fish tank or the kids outside. What do I do then? At that second I'm thinking, 'Oh, I am hearing the fish tank, the water, the kids.'" My answer was, "If you hear the water and you generated the thought, 'Oh I am hearing the water,' that defeats the purpose, but it is the monkey mind's natural behavior, at least at first." On the other hand, you cannot be upset with yourself because that will defeat the purpose even more. To achieve the external stillness and the internal quietness, continue the process, spend more time and energy in sitting, and allow the thoughts to move into emptiness or into the breathing. Patience is a virtue. Eventually you will sense the water (fish tank water) and you will not be judgmental on a thought level. Eventually, you will actually sense or hear farther away from your body as well as deeper into your body while being able not to think but just to be. That is when you will be still on the outside, empty and quiet on the inside.

At first, when you practice, the monkey mind, the thoughts are strong, disturbing, and distracting from the goal. Naturally, your mind will want to project and be a part of it and the monkey mind will want to come and give its opinion: "Look, it is so beautiful! Oh, it is so quiet! Wow, I can hear voices and sounds that I did not hear before!" and on and on. New experiences and sensations are exactly the time and the opportunity for the monkey mind to step in and interfere, and be part of the exercise. *Remember though, we do not want the monkey mind.* We want the monkey mind to be quiet and still, the same way we want to keep the external body still. Over time, you will learn to just experience the sensation around you as well as in you without having an opinion about it or thoughts about it. At that point or time you may experience, at first, physical 'transparency' then maybe you will find the 'emptiness,' and maybe at the end you will 'crush the nothingness,' as they say in ancient Buddhist documents.

The Most 'Quiet' Time in Our Bodies

Another strong experience that you may have when doing sitting or standing meditating occurs especially when you are lingering at the end of an exhalation, which is the time when your body is the quietest. This lingering happens at the end of an exhalation when the diaphragm does not move and the last of the air is still leaking out. It is so quiet and comfortable at this point that there is a tendency to want to stay there forever. If you stay there forever, that means you are dead. Take a deep inhalation in order to continue. When the need for air is an issue, you may generate more thoughts: "Oh, I need to take an inhalation." But, again, over time the breath will just happen; it is fine-tuning until fine-tuning is not needed. You will not need to spend any thoughts on this need for inhaling. Many of these sensations happen because this is the first time you are noticing them, and then when you notice them, the monkey mind automatically has an opportunity to come in and give an opinion. Experience will teach you to make that change between the end of exhalation and inhalation without generating any thoughts.

Fire Breath With the 'Ha' Sound

Some days, it will be very difficult for you to empty your mind. On those days, use the fire breath with the 'ha' sound. If this does not work, just let go and do it another day. This fire breath breathing is a breath with a slight sound but this time with the mouth rather than the nose.

On the inhalation, drag the air a little more quickly and strongly through the nostrils. When you exhale, exhale through the mouth with a quiet 'ha' sound. You can also have the air coming out of the nose a little more strongly with sound as described in the previous fire breath. By performing the fire breath breathing with the 'ha' sound, the need from the mind for creating and following the strong breath in and out will allow you to empty your thoughts more easily on those days that the monkey mind is unusually strong. Hopefully, you will not have many of those days. As soon as you can, go back to using the water breathing, which is a very silent and quiet breath with deep, long, and peaceful inhalations and exhalations. Your breathing is quiet, silent, and peaceful, and so will be your mind.

Cleanse

It is important to do a cleansing exercise first to be able to achieve the most from the nourishing exercises, or to relax at the end of your day. Cleansing is done mostly with your mind with a little help from your arms. Using the setting sun to help the mind to cleanse the entire physical and energetic body is a very powerful experience. When you can, you should take advantage of the special forces of this time, but do not wait only for this time to cleanse. When you do have an opportunity to cleanse while the sun is setting, keep the up and down forces as well as your deep breathing. A strong experience of physical transparency and dissolving your stored energetic impurities will bring you back to meditating during this unique time of the setting sun. Cleansing can be done while sitting on the edge of a chair, standing up, as well as just mentally, without using the arms. Repeat until you have a clear feeling throughout your body.

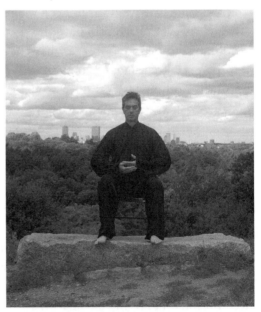

Scoop your palms while scanning the body for impurities (sitting).

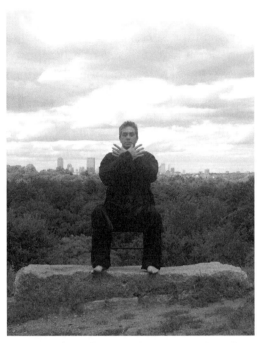

Cross in front of chest, collect impurities (sitting).

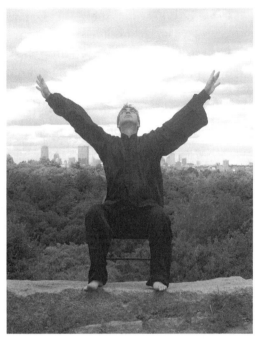

Lead and deposit impurities in the stars (sitting).

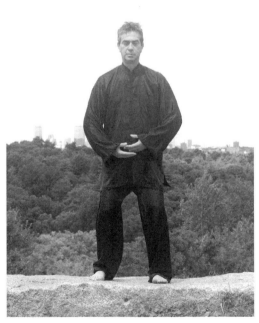

Cleanse. Ready posture (standing).

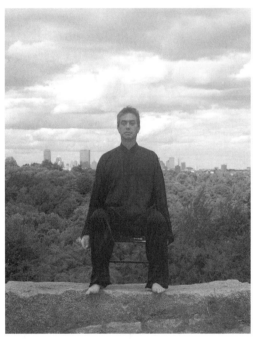

Mental cleansing (sitting).

To Cleanse While Standing

Stand with feet shoulder-width apart, slightly bend the knees, and tuck the sacrum in. Eventually you will want to drop the sacrum in, but at first you need to have a physical motion of tucking versus dropping. Once the muscles loosen up and lengthen around the pelvis and groin, the hip will open, and you will be able to drop the pelvis versus tucking it. Lengthen through the spine, extend the head, relax the shoulders, and close your eyes. The tongue touches the roof of the mouth. Sense the sensation from the soles of the feet, through the entire body, all the way to the top of the head. Scan your body with your mind and try to identify any impurities. Impurities could be anything from aches, pains, numbness, a tingling sensation of electricity, association with dark colors, hot, cold, something you know is there, something you feel is wrong. Look for any of these sensations throughout the body.

At first, just scan the body from the bottom up, two or three times, and just try to identify the impurities; then on the next inhalation bring your arms toward the lower energy center in a scooping motion.

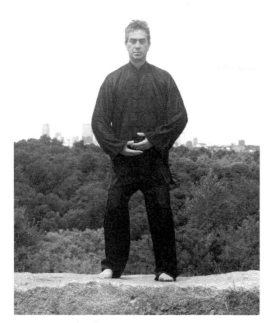

Scan and collect impurities, scooping motion.

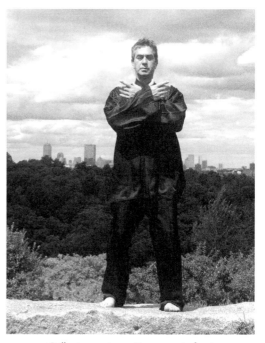

Collect more impurities, cross in front of your chest (standing).

Bring your arms up and cross them in front of your chest with the palms facing inward; then raise your arms straight over your head, and then open them wide.

Circle down pointing toward the floor and again in a scooping motion toward the lower energy center, cross in front of your chest, palms face in, move up straight over your head and around.

The motion of your arms represents the action of your mind: collecting and gathering the impurities and sending them up into the stars and depositing them there.

When the arms scoop toward the lower energy center that is when your mind gathers all the impurities from the legs and brings them up through the body. Also collect all the impurities from your abdomen, from your chest, from your spine, from your back, from every part of your physical

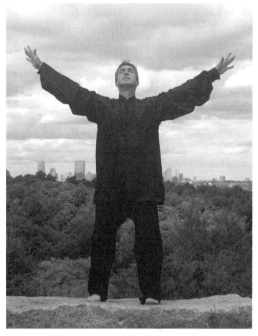

Deposit impurities in the stars, arms straight over head (standing).

body as well as your energetic body. Once you have collected your impurities, lead all the impurities up through the center of your arms and then out through the center of your palms, up through the face as well as out through the 'heavenly gate,' the soft part on top of your head, and send the impurities up into the stars, and deposit the impurities in the stars. Come back around, with your arms as well as your mind, into the earth and come up from the center of the earth all the way into the soles of your feet. Gather all the impurities from the legs, from the pelvis, from the trunk, from the head, and send them all through the center of the palm and the top of the head to the stars far away. Deposit the impurities in the stars (Figure 32). Come back around the earth, through the center of the earth, up through your body, collect all the impurities and cleanse the body.

Keep breathing softly through the nose. The tongue should touch the roof of the mouth. When inhaling and scanning for impurities, stretch the bows slightly. When exhaling and releasing the impurities, release the bows. In other words, when inhaling, empty moon, when exhaling, full moon.

Remember as you improve your mental visualization, when you send your mind to the stars and your arms are pointing up, you should also have your mind in the center of the earth and have a little bit of a sinking through the legs.

Also remember there is a nice, heavy feeling from the belly button down and a light sensation from the belly button up through the spine.

When doing the cleansing, stretch the bows to collect the impurities and release the bows to send the impurities to the stars. In the cleansing, we use the bows differently than when doing 'stretch the bows' in our program. When releasing and sending the impurities to the stars, do go further than regular bow breathing. Look up to the heavens and gently arch the spine back with just the beginning of a bend in the thoracic spine.

Try to notice the most yin physical point of cleansing and the most yang point of cleansing. The yin point is when the body is most relaxed. The yang point is when your arms, spine, and chest are stretched.

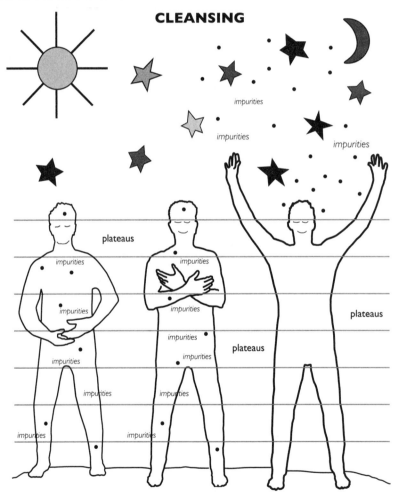

Figure 32. Scan plateaus, collect impurities, and deposit them in the stars.

Pause, every now and then, at the yin point and the yang point, just to experience the two physical extremes as well as the different experience of energy within each posture. Standing still in specific postures is a very common practice throughout the Eastern arts. In Chinese, it is called Yi Chuan or standing still meditation.

MEDITATIVE SHAKING AND PULSING

Western exercise starts with warming up by increasing the heart rate to saturate the muscles with blood and oxygen. Therefore, we can say that Western warm-ups focus first on the heart and muscles. On the other hand, Eastern exercise starts by charging and igniting the energetic system and then the rest of the body. You can charge the energetic system in more than one way. One of the ways to jumpstart our energetic system is by creating a gentle movement in the joints or in the ligaments. This skill of isolating the ligaments and creating movements in them is actually part of our natural day-to-day physical behavior. It happens whenever we use our arms and hands. It is helpful to refine this skill and train our ability to isolate this skill in whatever part of the body we choose.

In order to achieve this isolation, we need to first understand the various physical motions, and second, be able to put into action these motions: pulsing, pumping, and shaking. Each of these words is important because each one affects the body and the energy differently, which creates different sensations and experiences. Pulsing can be created through gentle up and down movements or gentle in and out motions, and with small side to side movements. It is a great way to loosen up. Pumping is a stronger movement than pulsing, although the actions of up and down, in and out, and side to side are similar. Shaking combines side to side first and then some in and out motion with a gentle up and down. All three have a gentle rotation that can be added to each one while they are happening. You need to understand that each one is different and over time, you will experience the differences as well. This exercise (meditative shaking) will activate your energetic system, remove some stagnation, and can also serve as a good warm-up. Even if you only have five minutes, doing this meditation will go a long way.

When you shake, you may notice that the fingers are tense. This next piece of information is essential for loosening this tension. Move the joint above the one you want to isolate. For example, if you want to loosen the finger joints, shake the wrist, but put your mind on the fingers. Try to isolate this gentle movement in your joints, rather than moving the muscles or tendons. To loosen the wrist, move the elbow. *Remember, your jaw is a joint as well.* When practiced correctly, you will begin to feel patches of warmth in your joints and some warmth in your the internal organs or lower energy center.

Using the Setting Sun during Shaking

Allow the warmth of the sun to caress your skin and especially your joint areas, and allow the drawing energy of the setting sun to pull the impurities away from each joint you are working on. Do not wait to do the meditative shaking only during this time. However, if you do have an opportunity to do it during the setting sun, your experience can be much stronger than at any other time.

We will go into detail with each of these exercises for those who do not easily feel a mind/body connection. The tiny details of stretching each body part in all possible angles are only a guide for you to develop your own body awareness. The ultimate goal is to completely loosen every part of the body deeply during this shaking, while maintaining a relaxed meditative mind.

Fingers

Stand with your feet shoulder-width apart. Start with the gentle movements of pulsing and some pumping through the ligaments in the fingers. *Remember to loosen the fingers and gently move the wrists.* You want to notice the sensation throughout the joints as part of the journey to develop awareness and sensitivity. How do you do that? You put your mind in the fingers while you are moving the wrists. Pay attention to the various sensations throughout the joints. For example, if I put my mind in the fingers, the first sensation that calls my attention is the thumb because it is the biggest joint. And then when I put my mind in my thumbs, I can feel that my left thumb is looser than my right thumb. This is a significant part of the exercise. Put your mind in the joint, sense the sensations, determine the differences, and find the similarities. Learn to focus and concentrate on each sensation. Over time, you will even be able to feel the differences between the smallest joints: the pinkies. Of course, at the same time, you want to take deep breaths through the nose while your mind is focusing in the joints. *Remember, you need to be between awake and asleep and in deep relaxation* in order to gain even more from this meditation.

Wrists

Now we move to the next joint, the wrist. To isolate the pulsing or pumping in the wrist, focus on the elbows. If you can integrate more of your skills, put your mind in the lower energy center. Some joints have more varied movements than others. The wrist has more range of motion than the fingers. When moving the wrist, notice the wide angles and various directions it can move: forward and backward, left to right, up and down, circles, twisting, and rotation. Feel or sense the difference between the right and left wrists, and between forward, backward, and sideway movement.

Elbows

Then we shake the elbows and move the shoulders in order to create the gentle shaking, pulsing or pumping in the elbows.

Shoulders

Next, focus on the shoulders. What is the joint above the shoulders? Well we do not have one and that is the reason at this point that we start pumping the feet against the floor. Do this very gently and just find the middle between pulsing and pumping: not too strong a pumping action but not as little as a pulse. By gently pumping up and down against the floor with the legs and the soles of your feet, you will be able to create the desired shaking and isolation of the shoulders. Of course, if you move the shoulders themselves, the movement would be too tense. This gentle bounce moves up through the body and reaches the shoulders, which will move gently up and down. They will just follow the motion from the ground up. To prevent knee problems and to practice the tai chi form, when bouncing and pumping through the legs, make sure that the weight moves through the knees into the floor and not into the knees.

Discovering Yin and Yang Layers in the Shoulders

Here is an example of how to discover the various yin and yang sensations. For the first major sensation, you simply pulse and pump the shoulders. To feel the second and third sensations, you try to tune into a clearer sense of the energy of the shoulders.

The shoulders have three major zones. In each zone, the sensations are different.

First Posture: Position the thoracic spine a little forward as in the turtle back posture. The shoulders move slightly forward. Pulsing the body in this posture creates one strong sensation, stretching the upper back.

Second Posture: Position the shoulders in the neutral middle position, straight up and down.

Third Posture: Thrust the thoracic spine forward, gently bend back and let the shoulders move backward, stretching the chest.

Alternatively, you can isolate one shoulder at a time. Close one side of your ribs and open the other. If you isolate the right shoulder, close the ribs on the right side, open the ribs on the left and allow the arm to hang like a noodle, and bounce on the right leg. This will allow the right shoulder to loosen further. Within each single shoulder focus, you still have the three major areas that change the sensation: back, middle, and forward. Because the shoulders are also connected to your neck, when you pulse or pump the shoulders, if you turn the neck to different directions or hold it in different postures, you will find again that the sensation in the shoulder changes.

Ankles

Once you finish with the arms, move to the ankles and try to pulse through the ankles. Pulsing the leg joints will create different sensations. The arms do not bear weight but we do bear weight through the legs, and that totally changes the sensations.

Obtaining Good Alignment through the Ankles

Alignment and weight distribution are the keys to accessing all ligaments in the ankles. First, we have four major ligaments that we want to create an even stress on between the foot and the bottom part of our leg; two ligaments in the front and two in the back (Figure 33). If you have the weight on the ball of the foot, you will feel the stress on the front ligaments while the back ones will be loose or free of stress. Now if you shift your weight to the heels, you will change the sensations of stress. The heels will now bear the weight that will generate stress on the back ligaments and will loosen the two front ones. If you allow the soles of the feet to collapse sideways, you will lose the alignments and lose the ability to isolate the pulsing those four ligaments.

Make sure you distribute the weight in the middle of each sole of the foot. Do not collapse inward or push outward. Maintain the alignment, and then enjoy the pulsing, pumping, and shaking to a much higher level. While doing so, you also will be preventing injuries. Alignment of the ankle is very important. Much practice and work in the different postures and movements needs to be done to understand and experience the ankles.

LIGAMENTS OF THE ANKLE

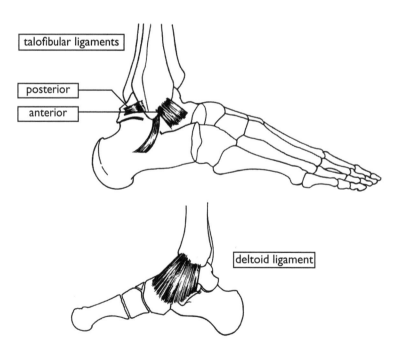

Figure 33.   Muscles and ligaments that support the ankle joint.

Knees

Next, move into the knees. Make sure you bounce the weight through the knees, right into the floor, and not into the knees. If you do it right, and your weight moves through the knees into the floor, you may be able to vibrate the whole floor of the room. You need wood floors to make this happen. If the weight moves into the knees, you will not be able to create that vibration of the wood floor. Moving weight into the knees is not good for them. The knees are not meant to be weight-bearing joints.

Hips

Then move to the hips. They, like the shoulders, have many strong and different sensations. The reasons are first, both the shoulders and the hips are the biggest joints in our body; second, the hips and the shoulders have the most range of motion in contrast to all the other joints in the body. The three major postures or positions that allow us to sense the various and different sensations in the hips are as follows:

First Posture: While pulsing and pumping, bring the pelvis forward by tucking in the tailbone.

Second Posture: While pulsing and pumping, stick the tailbone back and slightly out. You are coming out of alignment in this posture but in this case it is okay.

Third Posture: Once you pulsed and pumped with the pelvis back and in the front, find the middle between the two, dropping the tailbone down but not tucked in like the first posture and not pushed back like the second.

Of course, again, like the shoulders, each hip joint can be isolated by itself. By shifting all your weight to the left leg, you can isolate the right hip joint or you can direct the pulsing to the left hip joint with the weight on the right leg.

These exercises give you a way to create different sensations in the hips. Over time, you should find and explore other postures that lead to other sensations and new experiences.

Spine

After doing the hip movements, move up into the spine. As a beginner, rather than trying to pulse and pump each vertebra separately, start by dividing the spine into three major sections.

Create and isolate a pulse and a pump in each one of the three pieces you created. In the beginning, try to feel the pulsing or pumping sensation through the first section you choose to work with, for example, the lumbar area. For better isolation, find different ways to tense and relax muscles around the spine in order to isolate the area that you are trying to pulse, shake, or pump. Tensing and relaxing different muscles can help you learn to isolate the ligaments in desired areas, especially the small areas between the vertebrae. For example, let go of the abdominal muscles and pulse. This will create one sensation. Then, tighten the abdominal muscles and pump and shake. You should have more control over where you isolate the sensation. Sometimes you can use your hands to hold the abdominal muscles. Now there is some tightness but it is external. Pulse and pump. You may find that you are better able to isolate the desired area.

Here are some more ways to improve your skill of isolating the pulsing, pumping, and shaking: Let the shoulders go forward or backward by letting the ribs open and close, by holding the air in the lungs, and by emptying them out. Next, pulse the thoracic spine (the mid back). Adjust your hips and shoulders until you can isolate that chunk of your spine; then move up to the cervical spine between the shoulders.

Neck

You must be extra gentle and careful when pulsing the head. When pulsing the neck area, it is as if the head is connected by a spring to the spine. Pulse it in and out of the shoulders, and up and down, and have the head bob up and down with a gentle left and right, forward and backward movement as well. Shoulders and hips have a larger range of motion than the other joints, which allows for much more movement and sensations.

Do not rush when stretching the neck. It can take weeks of gently stretching to release tension that has built up for months or years.

The Jaw is Also a Joint

As you create the gentle pulse through the face, relax your jaw and let the jaw gently pulse. When you reach the jaw, you can close your eyes. At this point, if you have the tongue at the roof of your mouth, take it down and relax the tongue.

"I Already Know What I Am Doing"

I have seen it again and again. After students become familiar with the meditative shaking, they talk while they do it and their minds are not as engaged as when they first learned the motions. One of my teachers used to refer to this beginning time as the honeymoon period. We all tend to fall into this trap. After we become familiar with some exercise, we do not pay full attention to the sensations in the body and so we get stuck at that level for some time without experiencing more changes. It is part of the learning curve. That means that at first you will advance quickly. You see and experience many new sensations and you see quicker changes. As you continue in your practice, the changes and the experiences will subside and it will take longer to see and experience new things. Do not fall into this trap that so many people experience. It is important to keep fine-tuning your skills while you are in this plateau of learning and maintain a fresh and curious mind. The trick is to approach every day as if the meditation were new and every day we might just learn something. In order to reach the next peak, we need to keep going with an open, curious, and humble mind.

Sometimes, after finishing my three to five minute joint pulsing, I redirect the gentle pulsing into the rest of the soft tissue, especially the muscles and mostly the big groups of muscles: the chest, the abdominal muscles, the thighs. I especially enjoy this exercise because it is not easy to find a better massage than the one created by this meditation and pulsing. The gentle pumping creates a gentle vibration throughout the muscles and I am able to release lots of tension on my own. Over the years, I have learned to direct this gentle pulse to the skin, into the fascia, into the muscles, and then within the muscle, near the skin, or closer to the bones. As you practice the meditative shaking, you will discover how to isolate the various layers of soft tissue and direct the pulse and the gentle movement to the layer that you desire to massage.

Conclusion

Sense the pulse, the pump, and the shaking throughout the whole body. Scan the joints. Some people like to pulse, pump, or shake gently and others like to pulse, pump, or shake a little more strongly. Most people will find that at various times they may enjoy the two methods mixed, the slow and the fast, according to the time and the need.

When you do perform this mind/body prescription during sunset, allow the sun to warm your joints while drawing your aches and pains from the joints. When doing the meditative shaking, put your mind a few inches away from the joint you are working on. By putting the mind away from the joint, the impurities will be led away from the joint and the pulling energy of the setting sun will do the rest of the pulling and dissolving. When you practice the meditative shaking during sunset, you will experience a strong sensation that will be hard to achieve without the setting sun. This strong sensation is your guardian energy or what I call the energetic bubble. Do not wait only for this time of the day to perform the meditative shaking. This mind/body prescription needs to be performed at least twice a day.

Do the meditative shaking for three to five minutes every day. *Remember that when performing the meditative shaking,* keep breathing deeply through the nose, and keep the tongue touching the roof of the mouth except when pulsing the jaw. Once you finish the meditative shaking, you should stand still or sit on the edge of the chair, and for three to five minutes put your mind in your center of gravity energy center or lower energy center to allow the energy you built up to be led into the center and to strengthen and upgrade your lower energy center while still noticing the patches of heat throughout the joints. Lead your mind from the four gates, the tips of fingers and toes, into the lower energy center. You can also nourish the bones by leading the energy from the patches of heat inward into the joints and from there you can then move into the bones.

Once you are comfortable with this mind/body prescription, bring in the other building blocks: the breath, mind, energy, and spirit. Evoke spirituality by putting the mind in the three forces: heaven, human, and earth. It is a process that is called 'unification of the three forces.' There are other ways to evoke spirituality. You can use your own religious symbols or you can use the spirit of nature, such as a tree. Your arms can be the branches and they are shaking and becoming loose, gently in the wind.

Many individuals will testify how comfortable on both physical and mental levels they feel after performing this meditative shaking. They also express how relaxed they feel after this mind/body prescription. Pulsing, pumping, bouncing, and shaking are part of natural movements and performing them allows us to connect to nature in a new, interesting, and energetic way. In my personal experience with some of my students, the meditative shaking may have the strong effect of increasing bone density, but it is not scientifically proven yet. Some individuals get some of this pulsing and pumping motions while performing 'embrace the tree' (Yi Chuan) standing meditation.

SIGH SOUND

Maintain correct alignment, with the thoracic spine in and up, head suspended, and the face, neck, and shoulders relaxed. Close your eyes and breathe peacefully. Place the fingers of your hand gently on the solar plexus area. Use your mind to first scan the entire body, and then collect any impurities or stagnant energy from your entire body. Inhale and lead these impurities with your mind into the solar plexus area. Exhale and use your mind to move the collected impurities up and out your mouth. Sigh deeply while visualizing all the impurities releasing from your mouth toward the horizon.

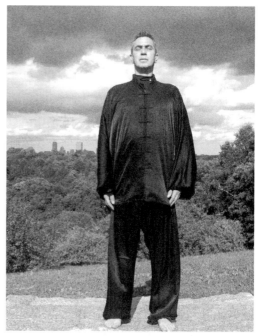

You can understand how special this cleansing is when performed with the setting sun. The powerful pulling energy of the setting sun just becomes one more force to achieve this cleansing goal. The sigh sound should be used throughout the day, many times. Waiting to do it during sunset is nice but it is only one of the times you should use this mind/body tool. When you release the impurities from your mouth, look toward the horizon, visualize the impurities getting pulled by the setting sun, half close your eyes, and continue releasing your impurities toward the pull of the setting sun. When exhaling, imagine yourself as a dragon and the impurities are like fire shooting from your mouth. Performing the visualization of collecting impurities and using the sigh

Thoracic spine in and up with the head suspended, and face, neck, and shoulders relaxed (standing).

sound to release them will offer a mental and emotional relief any time you need it.

Using the sigh sound has a few goals. One goal is to help release the muscles around the lungs in order to stimulate deep breathing and in order to bring as much oxygen as possible into the bloodstream, which upgrades the functioning of every cell in our body. Sighing helps the muscles around the lungs to relax and that allows more air to come in on the next inhalation. Inhale, breathe in to 80%, then exhale slightly, and then sigh. When you sigh, make a sound. Let go and physically move the thoracic spine forward, forming the turtle back. You do not need to do it every time you sigh, just every now and then. The rest of the time, you just sigh without bending the spine forward.

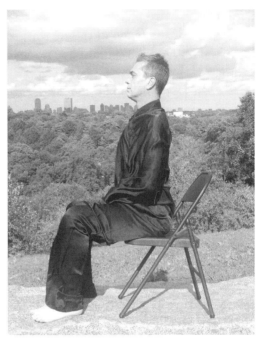

Thoracic spine in and up with the head suspended, and the face, neck, and shoulders relaxed (sitting).

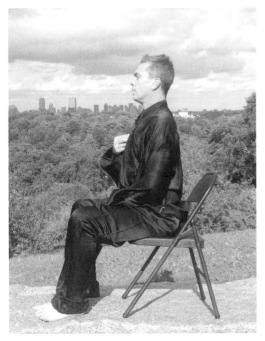

Place the fingers of your hand gently on the solar plexus area (sitting).

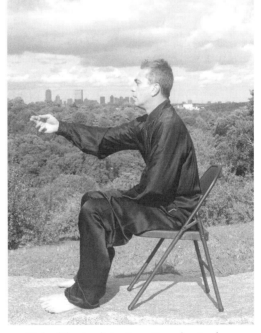

Sigh while visualizing impurities releasing from your mouth toward the horizon (sitting).

There are two ways to do the sigh. The first way is to sigh while keeping the spine upright. Sigh and let go of the ribs but not the spine. The second way is to sigh and let go of the ribs and the spine. That creates more slack in the smooth muscles, the muscles around the lungs.

When you sigh you also want to use a sound. The sound of sighing is "HHH …" There are two ways you can add a sound. You can sigh loud, high-pitched sighs using the vocal cords, which is not as good as the second way of sighing. The second way uses a deep, low sound from within, from the guts. It is not so much the sound you make; it is more the feeling and sensation of letting go and being able to relax the muscles around the lungs.

The second goal of sighing is to release the fire energy from the solar plexus area as well as the impurities throughout the physical and energetic body. The solar plexus area is related to our emotions and fire energy. The solar plexus or the sternum is the area that the fire from the food we eat and the air we breathe accumulates and is held. Using the sigh sound, the mental scanning, and the forward movement of the spine will cool down the fire not only from the solar plexus, but from the entire body as well.

Once More–Cleansing Impurities

Inhale and scan the entire body for impurities. Collect all the impurities from the body, using your mind, and lead them into the solar plexus area: the sternum. Then as you exhale, make a deep sigh. When you sigh, you let all the impurities you collected and gathered at the solar plexus come out of your mouth like a dragon shooting fire out of his mouth. Breathe in again, collect all your impurities, and exhale and sigh again.

You need at least three good sighs. The first sensation is more physical than mental. The second sensation is more mental or energetic. The skill of collecting the impurities with your mind is a process that will improve over time. As your inhalation becomes longer and longer and you have a more peaceful mind, it will allow you to collect more impurities and you will be able to do the visualization for longer periods of time.

Sighing While in Nature

I recommend that you try this sighing exercise while standing up on a mountain and looking down into a canyon. Close your eyes as you inhale and collect all impurities. Sigh and release all your impurities down into the valley. Standing on the mountain will give you a greater spiritual sensation as well as fresher air. If you think about it, our natural instinct is to use sound. If we are hit, what is the first thing we do? OOF! We use sounds to express many feelings and sensations. Certain cultures use sounds at specific situations more than others do. As a Jewish fellow, I can tell you that it is common among Jews to sigh and moan and to express feelings and emotions through sounds: 'oy vay.'

Sighing allows you to feel a deeper level of relaxation and cleansing. If you just exhale, it does not help you relax as much as if you exhale and sigh at the same time.

When you sigh with the exhale, you are mixing the mental and the physical. The mind follows the breath as you collect the tension and release it with a sigh.

Solar Plexus–the Last Stop

Pointing the finger to the solar plexus at the end of the mental gathering of all impurities is very important. It is the 'last stop' before the impurities leave the body. It also enforces the visualization of collecting and focusing the impurities at the solar plexus right before they exit our body. When expelling the impurities, move the finger from the solar plexus toward the direction you want the impurities to go. When you exhale and point the finger or the hand in the direction you want the impurities to go, also put the mind about 10 feet away from the body. You want to think away from yourself. In this way, the impurities will move out of your body. The action and the motion of the finger or the hand allow you to have a stronger experience of the impurities going out than if you just exhale. Some of my students like using both hands, moving from the solar plexus up toward the mouth and straight forward, then coming back to the solar plexus. Repeat the exercise three times.

This principle of putting the mind away from the place we intend to affect is often repeated in the world of martial arts. It is the same when we punch. You do not think of the person you punch, you think a foot or two beyond him. Then the power does not stop at the person but goes through him. This mental trick makes the punch much stron-

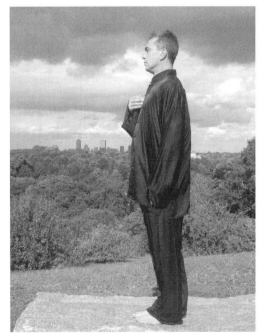

ger and more damaging. Also, when you put the mind in the lungs, you are building tension in the lungs. When you put the mind away from the lungs, the muscles around the lungs can be relaxed, which makes the lungs function more efficiently.

You can see why performing this exercise while standing on a mountain enhances this experience. You can also understand how the powerful pulling energy of the setting sun is an effective tool in boosting this process. When the sun is setting, we are getting two benefits that we do not get any other time. The first benefit is you have the setting sun to look at in order to move the mind away from the body, and the second benefit comes from the actual pulling energy of the setting sun that helps pull away your impurities.

Place the fingers of your hand gently on the solar plexus area (standing).

The Sound of Sigh

The sigh sounds themselves allow you to better empty the mind. By using the sound and the exhalation, they take over or capture our thoughts like the sound of a bell or gong, or the sound of music. The sigh improves our ability to empty the mind of thoughts and the body of impurities. Sighs with a 'ha' sound help to move energy and impurities from your body. Closed-mouth sighs hold energy in, which will hold the body impurities in, but you can sense a mental release or cleansing of impurities in the brain. Both are important for different reasons.

Different individuals like to sigh at different times and use a different number of repetitions. Finding the optimal time for the sigh sound is good for you, and how often, is up to each individual. Use the sigh throughout the program as well as your life. I found that deep breathing with sighing released my impurities. Lingering at the end of the exhalation is very powerful for me and is also effective for many of my students. Putting them together is a stronger experience and an essential tool in the mind/body journey.

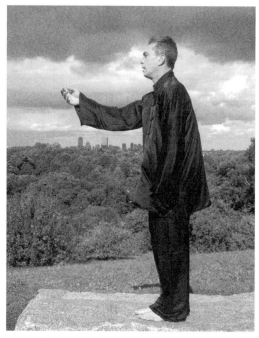

Sigh while visualizing impurities releasing from your mouth toward the horizon (standing).

BREATH WORK–AN INTRODUCTION

Working with your lungs and experiencing the breath work in the exercises introduced in this mind/body program is another method that will increase your lung capacity and oxygen intake. The increase of oxygen intake into the blood stream will allow every cell in your body to function better. Stronger lungs will improve your physical performance and will give you more success with your physical goals. Your immune system will become stronger and the function of this system will be in balance. When you hike or bike or do any kind of cardiovascular exercise, you will feel a huge difference. It will also help you stay relaxed, help you deal with anxiety, and help you deal with fears and stress. Most importantly, if you ever want to dive for pearls, like Japanese pearl divers without the aid of air tanks, working with the lungs and developing them will help you with this goal. Even if diving for pearls is not your goal, quieting the monkey mind and strengthening the immune system are two excellent benefits.

Physical Breath/Mental Breath and the Sunset

Practicing your physical and mental breath will allow you to enjoy the benefits of the sunset more efficiently. The pulling energy of the setting sun is only one part of the formula. Your mind and your other mind/body skills are the key to better use of the setting sun energy. For example, practicing the wing breath will give you larger and more developed lungs that will lead to a quieter monkey mind, allowing you to be more relaxed and quiet while the setting sun is helping with the cleansing of your physical and energetic body. The time you will need to spend to achieve your energetic goals will shorten through improving your breathing and mind/body skills. You can also actually practice your skills during sunset. The powerful pull of the setting sun will dissolve your stress, tension, and other impurities more efficiently and will allow you to practice longer mostly because your experience will be more energetic and definitely more spiritual. Of course, your main goal is to improve your physical and mental breathing skills so you can practice whenever you have time.

Linger at End of Exhalation

Close your eyes and breathe deeply. Observe the breath moving in and out of your lungs. Fill the lungs to 80% of their capacity, and as you exhale use your mind and the sigh sound to relax the muscles around the lungs. When you near the end of your exhalation, exhale much more slowly, and linger or pause as long as you can without holding your breath or turning blue.

When you are at the end of an exhalation, the diaphragm does not move very much. It is at the end of its movement, and the lungs are already empty of air that makes them quiet. The smooth muscles are relaxed and there is some slack in them. Because the lungs are empty, the heart, the pulse, all slow down. This time or space during our breathing is considered to be the quietest time in our body. Close your eyes, breathe in and out, notice the noise, and then linger at the end of your exhalation and enjoy the quiet. If your noise is very loud and you are suffering, you may need much practice and maybe some professional guidance.

I enjoy spending time lingering at the end of my exhalation. It is the quietest time in my life. I often say that I love being at the end of my exhalation, and I would not mind staying there forever, but that would mean that I am dead. Over time, your ability to linger at the end of an exhalation will improve, and you can stay there longer and longer.

Caution and Prevention

Some beginning students who are just starting to work with their breath may hyperventilate and experience dizziness. Because deep breathing is new to them, they have a tendency to work at 120% effort when breathing deeply. Groups of muscles become tense, and this tension blocks the flow of blood and oxygen to the brain leading to experiencing dizziness. Lingering at the end of the exhalation will prevent hyperventilation and dizziness by dragging large volumes of air over and over. Another benefit of lingering is the cooling down of the heart. You can monitor this cooling down by taking your pulse before you start, during, and after.

When you linger at the end of an exhalation, there is a tendency to allow the spine, the ribs, and the head to move down. Maybe it is because the eyes are closed or the lower back muscles are weak. Sometimes it is just the fact that we fall asleep for just a second. Balance the lingering by preventing the ribs from collapsing, lengthening the spine, and suspending the top of the head. Because during exhalation, there is a strong energetic movement downward and the rest of the body wants to follow. However, you want to balance the downward force of the lungs during exhalation with preventing the ribs, especially the front ribs, from collapsing or moving down and at the same time paying attention to lengthening of your spine especially the thoracic spine and suspending the top of the head. When paying attention to the ribs, spine, and head in relationship to the lungs that are moving down while you are exhaling, you are emphasizing the balancing action that will allow you to create and experience the up and down forces during exhalation and especially during lingering at the end of the exhalation. For more information about the major up and down forces, please see *Sunrise Tai Chi*, page 17.

To Hold or Not to Hold the Breath–That is the Question

When you linger at the end of the exhalation, are you holding your breath? No, you are not really holding your breath. What you are doing is exhaling the first 90% of your breath, and then slowly and quietly releasing the last 10% of the air that remains in your lungs, just as in releasing the air from a syringe. The air is still moving out, but it is moving so slowly and at such a low volume that it will look from the outside as if you are holding your breath, yet there is a slight motion. As your lung performance improves, your breaths will become longer and you will be able to linger longer at the end of an exhalation because you will have more lung capacity and your mind will be able to relax more deeply. Because your breathing is deeper and you are holding the oxygen in for longer periods of time, you are more efficiently oxygenating your blood and utilizing this source of oxygen. This in turn allows you to remain in this quiet space for longer periods of time (two to three minutes), which is important when doing the more advanced training. This is the process used by the deep divers in France. They have been reported as able to stay underwater for eight minutes. They oxygenate their blood before diving by doing fast deep breathing with lots of air swallowing and holding, and then they utilize that oxygen when they are diving.

The ability to linger at the end of an exhalation will improve over time as you become better with the skill of letting go of the muscles around the lungs as well as utilizing the power of the mind to achieve deeper relaxation. It is a combination of developing your lungs, having bigger, stronger lung capacity, as well as the mental skill that gives you the ability to let go and relax the muscles at the end of the exhalation, which will allow you to stay there longer. As you can see, this ability is divided into physical and mental. You always have to emphasize both.

Linger at End of Inhalation

Close your eyes and breathe deeply. Observe the breath moving in and out of your lungs. Fill the lungs to 80% of their capacity, and as you exhale, use your mind and the sigh sound to relax the muscles around the lungs. As you near the end of your inhalation, inhale much more slowly. Linger to the best of your abilities without holding your breath.

This work with the lungs, lingering and emphasizing different stages along our breathing path, is to get you familiar with various experiences on a mental as well as energetic level while stimulating different lung cells. When performing the skills in this mind/body program, you will experience the air moving in and the lungs expanding—your 80% capacity for exhaling while collapsing the spine and ribs and your 80% capacity without the collapse. You will experience the sigh sounds that help the muscles relax and the effect it has on tension and releasing impurities. You will also experience the special time of lingering at the end of an inhalation—this deep level of relaxation and stillness. You will also experience the time between inhalation and exhalation, the end of inhalation, when the lungs are 80% full.

When you try to linger at the end of an inhalation, you will find that it is not easy. You may find that you are not able to linger as long at the end of exhalation as you can at the end of inhalation. That is normal. A nice visualization that may help you while inhaling to 80% and lingering is to close your eyes and take the sensation of the expansion of the lungs and imagine that you and your lungs are an air balloon. Once you can experience the sensation of being an air balloon, try lingering on this experience and ride the air balloon as long as you can without holding your breath. When the time comes and you need to exhale, let go of the air balloon and land it safely.

When you are holding air in at the end of an inhalation, it gives your lungs and your body a chance to extract more oxygen, more than you would get when breathing your common shallow breathing. Slowing at the end of the inhalation will oxygenate more of your blood and will nourish every cell in your body with oxygenated blood, which allows every cell in your body to function and perform at higher levels. Breathing deeply is a conscious decision. Making that conscious decision is a large part of getting the full benefit of the exercise. That is the reason I keep repeating this information. It is to get you to make that decision to breathe deeply as much and as often as possible.

Yin and Yang in the Breath

The end of the exhalation is more yin, physically, compared with the end of the inhalation, which is more yang. At the end of an exhalation, you may notice that the mind is more active, more yang compared with the end of an inhalation, when the mind is more quiet, more yin. When the lungs are more yang, the mind is more yin, and when the lungs are more yin, the mind is more yang.

Many people are shallow breathers who tend to fill only the front upper part of their lungs. In the next part of the program, we will try moving air to different sections or compartments in the lungs to stimulate cells that may not get this stimulation due to shallow breathing. If you are doing cardiovascular work three to six times a week, you are probably not a shallow breather, but it is still rewarding to do these breath exercises. You may benefit from the science of breathing. These experiences and benefits will surpass the great experience of just having good lungs.

LATISSIMUS/SIDE LUNG BREATHING/WING BREATH

It is not enough to just breathe in and breathe out, or even sigh and linger. Next, we need to develop the skill of moving the air into specific areas within the lungs. Some disciplines call them chambers, some call them sections, and others call them areas, or rooms. I created friendly names and images for the different areas in the lungs—images that will help direct the air or the breath to wherever you desire it to move. For example, latissimus or wing breath represents the need to move air into the sides of the lungs. You want to move the air into the lungs sideways toward the area from the armpit down a straight line all the way to the hip, isolating air in our imagined wings, leading or pushing air to that area and moving the lungs laterally.

The latissimus muscles are the muscles that are next to the area of the lungs we are interested in stimulating and energizing in this next exercise (Figure 34).

Use the mind to draw air to the sides of your lungs and move the latissimus muscles outward. This skill involves being able to lead and isolate air into different sections of our lungs, in this case to the sides of the lungs. In this exercise, we focus on moving the air outward toward the latissimus muscles. Inhale deeply into both sides of your lungs, expanding the muscles and ribs outward toward the arms. Exhale and release the air, while using your mind and the sigh sound to relax the muscles around the lungs. Each time you inhale, try to fill your lungs to about 80% of their capacity, and surf the breath. Relax your shoulders, neck, and face. As you exhale, remember not to collapse the thoracic spine (Figure 35).

THE LATISSIMUS DORSI

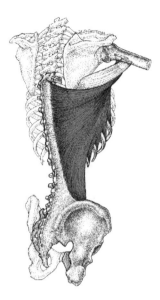

Figure 34. The latissimus muscle expands as you breathe into your "wings."

WING BREATH

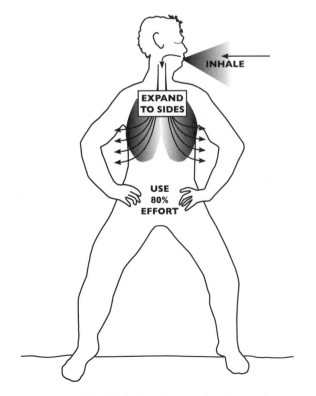

Figure 35. Inhale deeply, expanding the muscles
and ribs outward toward the arms.

You can actually monitor if you are doing this breathing correctly by placing the thumbs on the side of the lungs and the fingers toward the front of your ribs. When you exhale, your fingers will touch each other, and when inhaling, they will move and separate from one another. If you can have them move toward and away from each other, you are doing it correctly and you have mastered this wing breath breathing skill.

How can you actually expand the lungs in whatever direction you wish? One of my students is an expert in understanding the anatomy and function of the human body; he is one of the leading surgeons in the Boston area. After seeing what I can do with my lungs, he told me, "Rami the lungs are like balloons. When you breathe in, the whole balloon expands and when breathing out, it contracts. I do not know what you are doing and I do not understand how you are able to expand different parts of your lungs at will, but let me think about it and I will come back with an answer."

Theoretically he is right. You cannot expand parts of your lungs without moving air to the entire lungs. So how can you do it? How can you expand the sides or the upper back or just the front bottom of your lungs? A few days later, the same student came back, all smiles, "Rami, I know what you are doing!" I said, "Please tell me because I can do it but I do not know why." He told me, "Rami, it is through muscle control." The second he said this, I felt it. Some of the muscles I contract and others I let go. We have muscles around the lungs. You can learn to control them. You will learn through

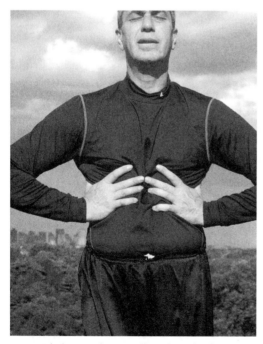

Exhale. Your fingers will touch each other.

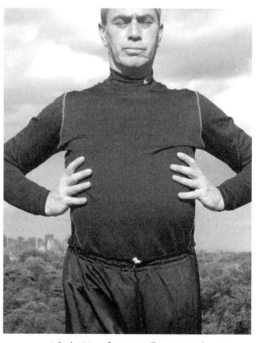

Inhale. Your fingers will move and separate from one another.

practice how to isolate specific groups of muscles and tense them, while allowing other groups of muscles to be relaxed. By achieving this muscle control, it will allow you to direct air to expand the areas in the lungs that you choose. By tensing and relaxing the various groups of muscles, you are restricting the air from moving to some areas and allowing it to move and expand in others.

Be the Eagle

Sometimes you can use the arms to help develop this skill as well as create the visualization, sensation, or illusion of having real wings and a spirit of an eagle. Sit or stand with your arms on your knees or hips and spread the armpits open. Move the elbows out and create the shape of wings; pretend that your arms are like two wings. Fill up your wings from back to front. Be aware that there is a tendency to get more movement in the front part of the lungs.

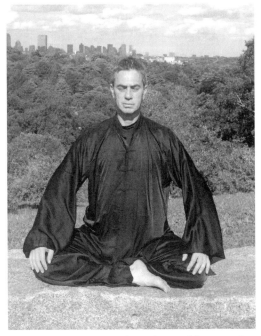

Inhale deeply into sides of your lungs while expanding ribs outward toward the arms (no support).

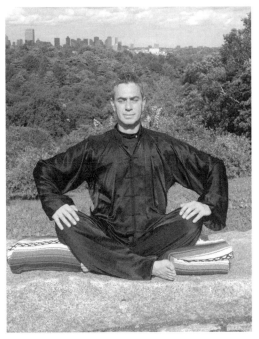

Inhale deeply into sides of your lungs while expanding ribs outward toward the arms (with support).

Partner Work

Person A uses the pointer fingers of both hands to gently clamp the latissimus dorsa muscle from the front and back. Person B attempts to breathe into that area and expand the clamped fingers of Person A. Work with the principle of the 80% effort. Sighing and lingering at the end of inhalation and exhalation adds tremendously to this exercise.

Finding Balance is Important

There is a tendency on exhalation, because the ribs and the lungs are moving down, to let go of the suspended spine. Balance the emptying of the lungs and the dropping of the ribs with lengthening of the spine and suspension of the head. Work with 80% effort or, with the lungs, you can work to 90% capacity because you want to bring as much air as you can into the lungs. Do not inhale all the way in and do not exhale all the way out. You are reserving 10% on each side: inhalation and exhalation. I call it the 'floating 10%.' It just floats from side to side between inhalation and exhalation.

Close your eyes and breathe in 90%. Sense the 10% that is left on the top. Back off and do not try to use this last 10%. Linger or just exhale but leave 10% at the end of the exhalation. Sense the 10% but do not *touch* it. If you do it slowly, it floats from side to side rather than jumps. When utilizing this skill, you allow your whole body to stay relaxed. You do not put compression against your nervous system at the end of

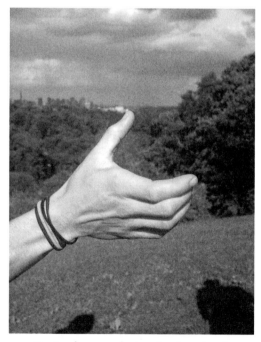

Use two fingers and set up the clamp hand.

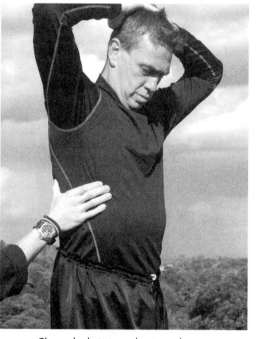

Clamp the latissimus dorsi muscle, one finger in front and one in back.

inhalation, and you are not running out of breath at the end of exhalation. This skill of using the 'floating 10%' will allow you to maximize the air and oxygen going into the blood stream while preventing the negative elements of breathing in and out using 100% effort. You can keep the breath, the mind, the energy, and spirit strong and in a smooth balanced circle of flow.

Another way to understand wing breath breathing, or the latissimus dorsi side breathing, is by practicing seesaw breathing, which we will explain in more detail later. When you perform seesaw breathing, you are performing half of the wing breath. You are moving air to one lung or wing at a time by lifting the shoulder and isolating one lung at a time. You may have a stronger experience of where that wing area is and how it feels to move air there. Lifting the shoulder may make it easier to tense groups of muscles that you were not able to control and tense when you were doing the wing breathing. When working with the lungs, you first experience the major areas, chambers, parts or sections, and later as you develop the skill of muscle isolation and control, as well as more sensitivity, you will be able to find other smaller points.

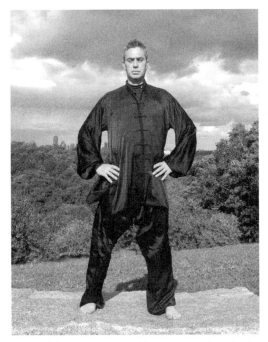

Pretend that your arms are like two wings (standing).

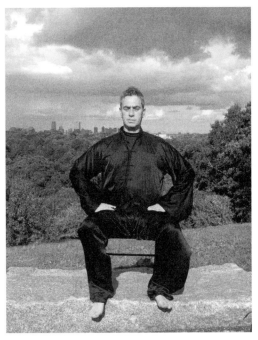

Pretend that your arms are like two wings (sitting).

TRAPEZIUS–UPPER FRONT AND BACK LUNG BREATHING

Once you have a strong sensation of the wings, you want to move into the next breath skill, mushroom breathing, or trapezius breathing. The trapezius muscles are a diamond-shaped group of muscles that go from the bottom of the thoracic spine, between your shoulder blades, out to the middle of each shoulder, and up the neck (Figure 36).

THE TRAPEZIUS MUSCLE

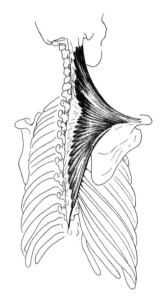

Figure 36. When performing the Mushroom Breath, the upper chest in
the front and the trapezius muscles in the back expand.

Inhale deeply and lead the air through your nose and into the upper parts of your lungs, expanding the upper chest and upper back area. Exhale, and lead the air out using your mind to relax the muscles around the lungs. Each time you inhale, try to fill the upper parts of your lungs to about 80%. When you can isolate, tense, and relax the various muscles around your ribs and lungs, you will be able to draw air into specific parts of your lungs and in this case restrict the expansion to the upper front and back of the lungs.

Ultimately, you want to be able to lead air into the entire lung in order to stimulate the maximum number of cells to keep the lungs healthy and to bring in as much oxygen as possible. We all breathe very easily into the upper front lungs. In fact, most individuals, when asked to breathe deeply, will fill up the front upper lungs. Ask several people to take a deep breath and you will see that most will expand the upper front. The harder part is to fill up the upper back part of the lungs.

I recommend that you first isolate the upper back part of the lungs because it is more difficult. Inhale and try to create movement on the skin in the upper back between the shoulder blades. After a while when you can get some movement in the back upper lungs, you can add the front part of the upper lungs. When you do both of them together, it is like the shape of a mushroom or an umbrella that opens up and widens as you inhale.

In my first few years of performing the mushroom or the umbrella breathing, the front part of the lungs would always steal my breath and my mind. I decided to trick my mind and my lungs, and I started with the back part of the lungs first and then I added the front. I gave the back a head start because it was weaker physically and I had less mental control of this back area. The back part of the lungs fills more slowly and by giving them a head start, you allow them both to reach the finish line at the same time. On the other hand, on exhalation, it is the back that has an easier time and the front that has more work and tension. To balance this, on inhalation, concentrate on your back; and on exhalation, focus on your front.

Seesaw Breath

Close your eyes and breathe deeply. As you inhale, lean to the side and close the space between the ribs on that side while opening the space between the ribs on the other side. Lead your breath into the opened ribs and fill that lung to about 80%. Then repeat on the other side. Once you can perform the closing of the ribs on one side while opening the ribs on the other, you will be able to emphasize breathing with one lung at a time.

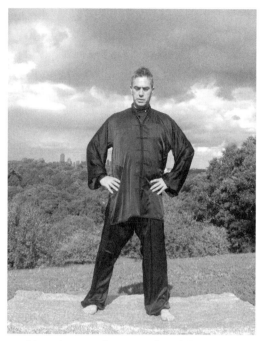

Neutral position for seesaw breath (standing).

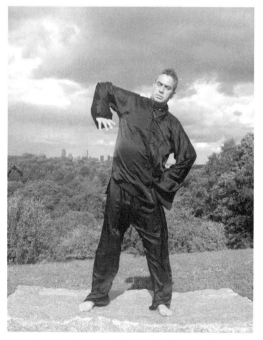

Open right ribs and close left ribs (standing).

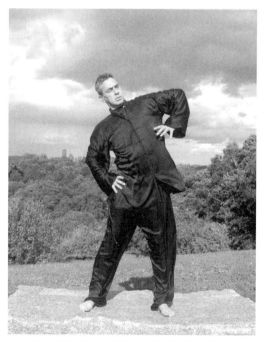

Open left ribs and close right ribs (standing).

Once you understand and can perform the wing and mushroom breathing skills, then you want to move to the next skill, which is to isolate and move air to one lung at a time using the seesaw breath. The seesaw breath breathing is unique because it allows you to experience one lung at a time. You use the ribs and posture to isolate one lung instead of tensing groups of muscles while sitting or standing still. Seesaw breathing will allow you to really feel the different sensations between the left and right lung and allow you to experience the lung that has three lobes and compare it to the lung that has two. It also allows you to experience the lung that has two lobes as wider and shorter rather than the lung that has three lobes as longer and narrower. After a while, you will be able to sense the unbalanced, unsymmetrical, sensation of your lungs. Once you know this sensation and you can experience it with your mind, you will want to balance this feeling and create an even sensation. Once you finish this specific training, move the mind away from the lungs and into the wings or the skin/bubble, a fist away from the body. That creates an even feeling throughout the lungs even though physically they are not symmetrical.

The seesaw breath demands that you lean from side to side and lift the shoulder of the lung that you are trying to activate or trying to stimulate. If you lean into the right, move the right rib and right shoulder down, lift the left ribs and shoulder up, and breathe deeply into the left lung. Exhale as you move the left ribs down, open the right lung, lift the right shoulder, and then inhale deeply through the nostrils into the right lung. Exhale, bring your lungs to an even position, move the right ribs and right shoulder down over the right lung, open the left, and lift the left ribs and shoulder. Inhale deeply from both nostrils and try to fill up the front and back parts of the lungs,

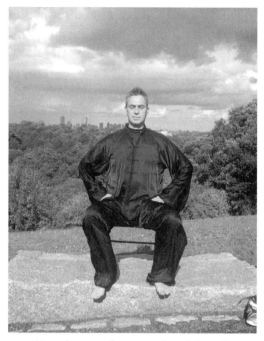

Neutral position for seesaw breath (sitting).

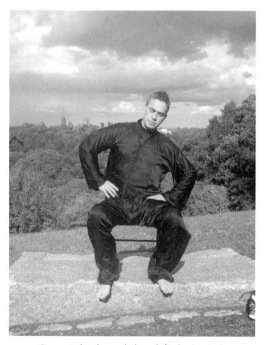

Open right ribs and close left ribs (sitting).

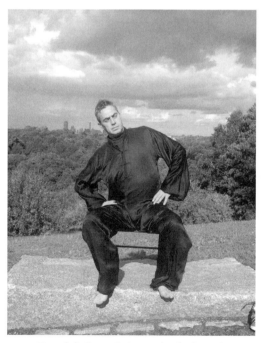

Open left ribs and close right ribs (sitting).

all the way from the bottom up. You can feel all the way down to the hip and all the way up to the armpit and shoulder. If you put your mind farther than your lungs, for example, at the ribs, skin or guardian energy, you will be able to move air all the way to the farthest edges of your lungs.

You can exhale at two different parts of this mind/body prescription. One time exhale while you are still in the bent position and the second time exhale while moving to the even position when moving the ribs and the shoulder down, like an accordion.

Once you feel comfortable with the different breaths, you should mix them and experiment with the various movements you know, and assess how these breaths and skills fit into your actions. The seesaw breath can be mixed with the other breaths. You can start with wing breath, move to the mushroom, and then the seesaw. Or you can start with the seesaw, go to wing, and then mushroom breathing. Improvise like a jazz musician.

Upper Energy Center

We discussed this area earlier at length. Now it will be used as one of the most important exercises in the cool down series. The pituitary energy center (i.e., the upper energy center) is located under the two lobes of the brain in the center of your head, in the area where the spinal cord connects to the brain (Figure 37). Hold your attention in this area, and build up a strong sensation or focus there. Do not allow the mind to wander while you focus your attention in the upper energy center. Once you can reside in your upper energy center for longer periods of time, more than 10 minutes, start visualizing this area as a golden or white ball of healing energy.

How to Get Started

First Steps: To cool the eye energy, close your eyes and drop the eyeballs into their sockets. Then you want to draw the feeling or sensation from the eyeballs backward into the brain, cooling down this path. Visualize the eyes as flashlights, and the switch for the flashlights is in the brain. Move back mentally, through the tunnels of the eyes into the brain. Once you reach the brain, you will find a switch. Just shut off the flashlight that cools the thoughts/brain energy.

THE PITUITARY GLAND ENERGY CENTER

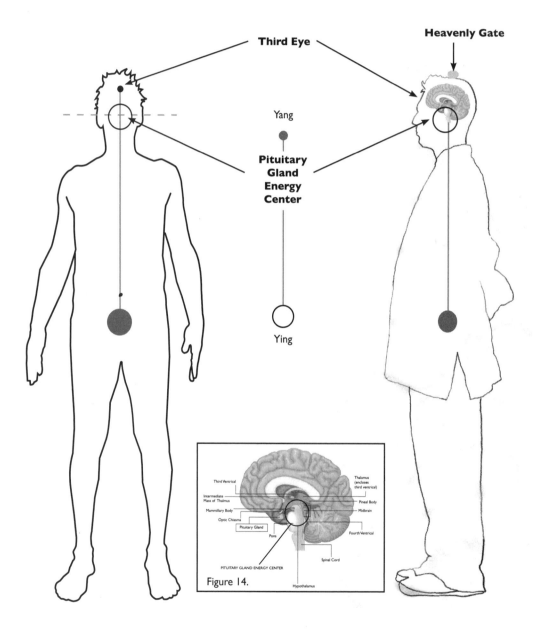

Figure 37. The Pituitary Gland Energy Center.

Next you want to cool the energy that is created from the millions of thoughts in our brain hovering over our head and over our hair. First, you just draw that energy down toward the brain, through the hair, and then the skull. Once it reaches the brain, allow it to sink down through the brain lobes into the spinal cord. A useful visualization for this part of the exercise could be that the energy at this point is like water going down the sink, which is the brain, and the spinal cord is the pipe that will take the water or the energy away from the bowl of the sink. Once you cool down the excess brain energy and the excess eye energy, you can reside in the upper energy center. Reside there as long as you can without losing the visualization. Every now and then, you may need to move away from the visualization and return to cool the brain and the eye energy. Work on helping them cool down some more and return to the visualization. The emphasis on cooling down the eye and brain energy will allow you to reside in and more strongly and clearly experience the upper energy center.

Second Step: Once you have cooled the eye and brain energy, put your mind in the pituitary energy center. Focus your entire mind into this area, as you did in the lower energy center exercise, using the same visualization of a point, or a ping-pong ball, or a marble of energy. Allow all your thoughts to dissipate, and focus only on this upper energy center. As you breathe deeply and peacefully, move your mind slowly into the upper energy ball. Other thoughts will steal your focus away from this energy ball. Gently refocus on the upper energy ball. Over time, your visualization will become stronger and clearer.

Training the pituitary gland energy center is a little more difficult because it is closer than the lower energy center to the active brain. Putting the mind in the upper energy center may spill over to the rest of the brain, leading energy into the brain itself. If energy does spill, the brain is likely to activate more brain cells, more thoughts. There also may be more distraction from the horse mind and less quiet from the monkey mind.

Third Step: Notice the characteristics of the upper energy center in comparison to the lower energy center. You may find out that the upper energy center is more active. The movement is more vibrant like electricity (yang). The lower energy center expresses the sensation of lava or mud (yin). You may also find it harder to visualize the upper energy center because it is closer to the brain and to the mechanism of activation of thoughts. Make sure you keep breathing deeply, and sigh and linger both at the end and at the beginning of the inhalations and exhalations. Maintain correct alignment. Do not collapse the spine or the head.

LOWER ENERGY CENTER

The lower energy center is located two inches below the navel and about three inches inward from that same spot. It is your physical center of gravity. Hold your attention in this area and build up a round physical sensation there. Do not allow the mind to wander while you focus your attention in your lower energy center. Once you can sense your energy center for longer of periods of time, more than 10 minutes, visualize a ball of healing energy there (Figure 38).

CENTER OF GRAVITY ENERGY CENTER
Lower Energy Center

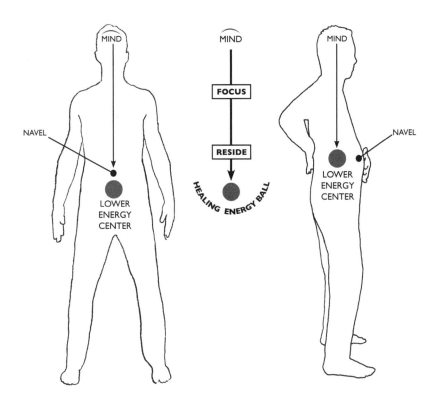

Figure 38. The Lower Energy Center is about
two inches below the navel and three inches inward.

How to Get Started

First Step: Sit on the edge of a chair or on the floor using a pillow as was discussed in the section about the small circulation. Focus two inches below the navel and a few inches toward the center of the body. Put your mind at this area, visualize a small ball the size of a marble or a cherry, and maintain your mind at the center. Start with a small ball. Over time, as your skills develop, you will be able to maintain your mind at the center longer and longer, and the ball will grow. You can visualize an energy ball, a magnetic field, or just a round feeling.

Second Step: There are a few tricks to maintaining the mind in the lower energy center: The first trick is to create a loose fist with your right hand and an open palm with your left hand; put the right fist on top of the palm. Line up both hands two inches below the navel. Then project this round sensation of your fist into the lower energy center. This fist or round sensation is used as a mental reinforcement, a physical tool to help the mental visualization. The fist that touches two inches below the navel will keep reminding you to keep the mind down at the lower energy center.

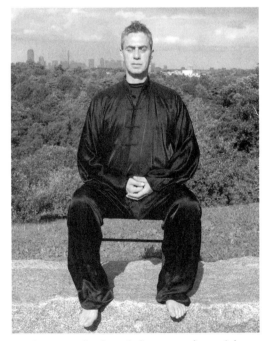

Projecting. Put the right fist on top of open left palm two inches below the navel (sitting).

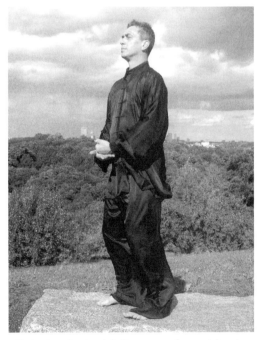

Projecting. Put the right fist on top of open left palm two inches below the navel (standing).

The second trick is every time you lose the visualization, loop the thoughts that you are having through the top of the head, through what is called, in qigong and tai chi, the heavenly gate (baihui) and send an imaginary string down through the heavenly gate with a weight or something round tied to the end of this string. Drop that string with the weight, slowly through the center of the body from the heavenly gate. Once the imaginary weight reaches two inches below the navel, the string stops and stays still. The ball that you have at the end of the string hangs and just swings gently two inches below the navel in the center of the body. Try to keep the ball still.

The third trick is holding the tai chi ball in front of your lower energy center (Figures 10 and 11) and projecting the round sensation between your hands to the lower energy center.

Third Step: At first you want to hold the visualization of a small energy ball maybe the size of a grape or a golf ball. Work with the small ball until you can hold the visualization constant and still for a few minutes. Once you feel comfortable with this size visualization and can maintain it for a few minutes, start increasing the size of the energy ball. Make it bigger and bigger—from a grape to an orange, from an orange to a grapefruit, and from a grapefruit to a watermelon until eventually you will feel it all the way at the skin of your trunk. Hold the visualization for 10 minutes at first and then slowly increase your time to 30 to 40 minutes per day.

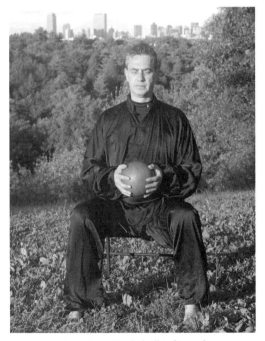

Projecting. Tai chi ball in front of
your lower energy center (sitting).

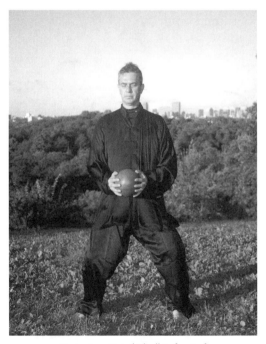

Projecting. Tai chi ball in front of
your lower energy center (standing).

Fourth Step: After you trained having it as a still energy ball, you will want to move to the next level. The next level is pulsing the energy ball. For example, pulse it from a grape to an orange, and back to a grape. When inhaling, grow the energy ball into a grape-sized ball, and when exhaling, expand into an orange-sized ball. This energy ball that you sense or visualize can have many different colors. Try to notice the various colors and sensation or characteristic that come along with this visualization of the lower energy center.

BOTH ENERGY CENTERS—THE ENERGETIC BATON

Once you are able to stay focused on both the upper and lower energy centers separately, connect the two with a straight line, like a baton. Pay attention to the sensations of both energy centers and the connection between them. This energetic core within your body is referred to in this book as well as in the *Sunrise Tai Chi* book as the energetic baton. A small reminder: Over time, try sensing the differences between the upper and the lower energy centers (Figure 39).

THE ENERGETIC BATON

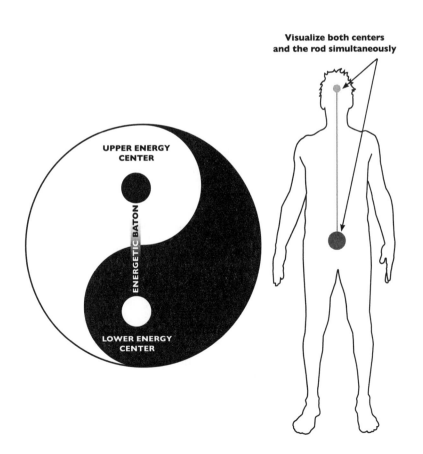

Figure 39. Connect the two Energy Centers.

How to Get Started

First Step: The External Baton: Hold the right hand fist in front of your nose and hold your left hand fist two inches below the navel in front of the lower energy center. Once you have your fists up in front of the two energy centers, visualize a line between the two fists. This line represents the path connecting the two energy centers and is an easy visualization. All you have to do is just visualize a line between the two fists outside your body. Once you emphasize and train for a while visualizing the energetic rod between your two fists, you are ready for the next step in the visualization.

Second Step: Once you can visualize the rod easily (this step could take a few weeks), move to the next visualization which is visualizing the whole external baton. At this point of the training, you may not need to hold your fists in front of your upper and lower energy centers. Keep practicing this visualization for a few weeks. Practice until you are able to close your eyes and visualize the external baton, and you can sense it right in front of you. Over time, the two energy centers will behave differently. When holding the visualization, you will have an external baton with two different heads because those two energy centers are totally different. Once you move into the center of the body, you have to visualize the two energy centers: the center of gravity energy center and the pituitary energy center, and then the internal energetic rod connecting the two. As you can see, steps one and two are just baby steps, a preliminary for the bigger visualization that allows the final visualization to be stronger.

The first two steps or visualizations will allow you to strengthen your mind before you move the visualization into the center of the body.

Third Step: Now you want to sit or stand still and move your mind inward into your body, the center of your trunk. First, start with the lower energy center. Build that visualization for a minute or two, then move up to the upper energy center and visualize that for a minute or two. Once you spend a few minutes on each separately, hold the two energy balls, lower and upper energy centers, as well as the energetic rod between them. When you are able to do this step, you can move to Step Four. If you cannot hold the whole visualization for 10 minutes, hold some of it and over time, you will be able to visualize the whole energetic baton. For example, you may sense the energetic rod and the lower energy center, and then when you move to the upper energy center, you may lose the lower energy center but not the energetic rod. Keep practicing your visualizations separately: the upper lower energy centers as well as the road that goes between them. Keeping the up and down forces while breathing deep will help you achieve these visualizations so you can move to the fourth step and hold the energetic baton for at least 10 minutes while noticing the various differences between the two energetic balls or energy centers.

Fourth Step: In the fourth step, visualize your internal energetic baton and see how long you can stay on the whole visualization. At the same time, see if you can notice the various differences in each ball's characteristic behaviors.

Drain the Energetic Baton

Because energy moves up and we use the upper energy center often throughout the day, I recommend that you cool down the upper energy center at the end of the day.

Focus your attention on the energetic baton within your body, and build a strong sensation or visualization of both energy centers and the connecting energetic rod. Observe the similarities and differences in the sensation of each energy center that are revealed to you during quiet observation. Once you are able to maintain a strong visualization of the whole energetic baton, try leading the energy from the upper energy center downward to the lower energy center. Enjoy the sensation of leading the energy downward and allowing it to gather and settle in the lower energy center. As you progress with this exercise, you may feel a spiraling energy moving downward. This practice or visualization can help you to balance and cool down your fire energy, which is stronger at the end of the day.

How to Get Started

First Step: To cool the eye energy, close your eyes. Drop your eyeballs into their sockets, and follow the sensation from the eyeballs backward into the brain. By following the sensation back, you soften and cool the flow of energy that shoots from the brain toward the eyes. Another thing you can do is imagine that the brain is like the switch of a flashlight. The energy that comes out of the eyes is like the 'light' of the imaginary flash light. Turn the switch/brain off and turn off the energy that comes out of the eyes. Then you follow this dark feeling backward toward the brain.

Second Step: To cool the brain/thoughts energy, move the energy from over your head, down toward the hair, and toward the skin of the skull. Continue to slowly move that energy down toward the two brain lobes and once you reach the lobes, use the visualization of the morning dew and just have the sensation of that energy dwindle through the brain lobes until it reaches the area where the brain is connected to the central nervous system/spinal cord.

Third Step: Once you have cooled both distractive energy elements, you are ready to start moving the energy down from the upper energy center to the lower one. Remember the physical action of sweeping? Keep going mentally backward and forward, gradually increasing your sweeps. Slowly move the mind down through the center of the body. Move with your mind gently, drawing the substantial energy sensation from the upper center to the lower one.

Fourth Step: Once you can move the energy from the pituitary energy center to center of gravity energy center, you can try residing at the lower energy center for 20 to 30 minutes. You will notice that at first when you do the drain the baton visualization, the energy will move down like the sweeping motion of the broom or the downward movement of a waterfall. This is great for now. You are pushing energy more than leading it, and that is fine at first. When, however, you are ready to move to the next level, you need to remain at the lower energy center and lead the energy down instead of pushing it. There is a big difference between pushing and leading. In qigong, it is said: "The yi leads the qi." Your intention, or wisdom mind (yi), leads your energy.

EMPTY MOON/FULL MOON–BUDDHIST

There are two kinds of full moon/empty moon breathing: Buddhist and Taoist. We use Buddhist breathing to relax and to help our energy to more strongly and smoothly circulate throughout our body. Inhale, and gently push your abdomen and lower back muscles out. Your diaphragm moves down while your lungs, abdomen, and back muscles expand outward. Use your mind to relax the muscles around your ribcage and take in more air. As you inhale, the entire abdomen expands. Exhale and release. Coordinating the muscular movements with the breath will also help you to regain conscious control of the muscles in your abdomen and make them stronger while constantly massaging your internal organs. When the muscles are pushed out, it is a full moon. And when they are drawn in, it is an empty moon. Try slowing your breathing and movement until you can count 30 increments, which symbolize the cycle of the moon.

EMPTY MOON/FULL MOON–TAOIST

Use Taoist breathing when you have a strong intention and when you want to manifest energy away from the body. When you inhale, gently draw in the abdomen and lower back muscles. And when you exhale, release them. Inhale, and the entire abdomen contracts. Exhale and release. This exercise will compress your mid-section, giving your organs a gentle massage, and will quickly build up energy in your lower energy center.

Once you can control both the abdominal and back muscles comfortably, with each abdominal breath try adding the movement of the pelvic floor, the area between the groin and the anus, as well as the entire trunk muscles, the muscles between the abdominal and the back muscles. Find them, and work toward coordinating their movement with every breath.

First Step: Either sitting or standing, use both hands to help the abdominal muscles to move. Inhale and move the muscles out, and exhale and move them in. Work gently so as not cause soreness in the abdominal area.

Then reverse the action of the abdominal muscles: draw them in on the inhalation and lead them out on the exhalation. Repeat a few times until you feel comfortable with the movement and can do it without your hands. Using your hands will always make the experience different. I recommend that you keep using this skill on a regular basis, even when you can move the abdominal muscles without the help of your hands.

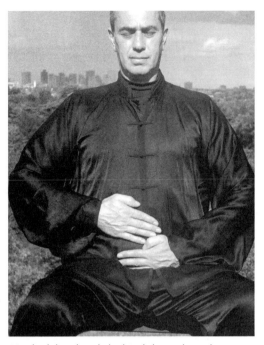

Use both hands to help the abdominal muscles move.

Second Step: Next, place the back of the palm on your back. Using the back part of the palm prevents tension in the shoulders.

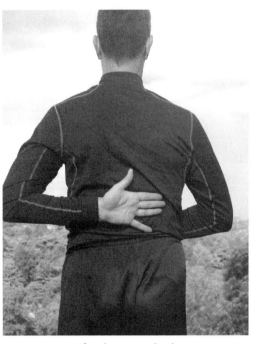

Left palm on your back.

Place the other hand with the palm on the abdominal muscles.

Start moving the front and the back abdominal muscles together: out on the inhalation, and in on the exhalation. Then reverse the order and when inhaling contract the moon, and when exhaling expand the moon. Practice for two minutes at first, and over time increase the training periods until you can easily move both the front and the back when doing either the Buddhist or the Taoist breathing.

Third Step: Now you want to master the movement of the abdominal and back muscles until you can move all the way from the solar plexus to the bladder area, and the back area from the tailbone to lower ribs, and eventually the pelvis floor, gently, like a pulse, as well as the entire trunk muscles between the abdomen and the back.

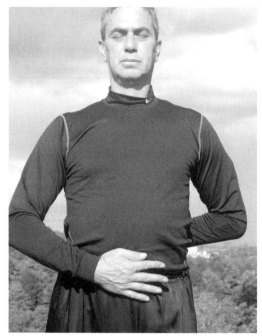

Right palm on the abdominal muscles.

Fourth Step: Moving in a wave is the next step. Again, use your hands to help at first, and then slowly start moving the abdominal and the back muscles in a wave verses just in and out. Yes, you are learning some belly dancing at this point. Try making your wave cover the entire space from the solar plexus to the pubic bone in the front and the smaller wave from the tailbone to the lower ribs area in the back. The front wave will be much bigger than the back wave. Make sure that you start and end both sides at the same time as well as performing them evenly and gently. Over time, your wave will be large yet quiet and gentle and you may experience a certain transparency.

Side Step: This step is what I call hardcore empty full moon. Either with or without your hands on the front and back muscles, for two to four minutes perform, at a fast pace, the empty full moon. Do the Buddhist breathing first for two to four minutes, and then do two to four minutes of the Taoist.

Fifth and Final Step: Very slowly, try to emulate the various stages of the moon; there are thirty. Move the abdominal and the back muscles out on the inhalation. Move them slowly and try creating, at first, five or ten stages of the various positions of the moon. This final step is all about muscle control. Do the same with the Taoist breathing. Your goal is to move the back and the front muscles so slowly that you can count 30 different stages between empty moon and full moon. The stages will be physically very small.

There are two standing exercises that help when practicing the empty to full moon, as well as when practicing residing the mind in the center of gravity energy center:

Exercise #1: Stand with your knees slightly bent, feet shoulder-width apart. Place your palms, one on top of each other, two inches below the navel. Use Taoist breathing and imagine drawing energy up from the center of the earth. Lead the energy up into the two gates in the soles of the feet, up through the center of your legs, and into your center of gravity energy center. Exhale, allowing the mind and this energy to expand from the point in your energy center outward into your internal organs (Figure 40).

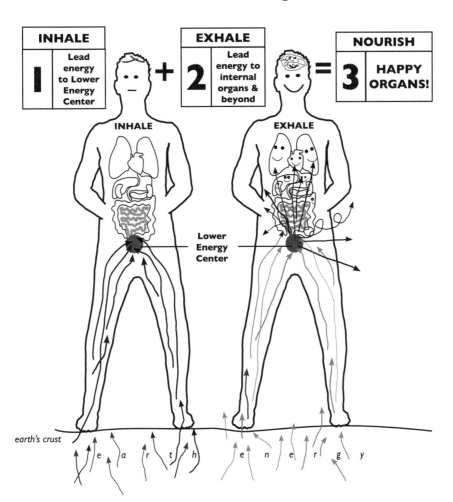

Figure 40. Inhale—Empty Moon. Exhale—Full Moon.

I like to call this mind/body prescription 'happy organs' because you are nourishing the organs with the energy you are bringing and leading from the earth into the internal organs, and at the same time massaging the internal organs from the outside, using the movements of the trunk muscles. This exercise also enhances the blood and oxygen circulation in the organs.

Exercise #2: Stand with a partner. Partner A places the center of one of his or her palms on the front of Partner B, two inches below the belly button, and the other palm on Partner B's lower back muscles, near the kidneys (or mingmen cavity in acupuncture).

As Partner A inhales, Partner B exhales and vice versa. One exhales as the other partner inhales. Both partners focus their attention on Partner B's center of gravity energy center. At the same time, both partners imagine they are circulating energy through the four gates of the body, both palms and both feet.

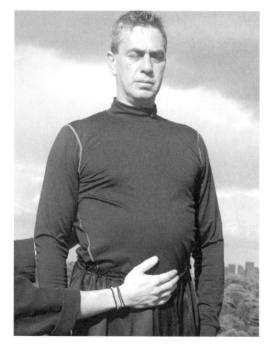

Partner A places his or her palm in front of Partner B's center of gravity energy center.

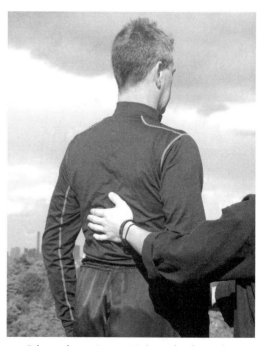

Other palm on Partner B's lower back muscles.

THREE FORCES

Close your eyes and breathe deeply. Observe the breath moving in and out of your lungs. Fill the lungs to 80%, and as you exhale, use your mind to relax the entire body. Maintain correct alignment. Notice the sensation of your entire body, and your energy centers. Use your mind to expand your sensation outward from your body, down into the earth, and upward into the heavens. Maintain your awareness of the three forces: heaven, human, and earth.

If this visualization is too challenging, start with maintaining awareness of one force at a time. Once you have a strong and clear sensation of one force, such as your entire body, you may then add the other forces. Sensing the three forces can evoke a deeply spiritual sensation and allow you to experience being one with the universe.

Three forces refer to the heaven, human, and earth forces. Those are the three forces that we are seeking to sense while we do all of our training. It is very easy to be stuck or pulled by thoughts that distract us from having a stronger sense of ourselves as well as the forces around us. We must keep trying to integrate into every mind/body pre-scription all five building blocks of our being as well as harmonizing them with the three forces: heaven, human and earth (Figure 41).

For example, if you are in a specific standing meditation physical posture, add the breathing to this posture, and then integrate the mind. The mind can then focus on the energetic system. Lastly, you need to evoke your spirituality. One of the ways of evoking spirituality is putting your mind in the three forces.

It is easy to put your mind in your energetic system. For example, when you visualize the internal baton, you can expand the mind up to the heaven and down deep into the earth. This energetic sensation of the baton will help the mind to move right into the other two forces around us. Over time, you will notice the different sensations that are associated with the different forces—the yin energy from the earth, the yang energy from the heaven, and your own human energy that combines them both.

I strongly recommend practicing each force separately over the training sessions. You can focus sometimes on bringing your mind deep into the earth and experiencing human and earth energy, then sending your mind up to the heavens and experiencing human and heaven energy, and then eventually putting the three together.

When doing tai chi or even when walking, we shift our weight from the heels to the balls of the feet, back and forward, rolling or shifting. You may experience the two different energies when the weight is distributed on the different parts of the sole of the foot. When shifting your weight to the ball of the foot, you allow the earth energy to rise up through the back. Over time, you will have a stronger sensation of this feeling or experience that will help you to identify the characteristics of earth energy. When shifting the weight to the heels, you allow energy from the heavens to drop through the

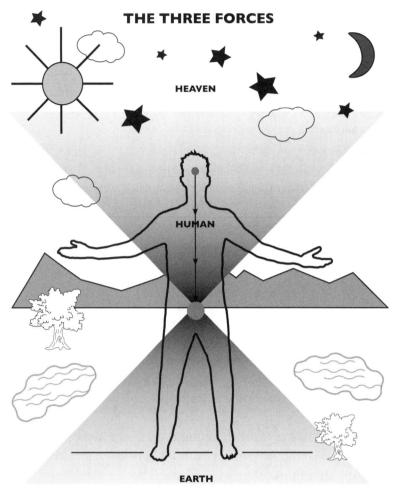

Figure 41. Heaven, Human, and Earth.

front. The sensation of the energy coming up from the earth through the back is a little more noticeable than the sensation of the energy dropping through the front. That may be different for some individuals.

The three forces also represent the three different layers of qigong. We have qigong masters who specialize in human qigong, qigong masters who specialize in earth qigong, and experts who specialize in universe qigong. Each one has its own mastery and its own masters. Sometimes, but not often, you will stumble onto a master who understands and trains two or all three of the qigong layers.

POINT TO HEAVEN

Point to heaven is the name of this mind/body prescription because you first point to the heavens with your index fingers when performing the stretch while also leading your mind up to the heavens. At the same time, you balance the movement with moving the mind deep into the earth. After doing this part with your mind, energy follows. Another trick to strengthen the spine energy is to sense the sensation of the straight index fingers and emit that sensation through your spine.

Keep your feet parallel and the weight distributed evenly between the ball of your foot and your heel, or sit on the edge of a chair.

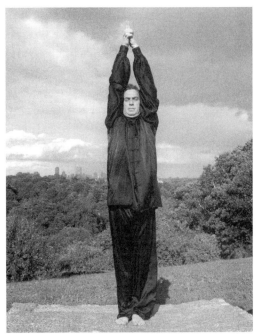

Interlock your fingers and lift arms toward heaven (standing).

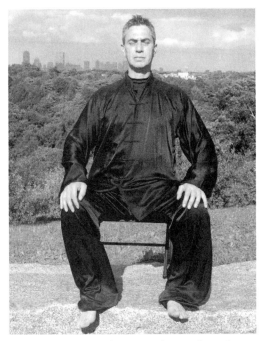

Neutral position for point to heaven (sitting).

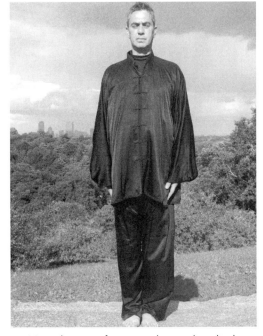

Neutral position for point to heaven (standing).

Maintain correct alignment: tailbone dropped, head suspended, face and shoulders relaxed, and a slight bend in your knees. Interlock your fingers and lift the arms over your head toward heaven, while relaxing the inner shoulders downward. Straighten your arms without locking your elbows. Tuck the tailbone in slightly. Bend the knees a little bit so there is some slack in the hamstrings, and you are able to more easily tuck the tailbone. Keep your feet flat and rooted while you turn and stretch. Do not collapse the inner arches of your feet. Breathing deeply can enhance the stretch from within the torso. Remember to emphasize lengthening upward through the spine as much as turning.

When you stretch up, around, or laterally, remember to keep breathing deeply and peacefully. Keep the sensation of a gentle smile on your face and in your body.

There is a heavy feeling through the legs from the belly button down and there is a light feeling through the spine that continues into the arms and up through the index fingers. Touch the tongue to the roof of the mouth. Inhale and exhale through the nose.

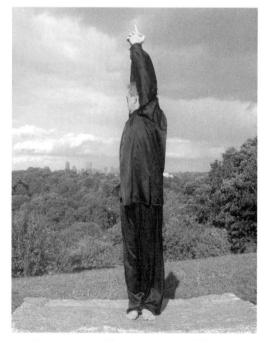

Turning right and lengthening upward through the spine as much as turning (standing).

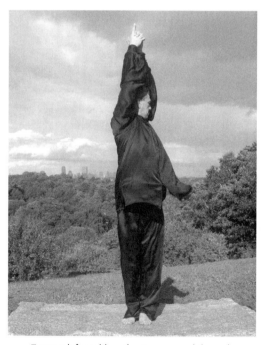

Turning left and lengthening upward through the spine as much as turning (standing).

Inhale and lengthen from the floor up. On your next exhalation, rotate to your right—do not lose the connection to the ground at the soles of the feet. Keep the inner arches alive; do not collapse the soles of the feet.

On your next inhalation, come back to the center and lengthen through the spine, and on the next exhalation, rotate to the left. Inhale and come back to the center. Every time you inhale, also lengthen through the arms, through the spine, and push down through the feet into the ground. On the exhalation, rotate while maintaining the lifting energy or force throughout the spine and arms and the sinking force through the legs. Inhale and come to the center, and rotate to the left. Do this breathing two times to each side: inhale, lengthen; exhale, and rotate.

Be aware that when you are standing straight with your index fingers pointing to heaven, you are not throwing the front ribs forward and collapsing or closing the ribs in the back. There's a tendency, in order to get the fingers straight over your head, to open the front ribs while collapsing the back ones. Don't do it.

Look for an equal feeling or sensation through the ribs, front and back. The movement of the palms and fingers moving over the head happens from the shoulder rotator cuffs, not from the ribs.

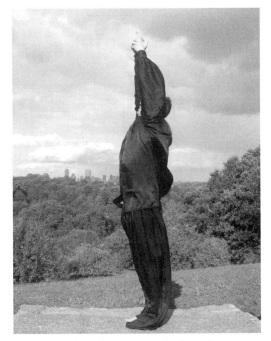

Don't do this. Opening the front ribs and collapsing the back one.

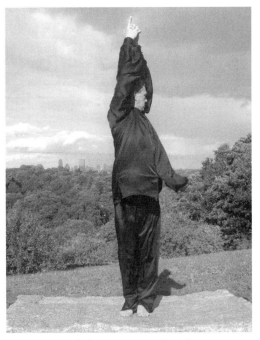

Exhalation. Rotate to the left.

RAINBOW OR HALF-MOON STRETCH

Hold your arms straight up, separate the grasp of your fingers, and grab the left wrist and gently lean to the right side. Then do the same on the other side. When you are bending to the left and right, you look like a rainbow or half moon. Do not just look like one, but actually be one, both with your mind as well as your spirit.

Inhale and lengthen through the core of your body. Exhale and bend sideways to your right like a half-moon or a rainbow.

Inhale, and come to the center. Grab the right arm with the left hand, lengthen and exhale, and bend. Bend but do not break the alignment.

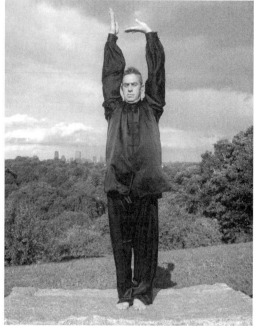

Left palm facing up.

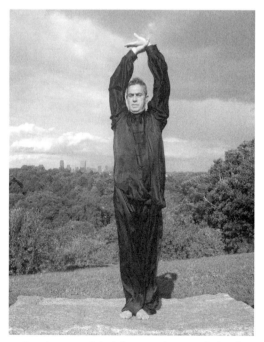

Grip the wrist of the left arm with your right hand.

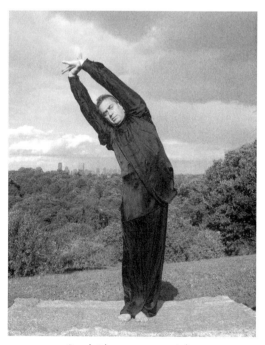

Bend sideways to your right.

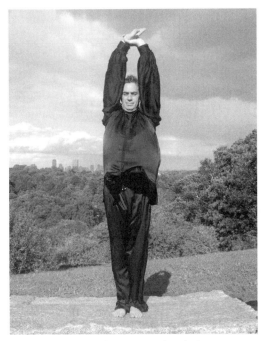

Come to the center and grab the
right arm with the left hand.

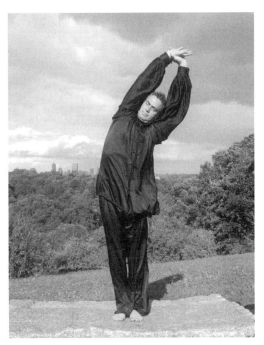

Bend but do not break the alignment.

There is one area around the ribs where you can bend too much, and this bending will break the alignment between the lumbar and the thoracic area. One way to test this alignment is to see if you can maintain a springy feeling between the pinky of the right hand, if you are bending to your left, and the small toe of your right leg.

If you imitate the picture that shows no alignment, you can see why you cannot spring sideways. If you imitate the one with correct alignment, you can see that you can spring sideways without leaning.

Move two times in each direction and then come to the center, grasp the fingers again, and point to heaven with your index fingers. Relax the face, the shoulders, and abdominal muscles, tuck the pelvis in, and sense the sensation from the soles of the feet to the top of the index fingers. Try to relax the whole body and breathe deeply, peacefully. When you are done, separate your fingers, put the palms together and slowly move both palms down the centerline all the way back to the solar plexus. Close your eyes and take three deep inhalations and exhalations. Use the sigh sound to help the muscles relax.

Sometimes you may find that holding the arms up and pointing the fingers to the heavens two times to each side is too difficult. You may feel sore in the shoulders, the neck, the rib area, lower back, or upper back. You will feel or sense tension in any of the soft tissues, which are short, and that may prevent you from maintaining

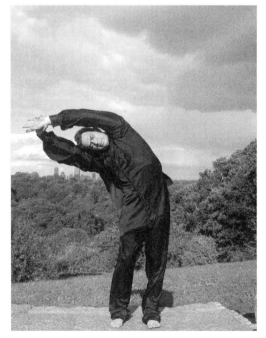

No alignment; you cannot spring sideways.

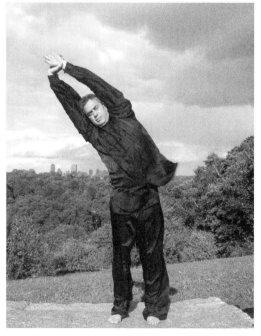

Correct alignment; you can spring sideways.

the posture for a minute or two. To alleviate some of the tension, hold the position of pointing to heaven, and then go by the wall or a tree and lean the forearms or the wrists against the wall or the tree. That will take some of the work off the soft tissue that holds up the arm and still will allow the stretching as well as the strengthening of the soft tissue. This posture is more passive, and it will get the shoulders ready and the ribs open while allowing you to hold the posture longer. Keep breathing deeply while you are at the wall or the tree, and try to integrate the other skills. Later, you will need to combine them with the rotation and the bending from side to side, the empty-full moon, visualization of the two energy centers, the baton, draining the baton down, as well as the bubble.

Throughout the rotation when pointing to heaven, you are massaging your organs. When turning to the right and left, you are massaging the liver and the spleen, the intestines, and the stomach. Sometimes it is advisable to hold the turn and inhale-exhale a few times so you get a good twist through the trunk, and the organs are held in a certain position and the muscles are tightened. The blood and oxygen is flowing but slowing at certain places because of the tension in the muscles. The tension is acting like a dam. When you release the turn by returning to the center, you release the dam. All that blood and oxygen rushes to areas in the body where circulation was weak and slow, and you bring flow, which leads to life. The flow will reach and nourish the entire body from the skin all the way to the bones.

There are two ways to do the exercise: rotate with each inhalation and return to center on the next exhalation. The other way is to inhale, move into the rotation, and then stay in the rotated posture and exhale and inhale a few times before returning back to the center.

When pulling on one of the arms and doing the rainbow or half-moon stretch, you will notice that maybe when you pull to the right your left lung is much more open. Try to get both lungs to open. You do not want to collapse the right lung just because you are bending toward the right. Lengthen through the right lung and ribs even though you are bending to the right. That means that you are not collapsing the right lung and ribs, but instead you are bending as well as lengthening. One trick is to lengthen through the hand that is pulling. If you are pulling with the right, the left lung is easy to lengthen because the right is pulling.

When you breathe deeply through the half-moon posture, you will find that you can lead more air into the left lung when bending to the right and more air into the right lung when bending to the left. The experience is a part of the seesaw breathing but instead of going from one lung to the other, you keep inhaling a few times into one of the lungs, while holding the stretch, and then you switch to the other. When you inhale into the lungs, when you are doing the rainbow or half-moon stretch, try to lead air to the bottom front as well as the back parts of the lungs.

BOW BREATHING

In this exercise, emphasize the stretching and releasing of the two major bows in our body: the chest, or cross bow, and the spine, or long bow (Figure 42).

Inhale and stretch the bows, slightly rounding the upper back, tucking in the tailbone, and drawing in the chest. Keep your knees bent throughout this exercise. Exhale and release the bows. For health purposes, you may also stretch the bows with the exhalation while releasing them with the inhalation. Remember to coordinate your breath with the movement and perform sitting as well as standing.

The body has six major bows and also has many minor bows. The six major bows are the two legs, the two arms, the spine, and the chest area.

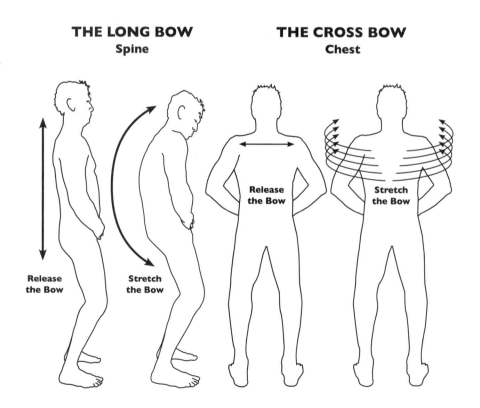

THE LONG BOW
Spine

THE CROSS BOW
Chest

Release
the Bow

Stretch
the Bow

Release
the Bow

Stretch
the Bow

Figure 42. Stretch and release the bow can be
done either on inhalation or exhalation.

We are going to focus on the spine (long bow) and the chest area (cross bow). You need to learn how to isolate these two bows and learn to create movement in them. This movement is called 'stretch the bows' and 'release the bows.'

First, isolate the bows. Sit on the edge of the chair, close your eyes, sense the sitting bones on the chair, lengthen the spine, and be aware of the shoulders as well as your chest area.

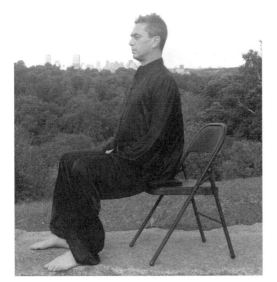

Bow breathing; release the bows (sitting).

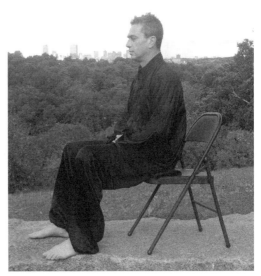

Bow breathing; stretch the bows (sitting).

By moving the tailbone and the head inward, you are stretching the long bow and when rounding the shoulders inward, you are stretching the crossbow. This position is also called turtle back. When you straighten up and bring the top of your head, the tailbone, and shoulders back to the original position, you are releasing both bows.

Once more, stretch the bow (this time standing): the spine curves, the shoulders round toward the front. Next, release the bow: lengthen the spine and send the shoulders backward until your body is aligned.

You can isolate only one bow at a time. Practice the spine bow without the chest bow, and then practice only the chest bow without the spine bow. You will notice that when you isolate the bows, you do not get as much movement as you would if you used both bows together. Both bows create a slack that helps each bow to get more movement.

Two Bad Habits: First, there is a tendency to round the shoulders too far forward. This tendency is much easier to fix then the second bad habit, which is the tendency, when stretching the bow, to move only the upper part of the spine from the solar plexus to the top of the head more than the bottom part of the bow, from the solar plexus to the tailbone.

It is very important to make sure that you get an even stretch or movement throughout the bows. The sternum or the solar plexus can be considered as the middle of both the long bow and the cross bow, which means that this area should be the peak of the curve inward. The solar plexus is the peak because that is the middle of the bows and if you were to tie a string between the forehead and the area between the anus and the groin area, and pull the string away from the body, that will be like stretching the long bow; and if you release that string that will be like releasing the long bow. If you stretch a string between the shoulders and stretch it away from the body that will be like stretching the cross bow and when releasing it will be like releasing the cross bow. Pull the string, stretch the bows, and release the string, release the bows.

When sitting on the chair, moving the sacrum will not be as easy, but this sitting version of the exercise will give you a taste or sense of the long bow, and then when you stand up you will find that it is much easier to tilt the sacrum area and to coordinate that with the top of the head and the shoulders, the cross bow, in order to create the posture. Sitting may make it more difficult to stretch the bows, but it is a good way to isolate the bows and experience them. Once standing, moving the whole pelvis and the tailbone will become much easier.

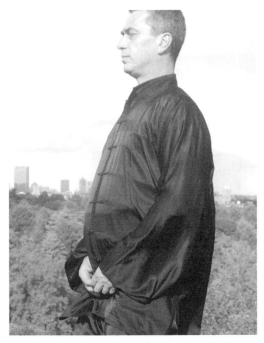

Bow breathing; release the bows (standing).

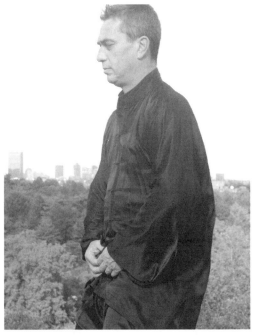

Bow breathing; stretch the bows (standing).

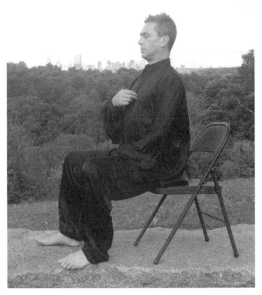

Release the bows. Pretend you are
pulling the string (sitting).

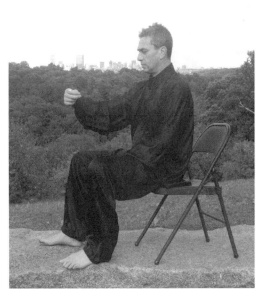

Stretch the bows. Pretend you are
pulling the string (sitting).

Once you understand the movement of the bows while sitting, stand up and practice moving the bows: first without using the arms, and then using the arms to pretend pulling the string that is attached from the third eye to your huiyin cavity.

This exercise is the long bow. Next, pretend you are pulling the string that connects from one shoulder to the other: the cross bow.

Slightly bend your knees and then stretch the bows. Tilt the pelvis in, the tailbone down and in, and allow the thoracic spine and head to move forward, and remember do not move the upper part of the spine too far. You should feel that there is a connection throughout the spine and you did not break the alignment or this connection.

Then release the bow and stretch the bow. Keep stretching and releasing the bow for approximately 15 times. When you stretch the bow, inhale, and when you release the bow, exhale. After 15 repetitions, change: when you stretch the bow, exhale, and when you release the bow, inhale.

Eventually, while working with the bows, you want to try to integrate the other skills you have learned: empty full moon, deep breathing, the sigh sound, as well as lingering at the end of the exhalation. When stretching the bow you can do Taoist breathing for a few minutes and then practice the Buddhist breathing while stretching the bow for a few minutes. Change between the two styles of breathing with the two different stages of the bows.

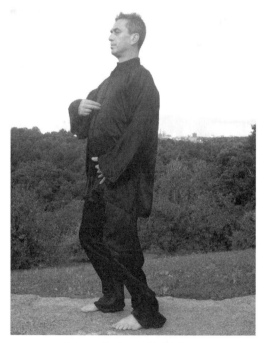

Release the bows. Pretend you are pulling the string (standing).

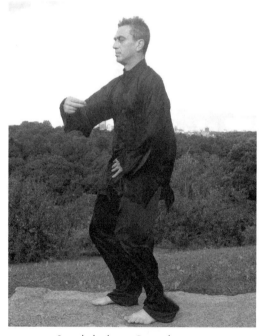

Stretch the bows. Pretend you are pulling the string (standing).

Warrior Spirit: Xena or Hercules Stretches the Spring

I chose the name Xena warrior princess or Hercules because I want you, when doing this mind/body prescription, to really have a spirit of a warrior. It is easy to just do the body, breath, mind, and energy and to forget the warrior spirit. If the name Hercules or Xena is in your mind when performing this exercise, the warrior spirit will also awaken as well. Once you feel comfortable isolating the two bows and creating an even stretch without breaking the alignment, then you want to add the other two bows—the arms—to the exercise. Hold your palms at about your eyebrow height, elbows pointing 45 degrees to the side. When your hands are by your eyes, that is when you stretch the bows.

You then release the bows and open the arms as if you are stretching a big rubber band or a spring right in front of your nose. On stretching the bow, as the hands come closer to the center toward your nose, inhale deeply. The bows are stretched, and the moon is empty. Then exhale, release the bows, release the moon, and open the arms sideways.

Once again stretch the bows. Inhale through the nose. The tongue should be touching the roof of the mouth. As you exhale, release the bows, release the moon, and open your arms to the sides. This exercise will give you an opportunity to coordinate the movements of the bows with the arms and see how the bows eventually are used in the tai chi form or in any of the qigong mind/body prescription exercises.

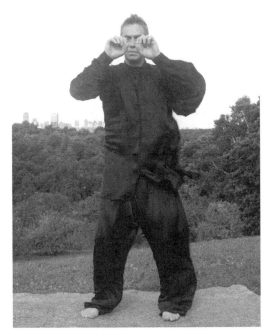

Xena stretches the spring. Stretch the
bows and close the arms (standing).

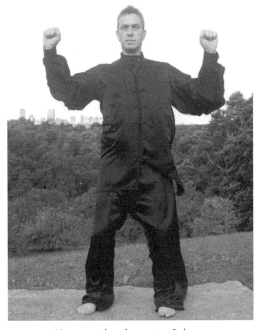

Xena stretches the spring. Release
the bows and open the arms (standing).

When Xena or Hercules stretch the spring, the elbows do not go beyond the line of the shoulders—they are actually a little bit in front.

If they had gone a little farther, they would have to break the alignment through the upper body and through the shoulder girdle.

Maintain this alignment. Open the elbows but do not push them backward farther than the front of the trunk. If you look from the side, the elbows actually will still be in front of the chest about an inch or two.

When you stretch the bow, you are in the turtle-back posture and the hands and fists are by your nose or eyes. You should sense a light stretched feeling in the skin and in the muscles in the shoulder blade area in the back.

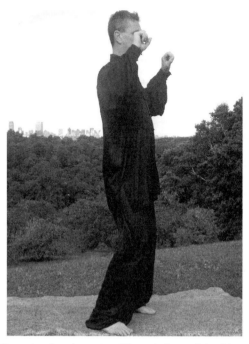

Xena stretches the spring. Elbows in front of shoulders.

When you release the spring, you should sense a gentle stretch through the chest or the shoulder area in the front. Your hands and fists are at shoulder height as well as slightly wider than the shoulder blades. The reason that the fists and the arms drop from the eye to the shoulders is not that the arms drop, as much as it is that the top of the head rises up.

Once you understand the movement of the bows, the long bow and cross bow, with simple movements like Xena or Hercules stretches the spring, then you want to try another movement that integrates stretching the bow as well as twisting the waist.

PUSH THE TABLETS

Next, we will learn the exercise 'push the tablets.' Have the right and left hands, palms up, in a 'reading the book' posture.

Imagine that there are two tablets, one in front of you touching your front left fingers and one behind you touching your back right elbow. You are now in the stretch the bows posture. We are going to push the tablets open on the next exhalation.

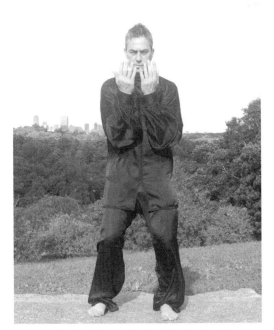

Push the tablets in the 'reading the book' posture (standing).

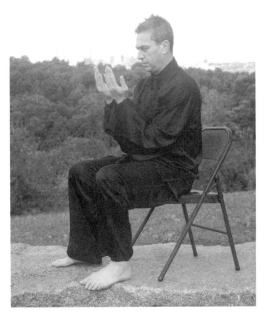

Push the tablets in the 'reading the book' posture (sitting).

The left palm is going to be the palm that pushes the front tablet and the right elbow will be the one that pushes the back tablet.

On your next exhalation, release the bows, rotate and push forward with the left wrist so the palm lies flat on the imaginary tablet, while at the same time, with your right elbow, push the imaginary tablet behind you. Push the two tablets away from your body.

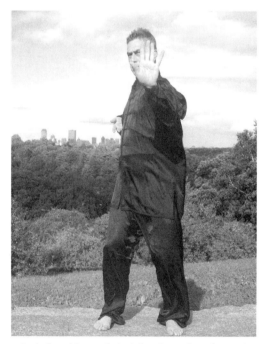

Push the tablets with the left palm pushing forward and the right elbow pushing back (standing).

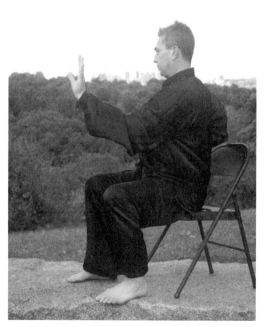

Push the tablets with the left palm pushing forward and the right elbow pushing back (sitting).

The left elbow is slightly bent when finishing the push the tablet movement, the same as you will do in any tai chi form. The right elbow that pushes back does not move to the right. It moves backward, in a straight line, in order not to break the alignment in the right shoulder.

Then inhale and come back to the original posture. The right palm moves through the waist. On your next exhalation, release the bows and push the tablets again, but this

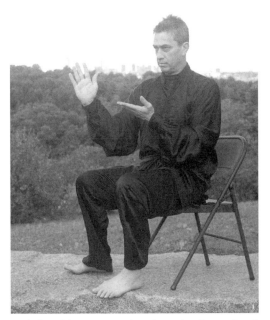

Push the tablets. Store, right palm pushes forward and left elbow pushes back (sitting).

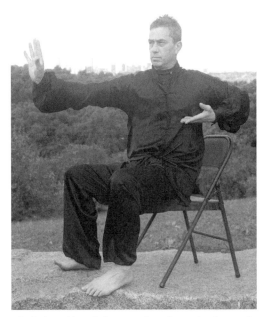

Push the tablets. Release, right palm pushes forward and left elbow pushes back (sitting).

time push the tablet in front of you with the right palm while pushing the back one with your left elbow. Move the right arm forward, while rotating the wrist so the right palm will lay flat on your imaginary tablet, while bringing the left palm through the ribs area so you can push the imaginary tablet, behind you, with your elbow.

Try to keep the knees bent throughout both exercises. Try to keep the same height. Do not bob up and down and just use the bows purely without using the leg bows. If you look in the mirror, you will see the head going up and down because when you stretch the bow you slightly shrink and when you release the bow you lengthen the spine and you slightly grow.

When performing pushing the tablets, there is a tendency, because of the turning of the waist, to collapse the inner arches of the soles of the feet. Try to maintain the area the Chinese call the kua, which is the space between the legs. The kua refers to the strong dome-like foundation of the legs and hips. Keeping the kua alive means keeping

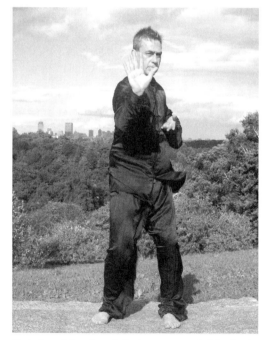

Push the tablets. Stretch the bow so you slightly shrink.

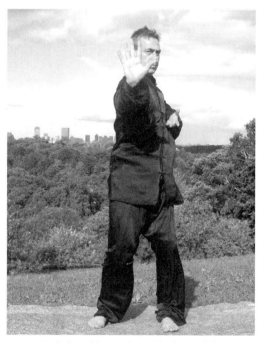

Push the tablets. Release the bow while lengthening the spine so you slightly grow.

alignment throughout the legs while performing the twisting of the waist and the stretching of the bows. When doing push the tablets, it is a little more challenging to maintain alignment throughout the legs, such as keeping the knees above the toes while the upper body turns side to side

Once you feel comfortable with the physical movement, try to add the internal visualization. When inhaling, stretch the bows and go to empty moon, focus your mind and condense it in the lower energy center, and at the same time the energy moves up to the shoulder blade area.

On an exhalation, you release the bows, and the energy from the shoulder blade area will be led into the outside of the palms into your imaginary tablets, while energy from the lower energy center or center of gravity energy center will shoot down into the earth, which is called four gates breathing.

At the same time, the energy from the bubble around your body, on an inhalation, while stretching the bows, and on empty moon, moves in toward the energetic baton, and then on an exhalation it moves out toward the bubble.

The third eye energy center, on inhalation, condenses and focuses, and on exhalation manifests or projects through the eyes. This energy is called fiery eyes. Integrating the internal visualization of the energetic system with the physical movement is essential and makes the internal arts into real internal work. It is the simple difference that changes tai chi from an external physical dance to an internal art.

Of course, this internal visualization should be trained slowly over time. Be easy on yourself, train when you feel comfortable, keep pulling yourself back to the basics, and over time you will be able to perform all the skills at the same time. The mind will be like the conductor that monitors the different skills of the different musicians.

BELT ENERGY VESSEL BREATHING

Stand in horse stance, close your eyes, and breathe deeply. Notice or sense the breath moving in and out of your lungs. Fill the lungs to 80%, and as you exhale, use your mind to relax the entire body. Maintain correct alignment, and sense the earth beneath you, and your energy centers within. Place the center of your left palm two inches below the navel on your lower energy center, while placing the back of your right palm a few inches below your kidneys.

Start circling your pelvis clockwise while visualizing a straight imaginary energy line between the two centers of the palms. It is very important to keep the knees as well as the soles of your feet aligned, and avoid collapsing them because of the pelvis circling. Also, circle in the opposite direction for the same length of time. As you rotate your pelvis, try not to move the knees or feet from their alignment. Practice in both directions. Keeping your waist loose and flexible is of utmost importance for your health.

This exercise also strengthens the energy circulation in your belt energy vessel, which some people refer to as a channel, around your waist (Figure 43). Once you feel comfortable with the lower energy center visualization, you can keep that visualization while at the same time visualizing the movement at the belt energy vessel. When circling clockwise, move your mind from the right to the back and around to the front. When

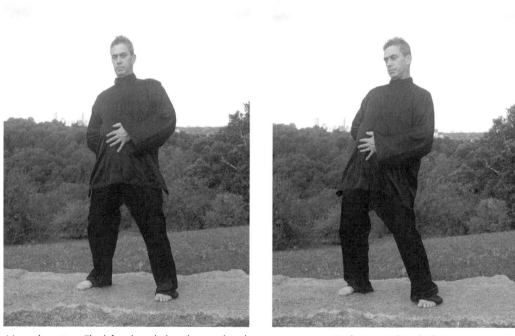

Neutral position. The left palm is below the navel and the back of right palm is below your kidneys.

Circle your pelvis clockwise.

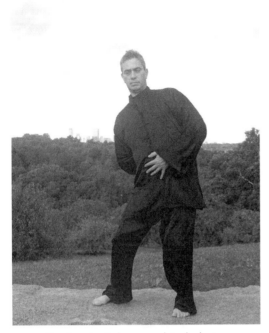

Continue to circle your pelvis clockwise.

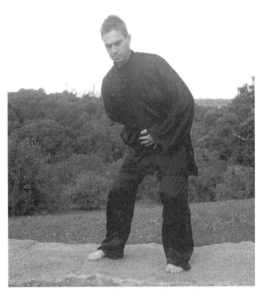

Continue to circle your pelvis clockwise.

circling counterclockwise, move the energy from the left to the back and circle to the front. Move the energy in the direction you are moving your pelvis. *Remember to maintain the visualization of your center of gravity energy center.* When you are comfortable with both visualizations and the smooth circulated movement of the pelvis, integrate some of the other skills. For example, physically add empty-full moon and deep breathing, and mentally integrate ones such as drain the baton and build the bubble.

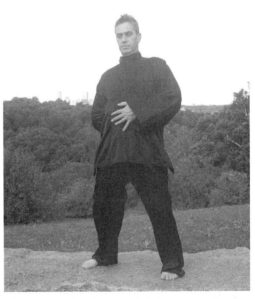

Neutral position. Left palm is below the navel, and back of right palm is below your kidneys.

BELT VESSEL

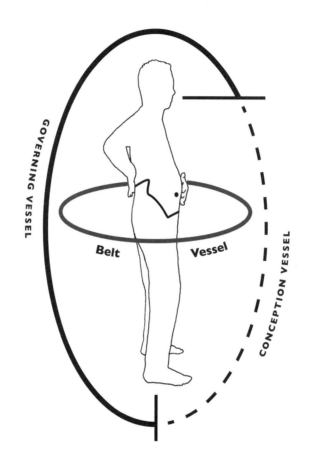

Figure 43.   The only horizontal vessel out of eight extraordinary vessels.

When you change the circle from right to left, you can also reverse the position of the hands. Switch the palms around. Put the left one in front, two inches below the navel, and the right one in the back. Many of my students, when performing this circling motion with the pelvis, feel uncomfortable with this sexual movement. To break the ice, I tell my students I am preparing you to do belly dancing or the samba. It takes time to open up the pelvis because of the tight soft tissue in various areas of the pelvis. We do not often stretch the muscles and ligaments around the groin, pelvis, outer groin, inner groin, hips, outer hip, and lower back. Circling the pelvis area and standing in a firm horse stance will also affect the pelvis floor as well as the leg muscles: quads, hamstrings, abductors, and adaptors. Over time, once you open the soft tissue, you will find that you can make the circles bigger and bigger as you move lower and lower.

Belt Energy Vessel Breathing with Hands

Hold your arms out with the palms down at belly button height, your elbows one fist away from the hips. Circle your arms and hands smoothly as if you were polishing a table. Coordinate the movement with your breath in an even rhythm. Practice both large and small circles. Try to feel the movement originating from your waist and lower energy center. Circle in the opposite direction for the same length of time.

Feel the connection of the entire body, from the feet to the fingertips. Work toward standing in a lower horse stance, while keeping your knees aligned and making larger circles with your hands. Repeating this exercise will help you to have a strong internal sensation when you perform the grind movement in the Sunset Tai Chi form.

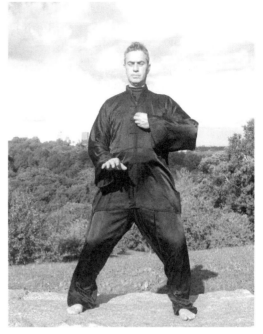

Neutral position. Arm out, palms at belly button height, elbows are a fist away from hips.

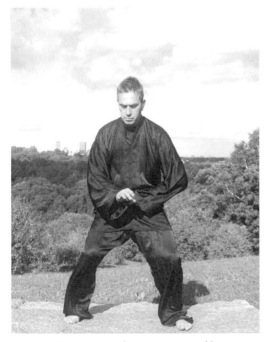

Continue to circle your arm smoothly as if polishing a table.

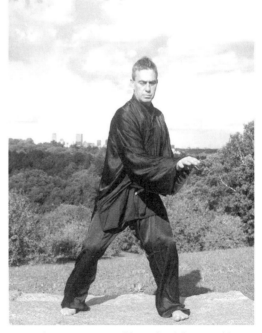

Circle your arm smoothly as if polishing a table.

Once you feel comfortable with the pelvic circle when your palms are on the center of the body, then you want to put both hands out in front of you and you want to allow the palms and hands to follow the pelvic circle. Make sure you maintain the alignment in the legs (kua). If you break the alignment of the kua, this energy flow becomes only an external physical exercise with no energy flow in it because for the energy to flow smoothly, strong alignment is the key point.

In order for the pelvic circles to become both external and internal, you must maintain alignment throughout the legs as well as in the spine. While performing the pelvic circles, you must still maintain correct alignment. Keep the head suspended and the alignment in the legs. When performing the circles with alignment through the legs and the spine, you will line up the heavenly gate with the huiyin cavity (the area between the groin and the anus), as well as activating the bubbling wells at the soles of the feet that will line up with the earth. When maintaining this alignment, you allow the energy to keep exchanging and moving between the three forces: heaven, human, and earth. Use a chair or a yoga block to achieve this skill of maintaining alignments through the soles of the feet, knees, and groin as well as keeping the kua alive.

Keep the wrist and the fingers relaxed, do not lock the elbows all the way. The elbows always stay slightly bent. This circling action of the hands is called in Chinese, "moo." Moo means grinding, as in grinding the rice. In order to evoke spirituality,

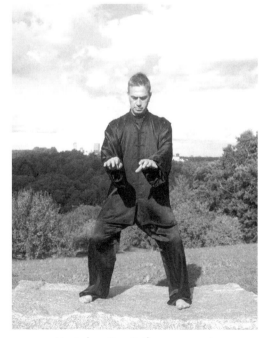

Neutral position. Both arms are out.
Strong alignment is key point.

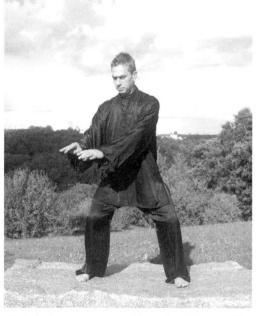

Circle both your arms smoothly as if polishing a table.

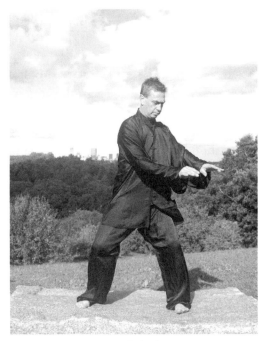

Continue to circle both your arms
smoothly as if polishing a table.

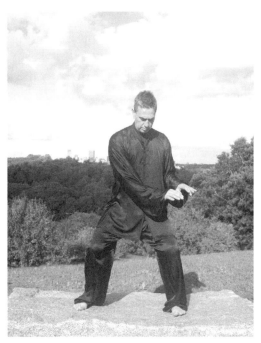

Continue to circle both your arms
smoothly as if polishing a table.

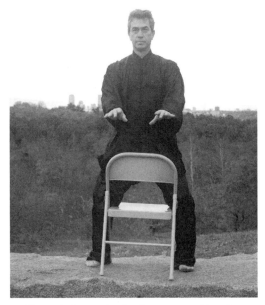

Use a chair to maintain alignments and keeping
the kua alive, especially when turning.

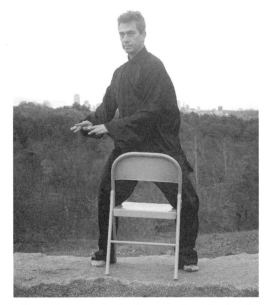

Use a chair to maintain alignments through soles of
the feet, knees, and keeping the kua alive.

pretend you are holding a stone grinder over a stone. You are moving the grinder along the edge of the stone and you are leading the grinding tool with the waist while keeping the legs aligned. The waist is the wheel that directs the motions of the arm. The power is generated from the floor through the legs into the waist, which directs the arms and the palms. It says in the *Tai Chi Classics*: "Power is generated from the legs, directed by the waist, manifested at the fingers."

Once you finish circling to one side, about 20-30 times, then change and circle to the other direction. The palm faces down, and the shoulders should be relaxed. Again, notice your trunk. The muscles tense and relax along the circle you are performing. When the muscles tense and relax, you are massaging your internal organs as well as creating more flow throughout the energetic and blood circulatory systems. The action of tensing and relaxing the muscles acts like a water dam. When the muscles tense, they hold the blood and energy and when they relax, they release the blood and energy. This release opens up areas where the blood and energy are not circulating smoothly, and the rushing blood and energy opens new channels of energy while the blood reaches and nourishes all parts of the body including the skin.

Once you feel comfortable with using the kua, rotating the pelvis, relaxing the shoulders, keeping the head suspended, then you want to integrate the long bow and the cross bow into the bow breathing exercise. To do that, start circling with one hand while the other is touching the solar plexus area, and pretend that you are holding the strings of the two bows, the long bow and the cross bow.

When your hand is right by your solar plexus, you can pretend to stretch the imaginary strings of the two bows. Next, when circling the pelvis, divide the circle into two—the back half and the front half. When you are circling and you are in the back half, stretch the bows while pulling on the imaginary strings of both bows, and when you are in the front half, release the bows and move your right hand back toward the solar plexus.

You stretch the bows when the hands are close to you and you release the bows when the hands move farther away. Once you understand this movement, switch and stretch the bows when you are in the front of the circle and release them when you are in the back part of your pelvic circle. Do about 20 of each. Start with the hands close to you. Use small circles and as you get better, make the circle bigger and bigger. The sacrum, which is part of the bow, and the tailbone, should not stick out at all. They go from straight to tucked-in or eventually they drop. Over time, when your muscles are open and relaxed you do not need to tuck, you can just drop the sacrum. If you run your hand on the back and you do not feel the tailbone sticking out, you are aligned.

The long bow, which includes the head, spine, sacrum, and tailbone, needs to be stretched evenly. There is a tendency to move the top part of the bow much farther than the bottom, which breaks the bow and the alignment letting the energy leak because of the broken alignment.

The two ends, the tailbone and the forehead, need to stretch in such a way that one does not go farther than the other; otherwise the bow is not stretched evenly. The same with the cross bow between the shoulder blades, The cross bow bends forward in such a way that when you do it correctly and you look at the shoulder blades, you will not see them sticking out. You should have a smooth round feeling through the shoulder blades that continues through the arms to the elbows and all the way to the fingers.

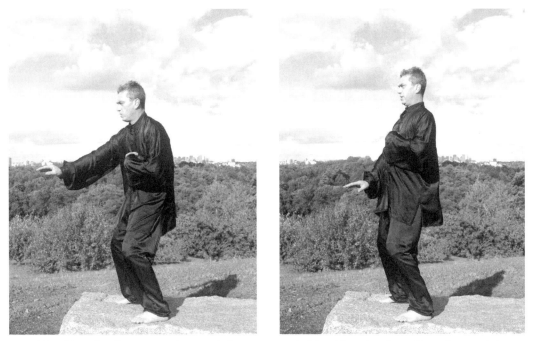

Left hand by solar plexus. Pretend to stretch the imaginary strings of the two bows, and then release the bows.

Left hand by solar plexus. Pretend to stretch the imaginary strings of the two bows, and then stretch the bows.

The two arms are another two bows and are part of the major six bows in the body. The long bow is the spine and the cross bow is the chest area. The four other bows are the legs and the arms.

Once you feel comfortable using the bows, keeping the kua alive, getting a large circle through the pelvis, then you want to add the skills of pulsing and pumping through the ligaments and through the joints.

For better understanding of bow breathing, look at the *Sunset Tai Chi* DVD in the Sunset mind/body program, after cleanse and before the sigh sound.

When your palm comes near your lower energy center, the joints are relaxed, and as you extend away from the body, you should also feel an extension through each joint. There is a pulsing, expansion, or growth locally within each joint when the arms are away from the body. When the arms are closer, a sensation of condensing, shrinking, or contracting should be felt in the joints. This pulsing or gentle pumping through the joints happens as the arms move away from the body and come toward the body. With repeated practice, maybe one day you will be able to pump and pulse the vertebrae in your spine; that is difficult.

SPINE WAVE SQUARE

The spine wave is the ability to create a wave moving through the spine all the way from the sacrum up through the top of the head, both backward as well as forward. This skill is very difficult for most people. It takes about three to four months for people to open up their muscles, tendons, and ligaments so they can perform this wave motion through the spine.

The wave starts at the pelvis and it moves up toward the thoracic spine, then continues all the way up to the shoulders, and finishes at the top of the head. Isolate the wave purely through the trunk, through the spine. Keep the knees still. Before you try to create the spine wave, first practice the square spine wave exercises that follow.

Spine Wave Square and Backward

Backward square spine waves: Stand with feet shoulder-width apart, straight knees, hands on your waist.

Push the tailbone backward. Your trunk is leaning forward. Bend to about 20 to 30 degree angle forward, knees still straight.

Then bend your knees while keeping the tailbone backward and the trunk forward.

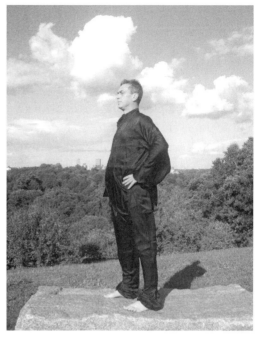

Neutral position. Stand with feet shoulder-width apart, straight knees, and hands on waist.

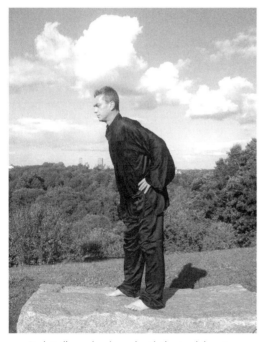

Push tailbone backward with the trunk leaning forward and knees still straight.

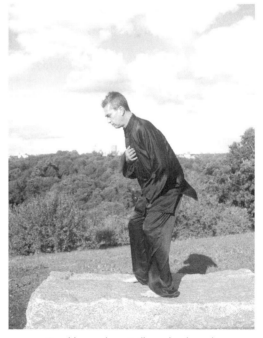

Bend knees, keep tailbone backward, and trunk forward.

Now you are going to move the pubic bone forward and the trunk backward while keeping the knees bent. Again, your trunk is leaning backward about 20 to 30 degrees while your knees are bent.

Next, straighten the knees while your pubic bone is still pushing forward and your trunk is leaning backward.

Now move the tailbone and the pubic bone backward to the original position where the tailbone is sticking out and the trunk leaning forward in a 20 to 30 degree angle. Keep the knees straight; you have just completed a full square.

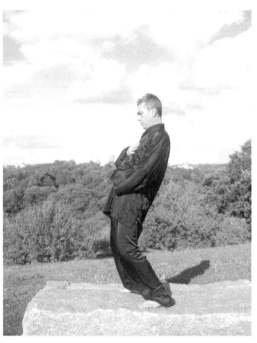

Move pubic bone forward, trunk backward, and keep knees bent.

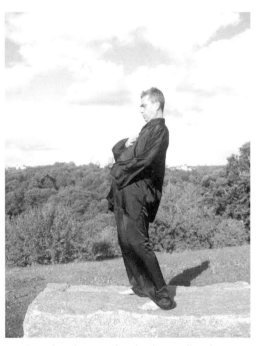

Straighten knees with pubic bone still pushing forward and trunk leaning backward.

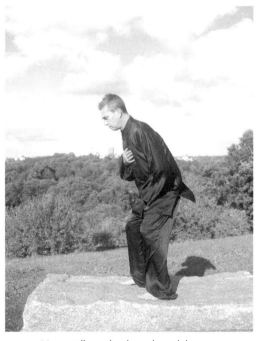

Move tailbone backward, trunk leaning forward, and keep knees straight.

Then you bend the knees. Move the tailbone and the pubic bone forward without straightening the knee. That is the difficult part of the square.

Straighten the knees while continuing to push the pubic bone forward and the trunk is leaning back. Move the tailbone back and the trunk forward, and then bend the knees. Move the pubic bone and the tailbone forward without straightening the knees. Once your pubic bone is pushing forward and your trunk is leaning back, that is when you straighten the legs. You just completed two full squares.

Once you have tried this exercise, you will find it is fairly simple. Here is a quick summary of the exercise:

1. Straight knees, tailbone back, trunk forward—20 to 30 degrees.

2. Bend the knees.

3. Pubic bone forward, trunk backward—20 to 30 degrees.

4. Straighten the knees.

In summary: Move the pelvis back and the trunk forward when the legs are straight and still, and move the pelvis forward and trunk back when the knees are bent and the trunk is still. Bend the knees when the pelvis is backward and the trunk is forward and still. Straighten the knees when the pelvis is forward and the trunk is backward and while it is still.

The up and down at the knees happens when the trunk is still, when it is either forward or backward. There is a tendency, when straightening the knee while your pelvis is forward and your trunk is back, to move the trunk instead of keeping it leaning back and still. Keep the tailbone tucked in and the trunk at a 20 degree tilt back when straightening the knees. Only after the knees are straight should you move the tailbone back and the trunk forward. Then bend your knees while the tailbone is sticking back. Over time, once you feel comfortable with the spine square backward, shave off the corners of the square and make this motion into more of a circle, or a wave.

Spine Wave Square and Forward

Once you are able to perform the spine wave square backward, performing the spine wave forward will be much easier. Start exactly the same as the backward movement—legs shoulder-width apart, straight legs, and hands on your waist.

The next step is different. Bend the knees first, and then move the tailbone forward while you move the trunk backward, about 20 to 30 degrees backward.

Then straighten the knees while maintaining the backward tilt through the trunk.

Next, move the tailbone backward while moving the trunk forward. The knees stay straight.

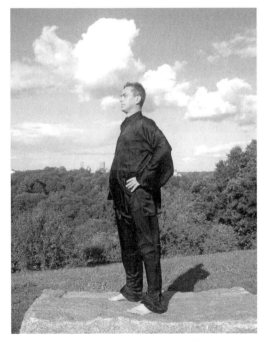

Neutral position. Legs shoulder-width apart, straight legs, and hands on your waist.

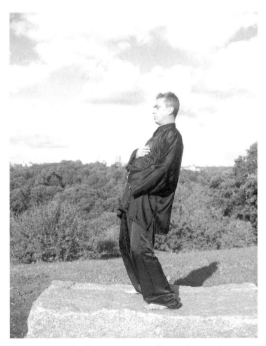

Bend the knees, move tailbone forward, and move the trunk backward.

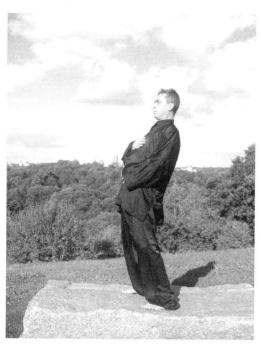

Straighten the knees, maintaining the
backward tilt through the trunk.

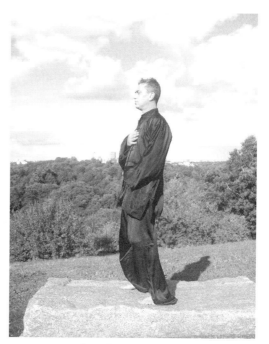

Move tailbone backward, trunk forward,
and knees stay straight.

Now, bend the knees.

You just completed a full square. Once
you can do both spine wave square backward and square forward in stages, try connecting the movement and make it move
faster while bending and straightening the
knees.

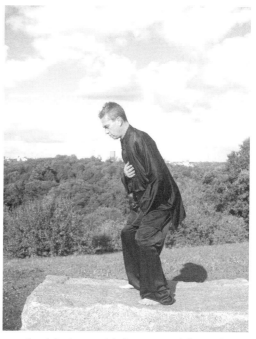

Bend the knees while keeping trunk forward.

Spine Waves Smooth and Round

From the square spine movement exercises, you will be able to round out the move-ment and make it into a circle or a wave, forward or backward. Place the fingers of your left, yin, hand an inch away or touching your solar plexus area, to cool the fire energy, while placing the fingers of the right, yang, hand an inch away or touching your center of gravity energy center to nourish that center. Do the opposite if you are left handed.

At first, you should use the knee movement of the square spine exercises to help you create the wave. Over time, try keeping the knees bent at all times. When you are ready for this step, try when manifesting the wave at the upper parts of the spine to sink into the ground through your legs. The ancient saying "When there is an up there must be a down."

Once you master waving and circling the bottom part of the pelvis and the lumbar area, then you need to move the wave higher up throughout the thoracic spine as well as the cervical spine and the head. *Remember, there is a tendency to just move the lower part of the spine, the lumbar, or just the upper part of the spine, the thoracic spine and shoulders.* For this exercise, perform the wave throughout the whole spine including the pelvis floor, the lumbar area, thoracic spine, cervical, as well as the head.

The reason for the difficulty of getting any movement in the pelvis is that this area is more dense and tight than the other higher parts. It is tighter because of the groin, hips, outer hips, and upper hips, as well as the hamstring and quads. The pelvis area is wrapped with soft tissues that prevent it from moving and creating a smooth circle or wave from the bottom all the way to the top of the head. That is the reason that many students just move the wave from the lumbar up while leaving the pelvis frozen and dead. The pelvis starts the wave, then the wave moves to the lumbar, continues to the thoracic spine and up through the cervical spine, and finishes with the head. Then, the wave moves down all the way to the huiyin cavity and back up the pelvis and spine. Many individuals do not move the wave through all these parts. Instead, some perform the wave starting from the lumbar, and oth-ers just wave from the thoracic area. The wave can be isolated in the various parts of the trunk, but make sure that you can first perform the whole wave through every part of your trunk. That is the reason it could take three to four months to open up all the soft tissue in the pelvis area and allow this circle, or wave motion, to happen smoothly.

When performing backward or forward spine waves, keep the shoulders dropped down at all times. There is a tendency to raise the shoulders when performing the wave. Allow your neck and head to be part of the wave. Close your eyes and touch the tongue to the roof of the mouth.

Divide the wave into two parts and inhale while moving through the first part and exhale when moving through the second. Once you are comfortable, add the other basic skills such as empty full moon, visualization of the energetic baton, as well as the bubble.

In the future, you will be able to visualize the small circulation while performing the forward spine waves. Touch your right hand fingers on the lower energy center and with the fingers of the left arm touch the solar plexus area. In this exercise, the purpose of the arm position is to slow the circulation to the arms because you are practicing only the small circulation. Having the arms loose by your sides will allow energy to go to the hands, which is considered working with the grand circulation.

After you have mastered the spine waves, you can drop the arms to your sides that open the path to the grand circulation. The arms will naturally follow the wave. As you move forward and up, your arms will follow and will naturally turn so the back of your hand faces forward. As the wave moves down and back, the arms will move backward, and the palms

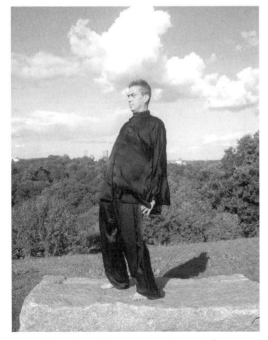

Neutral position. Arms are to your sides and legs are shoulder width apart.

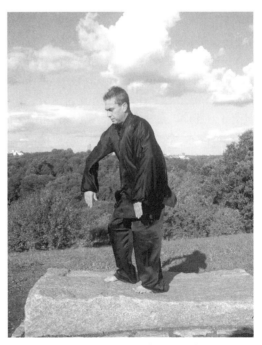

Wave moves up and forward while the back of your hands faces forward.

will face forward. Allow the arms to follow naturally, softly.

You might find that when standing on one leg, you can create more slack through the bows and experiencing the wave is a little bit easier or stronger.

Remember to add the internal skills that we teach in this book. When inhaling, perform the empty moon, and when exhaling, use the full moon. Use the lower and upper energy centers, and then drain the baton and build the bubble. Include four gates breathing and evoke spirituality.

SMALL CIRCULATION ALSO KNOWN AS THE MICROCOSMIC ORBIT

This ancient mental practice has been passed down from generation to generation for thousands of years. Leading the energy through the governing and conception vessels has many benefits on both physical and

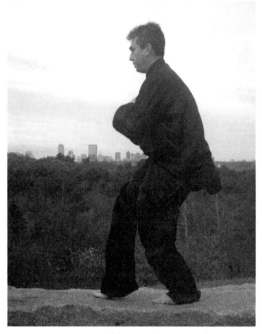

Spine waves while standing on one leg.

mental levels. Take your time, be patient, and yet persist. Eventually you will reach, experience, and explore many insights into your life as well as others.

Circulate your mind along the small circulation path. Start from the lower energy center and move down through the huiyin cavity, up through the back, between the spine and the skin, all the way around the middle of the skull, down through the front of the face, the trunk, and back through the huiyin cavity to your center of gravity energy center.

When inhaling, move your mind from the lower energy center to the huiyin cavity, up along the governing vessel, all the way to your upper lip, and when exhaling, your mind moves from the upper lip, down back into the huiyin cavity, and into the lower energy center. There are three paths that are very popular in qigong when talking about the small circulation: the fire, water, and wind paths. In this book, we focus only on the fire path: moving your mind up the governing vessel and down the conception vessel (Figure 44).

The ancient practice of improving the quality of the small circulation has existed for at least 3,000 years and has been used by Buddhists and Taoists. It is also known as the microcosmic orbit and acupuncturists refer to it as the small heavenly circuit rotation.

CIRCULATE YOUR MIND
ALONG THE SMALL CIRCULATION PATH

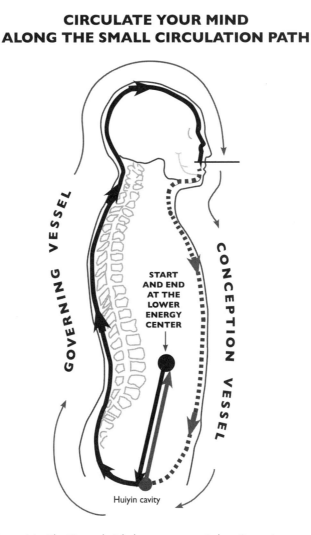

Figure 44. The Fire path: Inhale—move your mind up Governing vessel.
Exhale—move your mind down the Conception vessel.

The ancient documents advise you to practice this mental visualization with the legs crossed. You can sit comfortably on a pillow or a yoga block.

Sitting at a chair will work as well because this posture will slow down the flow of blood and energy to the legs.

Alternatively, you may stand and practice it while in horse stance.

There are reasons for crossing your legs or tensing them when standing in the horse stance.

1. Sitting with crossed legs or on a chair with bent legs will slow down and reduce the circulation of blood and energy to the legs. The legs are considered part of the large circulation. When this circulation is reduced, the mind is able to concentrate purely on the trunk and especially on the small circulation.

2. It will magnify the sensation and the experience of the entire torso.

This visualization is very important to build and balance our energetic system while nourishing our internal organs. It can help to strengthen the horse mind and quiet the monkey mind through the simple fact that the mind is focused on the governing vessel in the back and conception vessel in the front. This visualization is another way to capture the monkey mind.

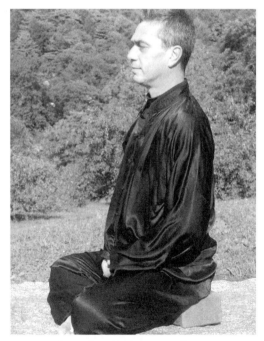

Sit comfortably, legs crossed on a pillow or a yoga block.

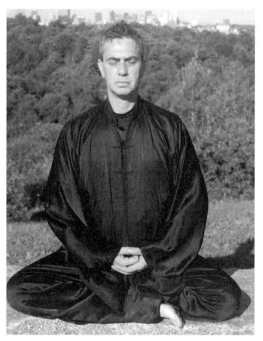

Sit comfortably, legs crossed on a pillow or a yoga block.

Before we start the small circulation, I would like to talk about the words 'push,' 'move,' and 'lead' in relationship to energy. Energy cannot be pushed. It is like water. If you have ever mopped the floor with a lot of water, you realize that you cannot push the water in one shot with the squeegee, but when you try leading, by pulling water, it works like a charm. Even though leading works the best, water and energy need to be pulled or led over and over—it is a constant collecting, gathering, and then pulling, and leading. Energy is the same; it needs to be led continuously and repeatedly, and the trick is very simple; put the mind ahead of the place you want the energy to go. Always stay in front of the energy, which is important when circulating the energy, especially through the governing vessel. There are a

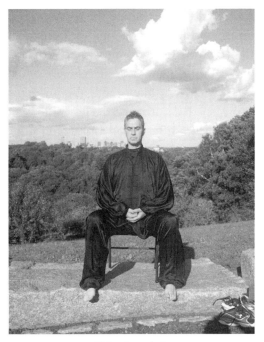

Sitting in a chair.

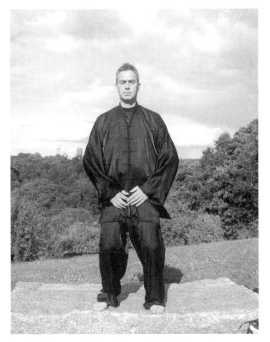

Practice small circulation while in horse stance.

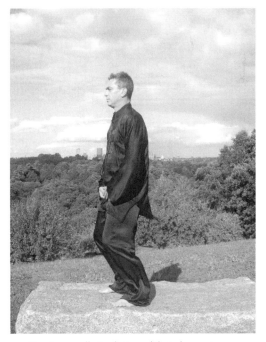

Practice small circulation while in horse stance.

few physical areas where the soft tissue is closer to the bones that are tighter along this vessel, and leading the energy using the mind is necessary to circulate through these tight areas. It is an essential trick to achieving the smooth flow of energy in the small circulation (Figure 45).

I would also like to talk about the tongue and the roof of your mouth. The tongue is the key to connecting the governing and conception vessels. Without the tongue, this circuit will not be closed and would not be as strong as it could be. Place the tip of the tongue on the roof of the mouth, very gently in the indentation at the roof of your mouth. Putting the tongue all the way to the teeth will be too tense, and if you put it too far toward the back you will hurt your tongue. The right place is at the indentation on the forward part of the palate of your mouth.

GOVERNING VESSEL: TIGHTER PHYSICAL AREAS

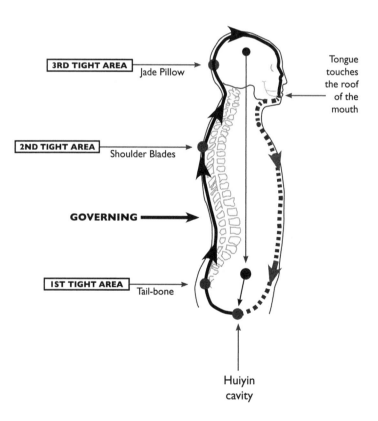

Figure 45. Circulate your mind/energy smoothly
and continuously through the tighter areas.

When you put the tongue at the right spot, your mouth will fill with saliva. When that happens, just close your eyes and swallow that saliva. Follow the saliva all the way down to your lower energy center. Use the sensation of the saliva to cool the fire energy around the solar plexus area.

Sit on the floor, on a block or a pillow. You may sit on the edge of a chair as well. Close your eyes, place one of your palms on the other one, and place them two inches below your belly button.

Put your tongue on the roof of your mouth, gently. On the next inhalation, lead your mind from the lower energy center out through the huiyin cavity and around the tailbone into the governing vessel. Keep moving your mind up the vessel, over your head, until you reach the area above your upper lip. Now exhale and lead your mind down the conception vessel to the huiyin cavity.

At this point you have two options. You can choose over time, which is the best for you. You can keep leading the mind around and through the vessels or you can move your mind in and back to the lower energy center. Then move your mind out of the lower energy center and circle it around again through the governing and conception vessels.

As you can see, you can either move out of your lower energy center and circle around and around the small circulation without going back to the lower energy center until you are done, or you can keep going back into your lower energy center every time you reach with your mind the huiyin cavity. Some people like to 'visit' the lower energy center during the visualization of the small circulation. At this point of my training, I stay in the governing and conception vessels with a two-breath cycle.

Often people cannot do the small circulation in a two-breath cycle. This is a small obstacle because the mind can move faster through the path of the small circulation to match the length of the breaths.

If you do want to move your mind slowly through the visualization and cannot match it with the length of your breath, you could use the five-breath cycles: inhale and lead the mind from the lower energy center to just above the tailbone; exhale, and keep your mind in the tailbone. Inhale again and move the mind up above the shoulder blade; exhale and stay at the shoulder blade. Inhale and move the mind to the upper lip, and exhale and lead your mind from the top lip back to the huiyin cavity.

Another method is the four-cycle visualization: inhale and lead the mind up above the shoulder blades; exhale, and stay at the shoulder blade. Inhale and lead the mind to the top lip; exhale and stay at the lip; and exhale and lead the mind down to the huiyin cavity.

As you can see, you can use the breath differently when visualizing the small circulation. You can divide the visualization into two, three, four, or even five cycles. Make sure that you lead your mind past the physical areas on the governing vessels that are tighter where the skin is closer to the bones.

The reason that I do the small circulation visualization without going to the lower energy center on every cycle is that I sit or stand at other times throughout the day and emphasize the visualization of the lower energy center as well as the draining the baton separately. When I do the small circulation visualization, I stay on the vessels until I am done. I always finish by residing in the lower energy center for a minimum of three minutes.

The different channels and energy centers are actually touching and overlapping while nourishing, interacting, and balancing with one another to the point that you experience being inside the body and outside the body at the same time. It is like an orchestra that plays in perfect harmony. The listener does not know and does not care if it is the piano or the violin that makes him or her feel good; the experience becomes spiritual.

The area between the groin and the anus is called, in Chinese, the huiyin cavity, which means the meeting of yin. The body has twelve meridians and eight extraordinary vessels. The twelve meridians consist of six yang and six yin channels and the extraordinary vessels consist of four yang and four yin vessels. The six yin channels are flowing primarily in the front of the body and are in charge of regulating and managing the yin internal organs in our bodies. The six yang channels flow primarily in the back of the body and are the regulators and managers of the yang internal organs in our bodies. The eight vessels are like reservoirs that manage and link the twelve channels or meridians. Three of the extraordinary vessels meet at the huiyin: conception vessel, governing vessel, and the thrusting vessel (in acupuncture, the penetrating vessel). The huiyin is considered the most negative yin point in the physical body. (If you are interested in earth qigong, the Dead Sea is the most negative yin or lowest point on our earth).

Repeat this visualization over and over. Start with five minutes and over time try to increase the visualization time to 30 to 40 minutes. You can also experiment with leading the mind slowly or quickly along this path. You may circulate as slowly or quickly as you choose, coordinating one orbit with a single breath, or as many as it takes for you to trace this path smoothly without skipping any place. As long as you do not hold your breath and you keep moving your mind along the circle, you are practicing correctly. To have more peace and quiet while you are meditating, I recommend eventually reaching a two-cycle breath with the visualization of the small circulation.

Over time, you will develop a strong physical sensation of the energy circulating along your vessels, just below the skin. Building the strength of these vessels will allow you to manifest more energy throughout life as well as when performing the tai chi drills or form.

Some people may experience a stronger sensation when the energy is flowing through the back, the governing vessel, versus the front, the conception vessel. That is normal because the front is the yin side and the back is the yang side. There is a tendency to experience or sense the energy through the yang side more easily than sensing the energy through the yin side.

Once you are able to lead the mind through the small circulation path, I encourage you to integrate this visualization while performing the spine wave or the tai chi form. Putting the two together is a unique experience but takes much practice. As long as you do not hold your breath and you play it cool, with not too much imagination, you should be safe. Of course, by having a teacher or an individual who has been through this journey to guide you through, your practice would be much better, easier, and safer.

TAI CHI BALL TRAINING

Tai Chi Ball–Grinding

The tai chi ball is a traditional training tool used to strengthen the muscles, joints, and bones. It is also a method used to open and strengthen the circulation in the belt vessel.

You may use any kind or size ball or any object that will fit between your hands for this exercise.

Stand with the feet parallel and the weight distributed evenly between the ball of your foot and your heels or sit comfortably on the edge of a chair. Maintain healthy alignment: tailbone dropped, head suspended, face and shoulders relaxed, and knees slightly bent.

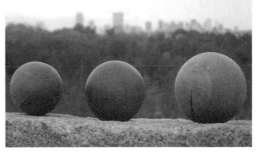

Use any kind or size ball, any object that will fit between your hands.

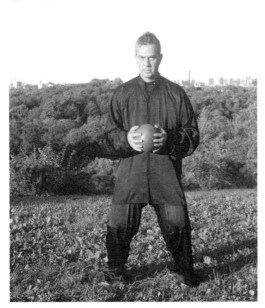

Neutral position, feet parallel, weight distributed evenly between the ball of foot and heels.

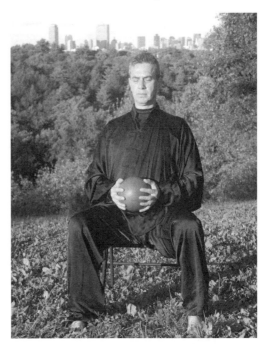

Grinding, neutral position. Sit comfortably on the edge of the chair.

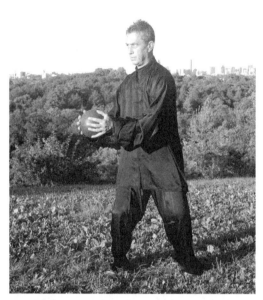

Visualize internal energetic circulation in body;
follow outer movements of ball in hands.

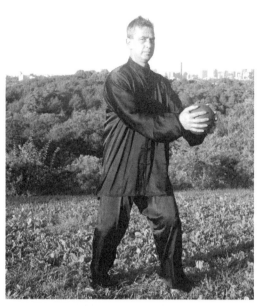

Visualize internal energetic circulation in body;
follow outer movements of ball in hands.

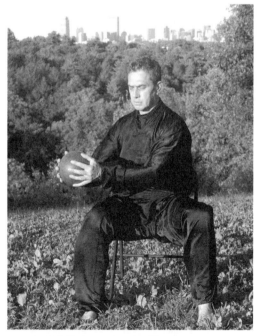

Grinding, maintain healthy alignment.

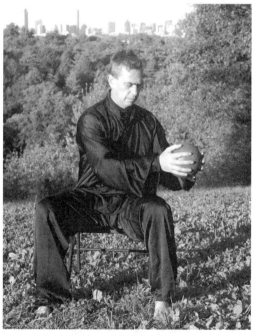

Grinding, head suspended,
face and shoulders relaxed.

Holding the ball can also strengthen our energetic visualization abilities by giving us physical feedback. Visualize that there is an internal energetic circulation in your body that follows the outer movements of the ball in your hands.

Tai Chi Ball Overhead

Take the tai chi ball and hold it over your head.

You can stand with feet apart or feet together. You can also sit on the edge of a chair, whatever is most comfortable for you.

Slowly, on an inhalation, move the ball down toward the neck and on the exhalation move the ball up as high as you can.

Do not lock the elbows straight up, keep them a little bent. This skill is like a typical weight-lifting exercise. The only difference is that we use the tai chi ball. Another

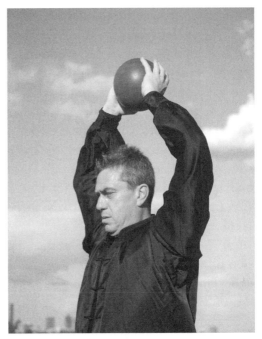

Hold the tai chi ball overhead.

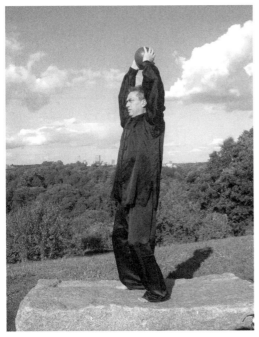

Stand with feet apart or feet together.

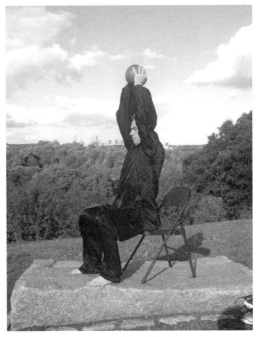

Sit on the edge of a chair.

difference is that we try to integrate some of the physical skills and mental visualizations while we are lowering and lifting the tai chi ball.

If you pump around 10 repetitions with an 8 to 10 pound tai chi ball, it is a good start. You may feel it the next day, but if you use a two to three pound tai chi ball, then you will not feel as much progress. Start with about 10 repetitions and gradually build up to 30 to 50 repetitions. If you raise your shoulders when doing the exercise or if you have weak muscles, you might use your neck muscles, which means you may get a sore neck the next day. If this soreness happens, balance this mind/body prescription by stretching the neck and the shoulder girdle. When my neck gets tight, I use the mind/body prescription, 'vitamin L' (*Sunrise Tai Chi*, page 51), or 'vitamin H' (*Sunrise Tai Chi*, page 57). You can also use the loosening the neck exercise (*Sunrise Tai Chi*, pages 60 and 61).

This up and down motion of the tai chi ball is used to help strengthen the visualization of the heaven and earth connection. When you move the tai chi ball up, extend your mind, and move and grow from the lower energy center through the baton out the heavenly gate in the top of your head upward, all the way to the heavens. Once the ball is at your shoulder blade level, exhale as you move the tai chi ball up.

Continue moving with your mind upward even when the tai chi ball stops. Do not straighten your elbows. Once your mind is in the heavens, you can feel a sensation of

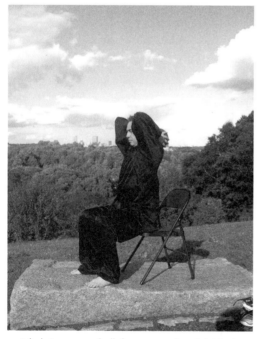

Inhalation, move ball down toward neck (sitting).

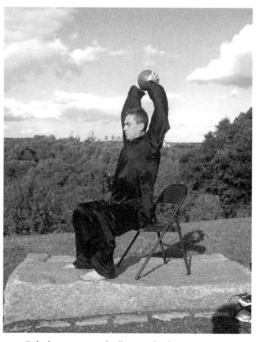

Exhalation, move ball up as high as you can.

expanding the baton from your lower energy center all the way up to the heavens. Maintain the visualization of your lower energy center when your mind is in the heavens. Be in both places at the same time.

Before you try this long energetic baton visualization, you may want to try visualizing the baton from the lower energy center to the tai chi ball above your head. When the tai chi ball is above your head, use your imagination to visualize it as your upper energy center. It will help you to extend your upper energy center by a foot or two above the real location, which is the pituitary gland area. It helps you have a sensation of a bigger internal baton. This exercise will prepare you for the visualization of expanding to the heavens.

Expand your mind between the lower energy center and the tai chi ball over your head.

You do not stretch or release the bow in this exercise. You just want to maintain alignment through the spine as well as the legs. This part is like weight lifting. You feel gentle compression through the spine and shoulders when the ball moves down and a light opening feeling when the ball moves up toward the sky. Do not lock the elbows and do the motion slowly.

To make the physical components different from just weight lifting, coordinate the movement of the ball with the empty-full moon technique. When the ball moves down

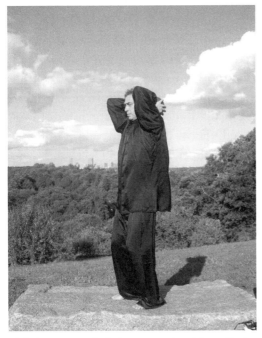

Inhalation, move ball down toward neck (standing).

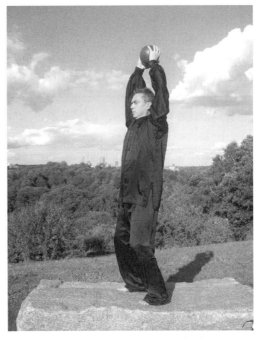

Exhalation, move ball up as high as you can (standing).

to the shoulder blade area, go to empty moon and when it moves up it is the full moon. Inhale on the way down—empty moon, and exhale on the way up—full moon.

Over time, try to improve your coordination of the empty-full moon with the movement of the ball. When the ball reaches the shoulder blades, it is empty moon and when the ball reaches over your head, it is full moon.

In the belt vessel exercise, tai chi ball belt vessel, and in many other qigong standing postures in which you physically move the arms, the ball, or a weapon, you want to make sure to balance the physical movement upward with a mental downward visualization or sensation. When the ball rises up to its extreme, over your head, you want to create a sinking feeling through the lower energy center into the floor and a light feeling through the spine. When the ball moves to the shoulder blade area, maintain that sinking sensation from the lower energy center to a few inches into the ground.

There is a tendency to lose the sinking sensation into the ground when your mind moves up with the ball toward the sky. Balance that upward physical movement of the tai chi ball with a mental visualization of sinking into the floor. You should always employ this concept of balance between the mind and the physical movements. I recommend starting with 'residing' in the lower energy center to avoid having the energy just rise. The upper energy center as well as the bubble will become stronger by sinking your mind into the ground. The more you sink through the legs, the more relaxed and balanced you will feel.

Regarding the elbows, you have two options when you hold the tai chi ball behind your shoulder blades. If the elbows are naturally moving toward the side at a 45-degree angle, you will feel the resistance more in the biceps, triceps, and in the shoulders.

If you move the elbows inward so they are pointing forward, you will strengthen your upper back and chest muscles as well as the biceps and the triceps. In this position, you will also feel it closer to the neck and more in the spine.

Training in both positions is recommended. Each position develops different muscles and will strengthen all around the chest, upper back, shoulders, and arms. Remember to balance this exercise with stretching the shoulders as well as the neck to avoid tension and stress around those areas.

Move the ball slowly to increase the time of resistance. Coordinate the movement with your breath. Exhale as you lift. Inhale as you lower the ball. You may use any ball, or any lightweight object. As with all of the exercises, once you are comfortable with the movement, add our other skills like empty-full moon, visualizing draining the energetic baton, four gates breathing, bubble visualization, as well as being one with the three forces. Over weeks and months of practice, you may gradually add weight or increase the number of repetitions.

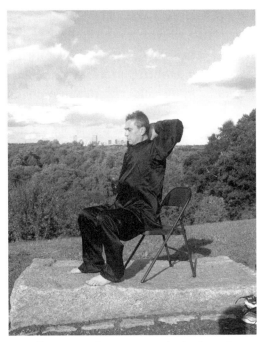

Elbows naturally going toward sides (sitting).

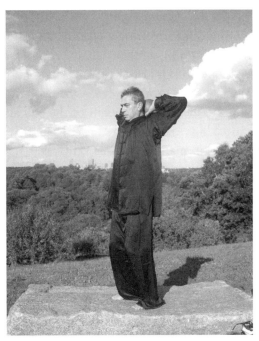

Elbows naturally going toward sides (standing).

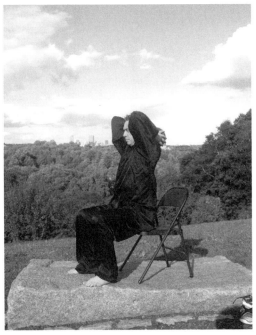

Elbows inward; they are pointing forward (sitting).

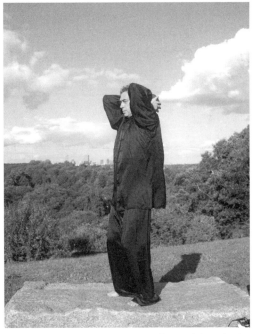

Elbows inward; they are pointing forward (standing).

Tai Chi Ball–Figure Eight

Stand with your feet parallel, and shoulder-width apart, with knees slightly bent, or sit comfortably on the edge of a chair. Move the tai chi ball slowly in coordination with your breath. Hold the ball at your solar plexus height and when performing the figure eight, do not drop the ball. Once you are strong and comfortable with this movement, you can increase the weight of the ball and bend the knees lower for more weight resistance, but still keep the tai chi ball at the solar plexus height. You may practice this exercise in many variations, either starting from the center of the figure eight, or moving out to the side first.

When moving the tai chi ball, the mind needs to sink through the legs, which creates stronger roots. You can perform this mind/body prescription at anytime, but when performing this exercise while the sun is setting, you will sense a stronger sensation of the sinking energy through the legs as well as the tai chi ball. If possible, you want to perform these movements facing the setting sun and allow the pulling energy of the setting sun to help your mind create a stronger sensation of the energy moving down through the legs as well as the tai chi ball.

Start with a basic horse stance, sink down and hold the ball in front of your sternum, the solar plexus area.

Then move the tai chi ball in a straight line out away from your body but do not straighten your elbows. Stretch to the point where your elbows are still sunk.

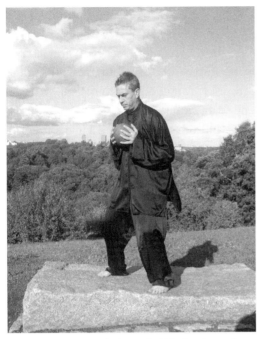

Horse stance, sink down. Hold ball in front of
sternum, the solar plexus area (standing).

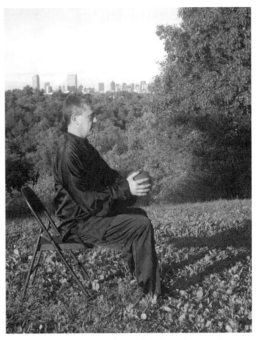

Sit on edge of chair. Hold ball in front of
sternum, the solar plexus area (sitting).

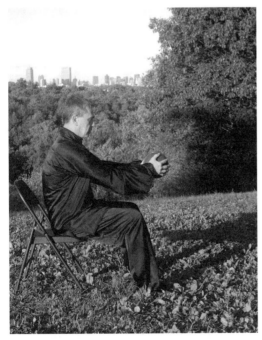

Move ball, straight line out away from
body; do not straighten elbows (sitting).

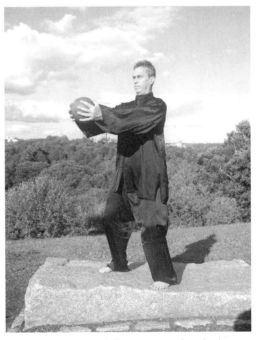

Move ball, straight line out away from body;
do not straighten elbows (standing).

Make a circle to your left, and come back to the center, the original position. Then move the tai chi ball straight and out from your solar plexus. This time make a circle to your right, and come to the center, the original position. As you can see, you are describing a figure eight or an infinity sign. Remember to start with a small figure eight and as you get better make the eight bigger, not just in front of your chest but to the sides as well.

Breathe in when holding the tai chi ball at the solar plexus. Exhale when you send the ball out away from your body. Inhale and bring the ball from the left around in a circle into the solar plexus area. Exhale and move in a straight line away from the body, and finish with an inhalation while bringing the tai chi ball back from the right to your original position.

You can mix in the long bow and the cross bow. Start with releasing the bow while in the original posture and as you go out in the straight line away from your body, you stretch the bow. As you lead the ball through the left to the original position, release the bows.

After you complete 20 repetitions, reverse the action of both the long and the cross bows. What that means is that when you do the figure eight the first time, you hold the tai chi ball at your solar plexus while your back is straight, which means that you are in the release the bow position. Once you move the tai chi ball away from your body, you use the stretch the bow position. To reverse the action, start with the tai chi ball at your solar plexus as before, but in the stretch the bow position. As you move out, release the bow instead of stretching the bow.

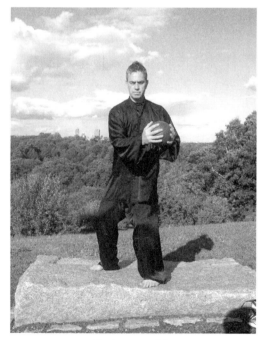

Circle to your left.

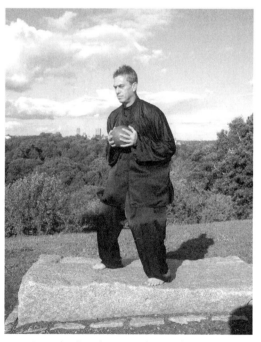

Come back to the center (original position).

The bows are used as a tool, the same as the breath; they are used differently, depending on your goal. Alternate the figure eight and move along it, but take different paths. You can go out straight, and then to create the figure eight you can move to the right or the left; that means that you are starting the circle of the eight from the top. You can also circle right away from the solar plexus to the figure eight, which means you create the eight from the bottom. Of course, the top and the bottom also have left and right. As you can see, you have at least four options for the path of the figure eight. Once you master this mind/body prescription, you may find other ways to perform this movement.

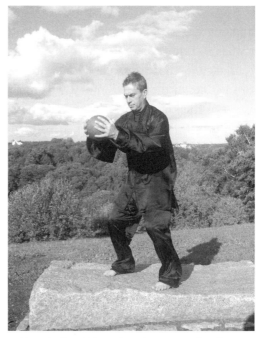

Move ball straight and out from your solar plexus.

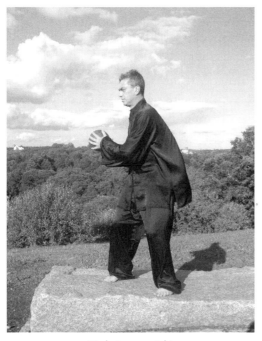

Circle to your right.

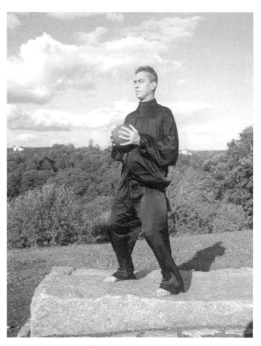

Come to the center (original position).

Make sure you do not break the alignment in the legs, especially the inner arches and the knees, as you circle the tai chi ball. There is a tendency to collapse the inner arches and the knees when circling the ball. When you turn toward the right, there is a tendency to collapse the left inner arch as well as the knee. By charging the outer edge of the soles of the feet all the way from the outer hips and paying attention to the alignment of the knees, you will prevent this collapse from happening.

The solar plexus is related to your fire energy. The food we eat, the air we breathe, and our emotions are all manifesting their energy at the solar plexus area or the middle energy center (dan tian). When you move the tai chi ball away from the solar plexus, use this physical motion to mentally send the fire out of your solar plexus, far away from your body. This mental visualization will cool the fire in our bodies.

Release and lead this energy from your middle energy center using the forward movement of the tai chi ball. This fire energy coming out of your sternum is like the "fire" that is shooting out of the dragon's mouth. This visualization will allow you to get rid of some of the fire energy in your body more effectively.

If you watch a burning candle, you will understand the spirit of fire. The flame is dancing from left to right and without warning, it shoots up or in. Imagine your arms are light and agile like the spirit of the candle flame, instead of the sinking heavy feeling through the ball you have when performing the tai chi ball belt vessel circles.

The trunk is still moving. One side of the groin area alternately closes and opens. The muscles around the internal organs are tensing and relaxing along the figure eight you are performing. Different groups of muscles, all around the trunk, are tensing while others are relaxing. Every time a muscle tenses, it holds blood and energy and when the muscles are relaxed, this accumulated blood and energy rushes to every part of our body. This tension is called the 'dam effect.' When the muscles are tight or tense, they behave like a dam and when they relax, it is the same as opening the dam's doors and releasing all the water to regulate the water flow. This strong flow that is created from the dam effect can reach farther to places where the circulation of both blood and energy is slow and low.

Notice which muscles tense or relax along the movement and sense which of the internal organs beneath those muscles are being massaged. Notice the feeling of your internal organs in front of the trunk: the lungs, stomach, liver, and spleen. Notice the internal organs in the back: the lungs and kidneys.

SPIDER CLIMBING

Spider climbing stretches the sides of the body in opposite directions. This exercise releases tension around the lungs and allows you to increase your lung capacity.

Inhale deeply and point the fingers of the right hand down toward the floor, while the left points toward the ceiling; both palms face forward.

As you exhale, bring the arms to your centerline: right palm at your belly button, front palm facing up, and left over your forehead with the palm facing down.

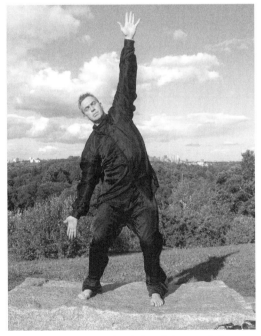

Inhale. Point fingers of right hand down. Left fingers point to up, and palms face forward.

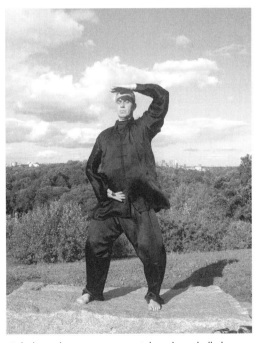

Exhale, with arms to center, right palm at belly button facing up, and left palm over forehead facing down.

Move the palms slowly closer to each other closing the gap between them.

Then point the left fingers down toward the floor and point the right fingers up toward the ceiling.

Now move the right arm up toward the ceiling. At about two-thirds of the way up, rotate your arm and the front of the palm forward. At the same time, move the left arm and palm downward, and rotate the arm and the palm so it will be facing forward. You are back in the original position; only this time your right arm and palm are up while the left is down.

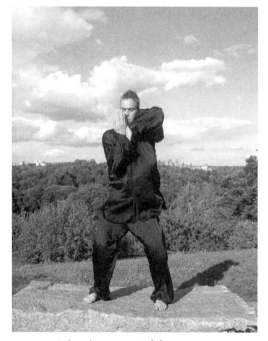

Solar plexus area. Left fingers point down, and right fingers point up.

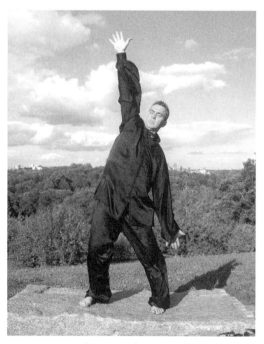

Original position, this time right arm and palm are up, and left is down.

Repeat the movement from side to side. Over time, you will be able to open and close ribs and emphasize breathing into one lung, as in the seesaw breathing exercise.

The setting sun gives this mind/body exercise a unique energetic and spiritual sensation. The arm that moves down imitates the setting sun and the one that moves up symbolizes the rising of the moon. Try coordinating the ribs and arms like the moon and the sun; one rises while the other is setting. When performing this exercise while the sun is setting, you will experience much stronger energetic and spiritual sensations. Try creating the same sensation when performing it at other times throughout the day.

Spider climbing can be done both sitting on the edge of the chair or standing up.

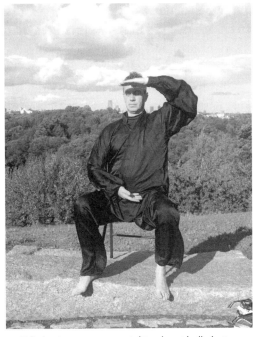

Exhale. Arms to center, right palm at belly button facing up and left palm over forehead facing down.

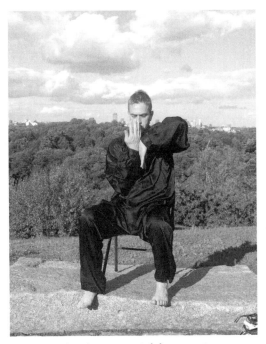

Solar plexus area. Left fingers point down and right fingers point up.

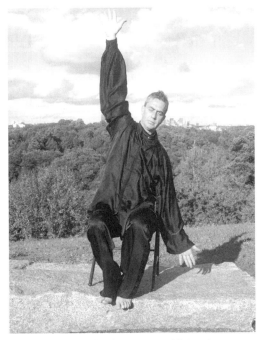

Right arm and palm are up and left is down.

When standing, I recommend you first practice a few inches in front of a wall or a tree. Face the wall or tree, with knees shoulder-width apart, slightly bent, sacrum tucked in, right arm and palm are up facing the wall or tree while the left arm and palm are down facing the wall or tree.

Both arms are opened to the sides of the body. Using the wall will give you a stronger sense of your breath, your energy, and the surrounding energy. The wall will also force you to use the long and the cross bows.

If your right arm is up and the left is down, your right ribs are open and the left are closed. One lung is stretched and open, and the other is closed.

On the next inhalation, bring the right palm facing down along the centerline so it goes above your head, the heavenly gate, or the forehead, and bring the left hand in, in a scooping motion, palm up. The movements should be kept in front of your centerline.

At this point, the centers of the palms are facing the centerline. The left is at your pubic bone height and your right is above your head. Do not straighten the elbow.

With the elbows slightly bent, the right palm is above your head as if you are pretending to create a roof over your head, and then continue by bringing the palms toward each other along the centerline. Once the hands reach the solar plexus area and almost touch, the left fingers point up while the palm slightly rotates and faces left. The right hand fingers point down toward the floor while the palm slightly rotates, to point outward toward your right.

Continue pointing up and down with your fingers along the centerline, and then when your right hand reaches the pubic bone, turn the palm toward the front. Rotate clockwise. When the left arm reaches over your head, turn the arm and the palm so it faces forward.

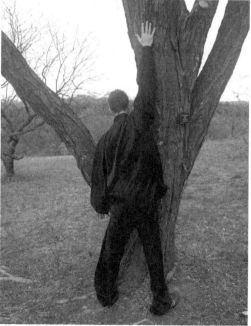

Few inches, in front of a wall or a tree.

Notice that when moving the right arm up, you open the right ribs and lungs. With the left arm moving down, you close the left ribs and lungs. Open the left rib, close the right rib, reach down toward the floor, and reach up toward the ceiling. On the next inhalation, close the left rib, bring the palms to face each other while the right palm, this time, is at the pubic bone height and your left is over your head pointing the palm face down. Previously, your right was over your head and your left was at the pubic bone. Inhale, move the palms toward each other. When they reach the solar plexus area, point the left fingers down toward the floor and the right up toward the ceiling. Continue until the left fingers reach the pubic bone and the right fingers reach the forehead, and then exhale, rotate the right palm forward and the left down toward the floor but forward as well; both palms should be facing forward at this point. If you are facing the wall or tree, the palm will be facing the wall or tree at this point; right rib open, left closed. You just performed a full cycle.

Try to keep the movements soft, relaxed, and agile. Coordinate the movements with the breath. Inhale all the way until the fingers are pointing up and down, and then exhale as you move the arms down and up. Keep your face relaxed. Do not lose the alignment in the legs and do not collapse the inner arches of the feet. When bringing the arms and palms in, stretch the bow, and when pushing the arms and palms up and down, release the bow.

Try to coordinate the timing of the right hand and the left hand. When you reach the peak with one hand, you also reach the bottom with the other hand. There is a tendency when crossing the palms, fingers, and the arms, to tense and crunch the shoulders. Try to maintain a widening through the shoulders as well as a dropping down action, especially when the palms come together.

Once you feel comfortable with the physical movement, add the mental skills as well. When inhaling and bringing the palms toward each other, perform the empty moon, bring your mind into the lower energy center, and move your energy from that center up the governing vessel into the shoulder blade area. When exhaling, perform the full moon and expand the mind from the baton into the bubble, and at the same time lead your energy from the shoulder blade area into the palms, as well as from the lower energy center into the soles of your feet or a few inches into the ground. When inhaling, condense the third eye and when exhaling, expand it like fury eyes. Maintain a heavy feeling from the belly button down and allow a light feeling throughout the spine.

Once you feel comfortable doing the exercise with the wall or tree, move away from the wall or tree and try to perform the movement without the wall or tree.

You will find that when performing this exercise without the wall or tree, it is a little bit harder because there is a tendency to push the palms and the arms backward away from the front part of the body. The idea is to do the movements along your centerline, about a foot away, in front of the body.

Make sure that you create the maximum movement through your ribs. When you are doing the exercise at a wall or tree, the wall is an indicator that helps and encourages you to reach up and down along the wall or tree. When you do it in the air, there is a tendency to forget to keep reaching. The arms do not work as hard if you move from the ribs. Drop the left ribs, the left arm will reach farther down. When you open the right ribs, the fingers of the right will reach farther up. Make sure that the movement of the arms is mostly generated from the ribs.

Eventually when utilizing the ribs to their fullest, the arms will line up in almost a straight line.

Being able to maintain a straight line between the two palms means that you are creating optimal movement in the ribs. Remember, you want to reach as high as you can with the right arm and palm and as low as you can with your left arm and palm.

Deep breathing, sighing, and lingering at the end of exhalation are very important. Keep your mind relaxed and open to experience various old and new sensations. Change the breathing technique you use from time to time: Taoist to Buddhist or vice versa. This change will allow you to experience the different sensations when training for martial arts or for health.

Martial artists most often use Taoist breathing because it is the strongest way to manifest energy. The martial artist will inhale when storing energy before an attack and will exhale when moving the arms up and down as he manifests energy or attacks the opponent.

When used for health reasons, use the more relaxed method of breathing, which is Buddhist breathing. Exhale when changing the position of the arms and inhale when moving the arms and palms up to the sky and down into the earth.

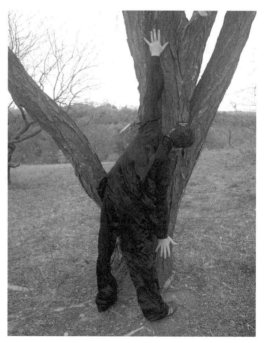

Utilizing the ribs to their fullest, arms will line up in a straight line.

I strongly recommend performing spiderman (or spiderwoman) sitting on the edge of the chair. Isolating the torso will allow you to experience many different sensations and elements of the movement that will make the movement much stronger when performed standing.

When one of your arms is up and the other is fully down, which is considered the peak of the physical motion or the yang part of the movement, you can look either up toward the fingers that are pointing to the heavens or down toward the fingers pointing to the earth. This exercise will also allow you to stretch and open up the neck. For example, if you do 20 repetitions, do 10 looking down and 10 looking up. You will be surprised how the turning of the head to different directions changes the whole sensation of stretching throughout the various layers of soft tissue.

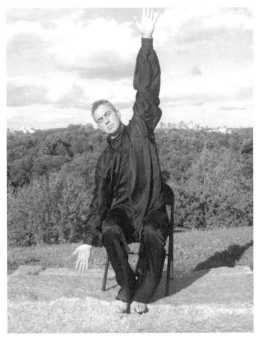

Left arm up, left ribs and lung open, right arm down, and right ribs and lung closed.

When sitting on the edge of the chair, you will discover that your legs are a little bit in the way. The hand that is going to go down toward the floor needs to move a little bit away from the leg and then point down to the floor.

WALL AND TREE PUSH-UPS

Face a wall or a tree, with your feet together and your toes about two to four feet away from the wall or tree, depending on your height and how much resistance you are looking for. The farther away from the support you are, the more resistance you will add to the muscles.

Place your palms on the wall or tree with the fingers pointing upward at shoulder height.

Practice these wall or tree push-ups while keeping your elbows close to your ribs.

As you straighten your arms, first lift your palms off the wall and or the tree, and then your fingers.

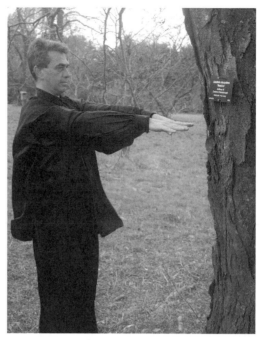

First set. Keep your elbows close to your ribs.

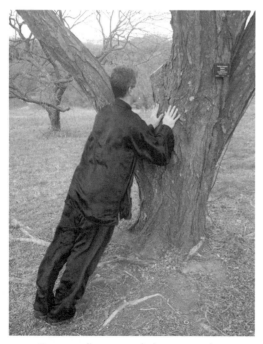

Face a wall or tree and place your palms on the tree with toes four feet away.

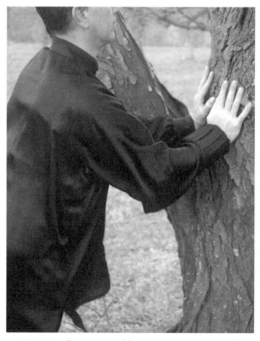

First set. Elbows in and fingers pointing upward.

Be careful, especially at first, not to overstress the fingers and their joints. Inhale as you move toward the wall or tree and exhale as you push away.

Land with your fingers softly when moving toward the wall or tree, and push with your fingers softly when leaving the wall or tree.

These push-ups will strengthen your wrists and fingers as well as the arms and upper body.

Practice a second set, this time with the elbows turned out and fingers pointing toward each other.

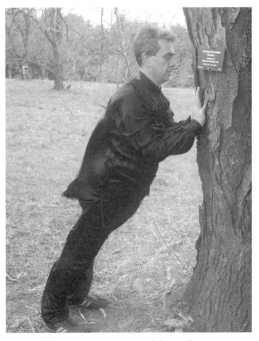

Inhale as you move toward the wall or tree.

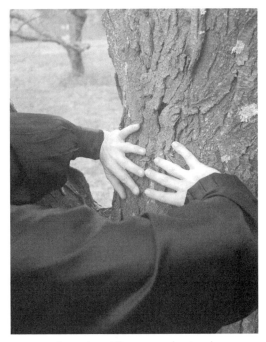

Second set. Elbows turned out and fingers pointing toward each other.

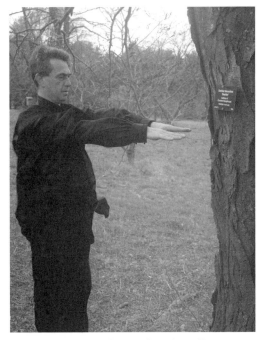

Exhale as you push away from the wall or tree.

Be careful, especially at first, not to overstress the elbow joints by trying to bring the head or the elbows themselves to the wall or tree instead of the chest.

Inhale as you move toward the wall or tree and exhale as you push away.

Some days you can practice the wall or tree push-ups closer to the wall or tree with the palms higher, and other days you can move your feet farther from the wall or tree and place your palms lower down.

Practice only as much as is appropriate for you, and gradually increase the number of repetitions.

Why Two Sets?

Each set will activate and strengthen different groups of muscles. For example, when the elbows are in by your ribs, you will develop many small groups of muscles, especially the biceps and chest muscles. Doing the push-ups with the elbows out will develop your trapezius and deltoid muscles. Both will strengthen the forearms, wrists, and fingers.

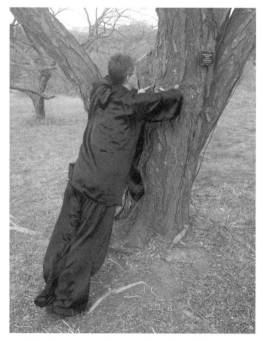

Exhale as you push away from the wall or tree.

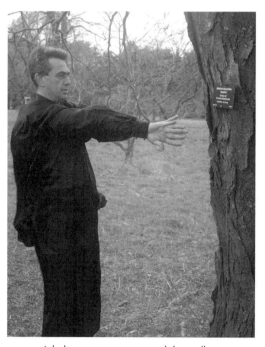

Inhale as you move toward the wall or tree with back palms facing each other.

Why on the Wall or Tree, and Not on the Floor?

To understand this question, we first need to talk about the chicken and the duck. The chicken has white breast meat while the duck has dark meat. We call it meat when it comes to what we eat but we call it muscles when we refer to ourselves; just a matter of mental convenience. The chicken's muscles allow it to move very fast so that the chicken can jump very high and even have bursts of flying for very short distances. The developed muscle fiber is not strong enough to allow the chicken to really fly. The chicken does have dark meat, which is in the leg muscles that power the high jumps and the almost flying. On the other hand, the duck uses its muscles for long-distance flights. The duck is stronger but slower. Our muscle fibers are not white and dark like the chicken leg or the duck chest and wings, but we still have fast and slow twitch muscles that behave exactly like the dark and the white muscle fiber in the chicken and the duck. If you want to develop more strength and bulk, use heavier weights or resistance with limited repetitions. If you are looking for speed and a trim physique, use lighter weights with lots of repetition. Now that you have this information, who do you want to be? What body type are you striving to have—the chicken's or the duck's?

As a martial artist, I do not want to be slow and bulky. I need to be quick. Performing the push-ups on a wall develops the fast twitch fibers of the muscles that are in charge of performing with speed. Performing push-ups on the floor develop strength in the same muscles, but it will make you lose speed. Now the question is, do you want to be a duck or a chicken? Of course, a balanced approach will be the best answer.

Can They Be More Than Just Physical Push-ups?

Yes. Inhale deeply when moving toward the wall or tree. Move to empty moon, breathe out, and sigh. Linger at the end of the exhalation. The bows are still but the mind is active. Visualize four gates breathing. When inhaling and moving toward the wall or tree, condense your mind in the lower energy center and lead the energy up through the governing vessel to the shoulder blade area. On an exhalation, move away from the wall or tree and expand your mind out and down through the legs, a few inches into the ground, while leading the mind through the arms, fingers, and even through the wall or tree. When your mind expands into the earth beneath you and to the wall or tree in front of you, visualize the bubble around you. The more you move your mind down the energetic baton, the stronger your bubble will be. Connect to the three forces: heaven, human, and earth.

The setting sun will help the visualization of moving the mind down the energetic baton; it reinforces the sensation. When doing the push-ups, inhale when moving toward the wall or tree and exhale when pushing away. When you push, you can also sigh and expel impurities from your entire body through the mouth. The impurities will expel from your body and the tremendous force of the setting sun will pull the impurities away from your body and energetic space. You may sense the whole body becoming transparent when performing this mind/body prescription with the sun setting. If, however, you do not have the luxury of doing this exercise outdoors, during that time, still do it and use your mind to expel the impurities away from the body and your energetic space. If performing on a tree, the tree will help drain the impurities as well.

How Many Push-Ups Should I Do?

You should always use the concept of 80% effort as well as placing your arms at various heights on the wall or tree according to your soft tissue condition. Some days, when you are sore or just want a light workout, perform the wall or tree push-ups with your palms and fingers at your shoulder height. On other days, when you want more challenge and resistance, place your feet farther away from the wall or tree, and the palms and fingers lower down at the solar plexus height. Remember, you have two sets. Some days, you can do them quickly and on others, go slowly. My personal experience is that if you can do the two sets, elbows in and elbows out up to 10 repetitions per set, you are at a beginner level. If you can do up to 30 per set you are intermediate, and if you can do more than 30 per set, you are advanced.

What Should I Be Careful Of?

The neck and the elbows: If you push through the elbows and move them when doing the wall or tree push-ups, you will experience pain in them. Keep the elbows away from the wall or tree and do not move them. It is your chest that moves, and the rest of the body is like a stiff board that just comes along for the ride. If you do too many repetitions too soon, this resistance exercise, which targets the upper body, could cause strain, especially in the neck. The only way to prevent that is to train at 80% of your capability and use the next mind/body prescription of balancing the upper body every time you perform your wall or tree push-ups. Make sure you keep your face relaxed throughout the entire movement. Your tongue should be touching the roof of the mouth.

BALANCING THE UPPER BODY

Many individuals engage in building their upper body using weights or other methods of resistance, but not enough individuals balance this act with an effective routine of flexibility. Balancing the upper body is a method of opening the upper body or the shoulder girdle. If deep breathing and visualizations are added, the results increase. Your goal, on a physical level, is to free the upper body skeleton from being a prisoner of the soft tissue. This goal will also lead to better physical performance as well as serve as preventing injuries to the entire upper body.

Arms and Elbows above Your Head

Hold the elbows over your head while relaxing your shoulders, neck, and face.

Use the setting sun to encourage more sinking through the shoulders and neck but especially through the face. Face the setting sun and allow it to caress and relax your face; relax the face layer by layer. If you are not doing this exercise while the sun is setting, use your mind to create the downward sensation. To facilitate this downward feeling, I like having moving water around when I practice. In order to achieve a stronger sensation, I use the sound of the moving water instead of the setting sun to help the mind to move energy because the sun sets only once a day and takes only a short time to set. Through this program, you may want to also practice near a source of water

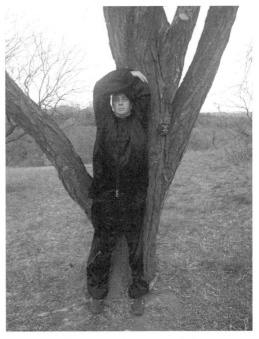

Elbows over head, and relax the shoulders, neck, and face.

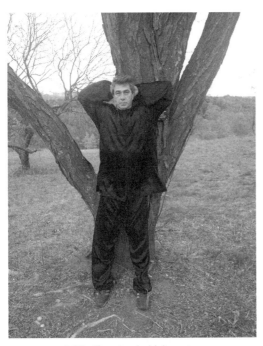

80% effort. Just hold the wrists over the head (standing).

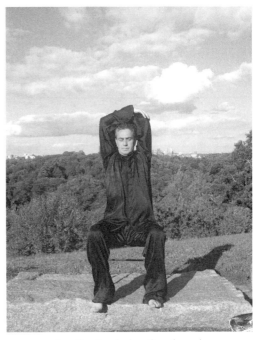

Breathe deeply, lengthen through the spine, and drop shoulders (sitting).

for the times when you are doing the exercise without the benefit of the setting sun's energy. Some individuals will need to start just holding the wrists over the head and then gradually bring the elbows closer together.

Remember to use the concept of 80% effort to avoid injuries. Stretch gradually. Try standing with your back against the wall or tree with the heels a few inches away from the wall or tree. Touch the sacrum, shoulder blades, and back of the elbows to the wall or tree while relaxing your shoulders and your face. Breathe deeply and lengthen up through the spine and drop down through the shoulders.

If you can, touch your sitting bones, shoulder blades, back of the head, as well as the elbows to the wall or tree behind you. If you cannot, work your body gradually toward that goal. First, you can move your heels farther from the wall or tree. Start with the sitting bones and sacrum. Next should be the shoulder blades. You may get stuck here for a while, but over time you will be able to put the back of the head against the wall or tree and eventually the back of your elbows. At that point, you can move the heels back closer to the wall or tree. When you are in the final stage, right before bringing the elbows to the wall or tree, move from the thoracic spine. Lift the thoracic spine in and up but keep your lower back and the sacrum against the wall or tree. If you put your hand at the lumbar spine, you should feel a small open space. The lumbar does not push to the wall or tree.

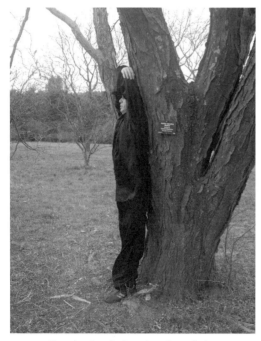

Breathe deeply, lengthen through the spine, and drop shoulders (standing).

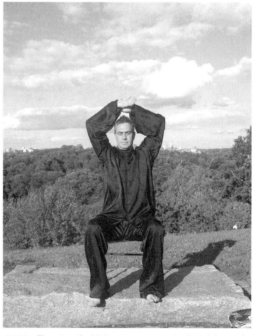

80% effort. Just hold the wrists over the head (sitting).

To help with the last stage of balancing the upper body, we will use the stretch called Iron of the Wall/Tree. Straighten the arms up along the wall or tree, lean your forehead gently on the wall/tree, bring the armpit and elbows to the wall or tree, but make sure you relax and drop your shoulders.

Start with your toes five to ten inches from the wall or tree, lean forward and gently place your forehead and elbows on the wall or tree. Relax your neck and shoulders and melt every muscle in your face. Breathe deeply and spend two to three minutes in this posture.

Once you can keep your shoulders, neck, and face relaxed, move your toes closer to the wall or tree until you can just touch the wall or tree with your entire front while breathing deeply and sensing total relaxation in the whole body. Next, move your head up and touch the chin to the wall, while still working on dropping the shoulders and relaxing the neck and face. Maintain this position for two to three minutes and breathe deeply.

Try putting your outer edge of your left ear on the wall or tree while keeping your elbows and chest area touching the wall or tree. Then turn your head and put the right outer edge of the ear on the wall or tree. Notice which side can turn farther and work toward getting the full turn on both sides. If you cannot perform some of those tasks because of restriction from your soft tissues, work your way slowly. Over time and with practice, you will open the soft tissue and will 'free your skeleton from being a prisoner of your soft tissues.' Finally turn the

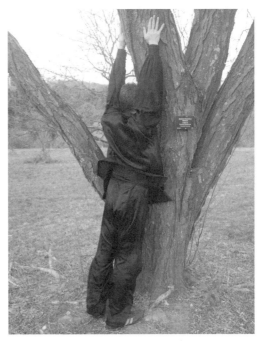

Arms up wall or tree with forehead and armpit gently on the wall/tree, and relax the shoulders.

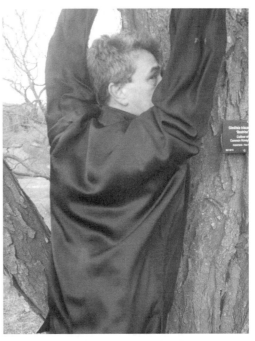

Left ear on wall/tree while elbows and chest area touch the wall/tree.

head to the left and stay there for about a minute. Then turn the head to the right and do the same.

Next, stand sideways and use the wall or tree to push gently on the elbows. Spend two minutes on each side. Make sure your front and your back ribs are evenly open. There is a tendency to open the front ribs and collapse the back ones due to tightness in the shoulders that prevents bringing the forearms over your head when grasping the elbows. Because the shoulders restrict this movement, the body finds ways around them. In this case, it is done through the front and back ribs.

Breathing deeply while your elbows are over your head will give you a special, unique light sensation because you are taking the weight off the shoulder girdle. The lungs are in a relaxed position when the

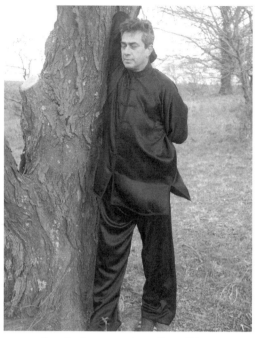

Stand sideways and use the wall/tree to push gently on elbows.

elbows are over the head. When breathing deeply in and out, there is a sensation in the lungs that we do not experience regularly. While breathing deeply when your arms are over your head, try performing wing breathing and mushroom breathing. Spend a few minutes on each one. Once you are able to lead the air to different parts of your lungs, mix the two.

Start with inhaling into the wing and continue directing the air into the mushroom. Breathe into the sides of the lungs. Then lead the air to the upper back and front parts of your lungs. Then lead the air to the upper front and back of the lungs, and then change the order. Lead the air to the upper front back lungs first and second to the wings, the side of the lungs. Focusing on these muscles helps to improve your mind/body connection and increase lung capacity.

When your arms are over your head, it is an opportunity to stretch the neck. When the arms are over your head, many of the muscles that are connecting the head to the shoulders are tensed, which moves the fix point closer to the neck. By turning the head to the left or to the right, you will sense a pleasant stretch through the neck.

Drop your shoulders and turn the neck to the left. Relax your shoulders and your face. Maintain the alignment in the neck. If your neck muscles are too short, the head will come out of alignment in order to achieve the distance.

When we try to stretch, the mind has the tendency to find ways to achieve the task even if it means breaking alignment. It may be more difficult to stretch and you may not get as much distance when keeping the correct alignment.

To make sure you are not breaking the alignment in your head and neck, you may need to use a partner to check your alignment. You could use a mirror but another person is the better choice. Spend one to two minutes stretching to each side. Breathe deeply while in the posture, close your eyes, relax your shoulders and your face. If you are stretching alone, you could use the wall or tree to help keep the correct alignment or you can use the floor.

Arms and Elbows Behind Your Back

Bring your arms behind your lower back. Start by grabbing one of your wrists with the other hand.

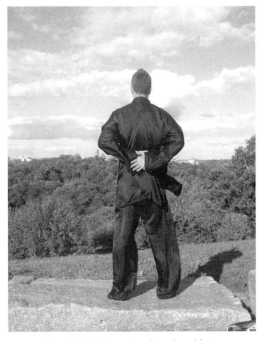

Arms behind lower back and grabbing one wrist with other hand (standing).

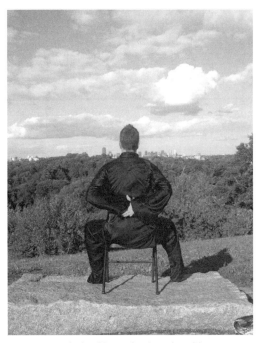

Arms behind lower back and grabbing one wrist with other hand (sitting).

Gradually work toward grasping both elbows with your palms.

Continue breathing deeply. Relax. Repeat the various angles and postures used in the exercises with the elbows over your head.

Push each elbow gently against the wall or tree, about a minute on each side.

Breathe deeply and relax your shoulders as well as your face.

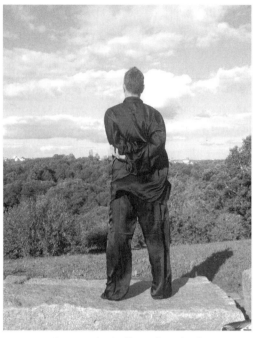

Grasping both elbows (standing).

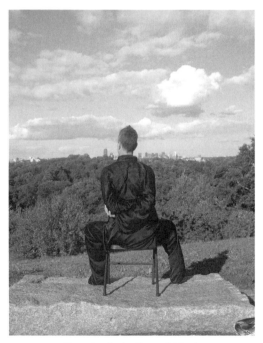

Grasping both elbows (sitting).

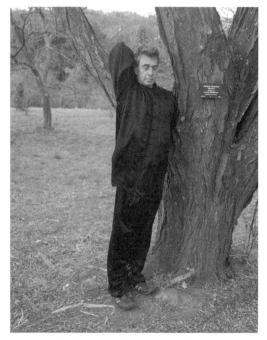

Push elbow gently against wall or tree.

For extra points, see if you can move your forearms up the spine while they are facing one another.

Holding both the arms over your head and the arms behind your back will be harder to perform if your upper body is more developed. The strong muscles on body builders will be more of an obstacle than that of an individual who does not lift weights regularly. On the other hand, I found that teens and elders can move in the full range of motion, from the shoulders and neck, that is, if they have no arthritis or any other upper body issues. Often they can do it more easily than individuals with strong upper body strength. This is all about balance. If you are strong and you developed your soft tissue, that soft tissue may serve as a restrictive force on the skeleton. On the other hand, if you do not have any restriction, you may be able to have a wide-open range of motion, but it may be that when it comes to performing strength tasks you will not be as capable. An individual with a flexible upper body should balance this with strength exercises and the strong upper body individuals should balance this with extra flexibility exercises, which is easier said than done. In order to balance this pattern, each individual needs to determine which skill is needed for his or her body type. Individuals with stronger upper bodies, which restrict flexibility, should focus on the stretching skills, while individuals with open and flexible upper bodies should focus on the wall or tree push-ups and other upper body strengthening skills.

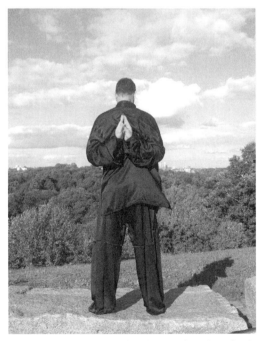

Forearms up the spine with palms touching (standing).

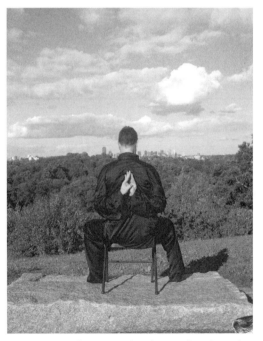

Forearms up the spine with palms touching (sitting).

Mix the Two–The Pretzel

Hold your right arm over your shoulder, with the hand hanging behind your back; reach for it behind your back with your left hand.

This is a difficult position to hold. Follow the principle of 80% effort. Use a yoga belt, a strap, belt, or towel for assistance.

Gradually over weeks and months, you may inch the fingers closer together. Because we are not symmetrical, you may feel the dominant arm has more difficulty reaching from the bottom. When the arm goes over your shoulder and head, the resisting muscles are only the biceps and the triceps. Reaching from the bottom involves other groups of muscles. Because the dominant side is more developed, when reaching from the bottom, there is more resistance that leads to even more restriction. Train both sides until they are both fully stretched.

Use the wall or tree to push gently on each elbow while breathing deeply and mixing in the use of the other mental skills that you have learned in this book as well as in *Sunrise Tai Chi*. Again you will find that when turning the head to the left and right, you will experience totally different sensations.

When you do work with the neck, spend the time needed to relax and lengthen the muscles. Be careful and stretch only 70%. The neck is very sensitive and has many groups, and layers of muscles and other soft tissues. If you push or pull too much and

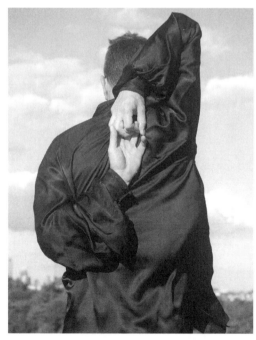

The pretzel. Fingers meet behind back.

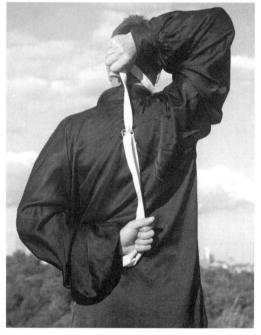

80% effort. Use yoga belt, belt, or towel for assistance.

too far, you will end up with neck pain and sometimes even migraines. Find the balance within balancing the upper body by backing away from looking for strong sensation when performing the upper body exercises. Generally, you are looking to find the 80% effort. When working with the neck, work with 70% effort. Always practice evenly on both sides to develop symmetry. Stretch often and use the props and tools we have recommended. If you are consistent and patient, you will achieve success.

QUADRICEPS STRETCH

The quads are important to stretch for strength and for better and longer performance, as well as to prevent injuries to both the lower back and the knees. For energetic purposes, we want to stretch the quads to create the potential environment for the energy to flow. If the quads are too tight or too weak, the energy flow will become stagnant. An approach that balances between strength and flexibility will lead to smarter quads. In the Eastern arts, there is a strong belief that by using a correct approach, you can actually change the intellect of the soft tissue. Stretching the quads on a daily basis is a part of this plan and also a goal.

This exercise works to stretch the quadricep muscles and tendons between the knee and the hip to prevent knee injuries and allow a higher level of performance with your legs (Figure 46).

QUADRICEPS FEMORIS

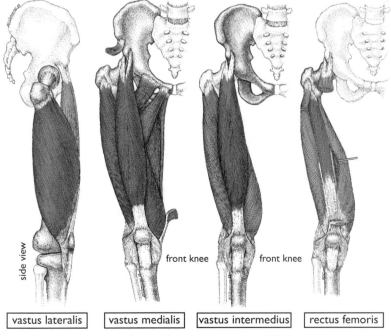

side view — front knee — front knee

| vastus lateralis | vastus medialis | vastus intermedius | rectus femoris |

Figure 46. The quadriceps are made up of four parts.

Keep your spine straight. Adjust the height as needed so that you get a good stretch without stressing your knee. Eventually, you can work toward using the back of a chair or an object at a similar height.

Stretching the quads is essential to protect the knees from injuries but also to upgrade any physical performance using the legs. The typical stretch, usually used by runners, is holding your foot with your hand. Most of the time, this stretch is not done correctly. Often people tilt the pelvis, which creates slack and defeats the purpose.

Even if you are able to perform this stretch with correct alignment, holding the leg is not comfortable and creates tension in your lower back. Holding the leg also discourages you from holding the stretch for the necessary amount of time, two to three minutes, as well as discourages breathing deeply and performing your visualizations.

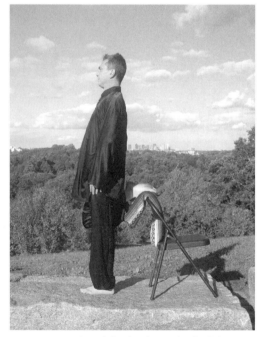

Spine straight with leg back. Use back of chair.

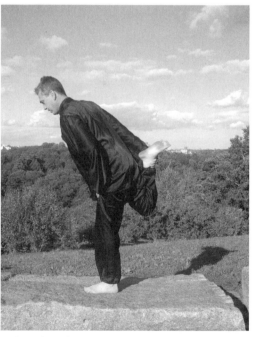

Tilting the pelvis creates slack and defeats purpose.

To identify your range of motion through your quad, start by standing on one leg with the toes pointing straight forward and the other leg bent back and placed on a chair. This is about halfway to the final goal, which is touching your right sitting bone with your right heel. Do the same stretch with the left leg. Once you are comfortable and ready to progress, use a yoga block or any other object to build the height under your foot.

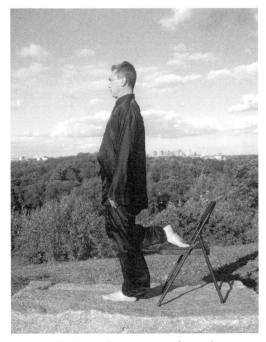

One leg with toes pointing forward, and other leg bent back placed on chair.

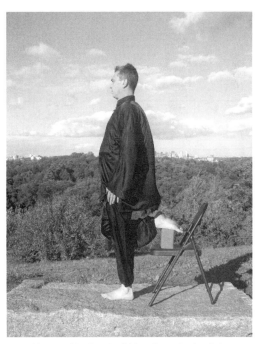

Add yoga block to build height under back foot.

Remember to keep your pelvis aligned while lifting the heel behind you. You can check yourself every now and then by facing the wall or tree with your pelvis, and then lifting the leg. The wall or tree will restrict the movement of the pelvis and will make the stretch purer. Once you are comfortable with each of the exercises, you can mix the mind/body prescriptions.

Make sure your knee is pointing straight down.

I recommend that you hold on to the wall or something stable to help you keep your balance while performing the stretch.

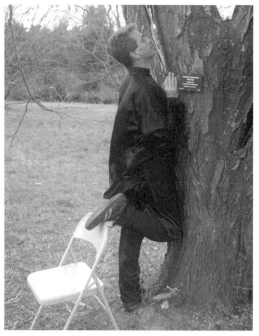

Wall/tree restrict movement of pelvis; make stretch pure.

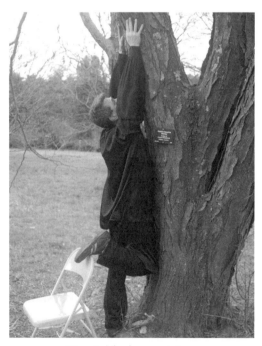

Mix mind/body prescriptions.

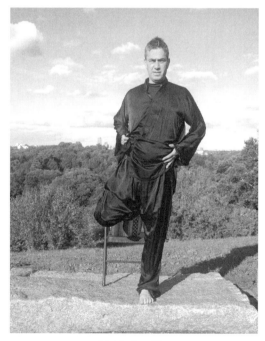

Not to the side.

If you would like to develop your balance as well, you can perform the exercise by standing with no support.

If the front of your foot hurts because of the object you are putting it on, use a pillow or something soft to cushion the front of the foot. Once you eliminate the support and you are practicing both the stretch and balance elements, make sure you distribute the weight on the standing leg between the heel and the ball of the foot. Make sure your inner arches are activated and alive, your spine straight, head suspended, face relaxed, and shoulders dropped. See if you can integrate your other physical and mental skills.

This mind/body prescription is especially effective when the sun is setting. This experience of standing on one leg and sensing the energy of the setting sun on your face and the rest of the body brings you to higher

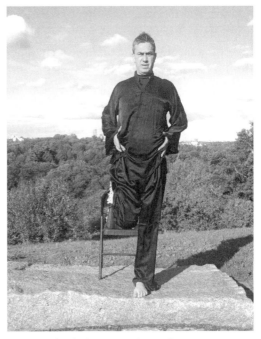

Develop balance; standing with no support.

spiritual places. I have been doing this stretch since I was 10 years old. When I did it, a few years ago, when the sun was setting, I experienced through my entire being the spirit of the heron.

This stretch is done in a stationary position but if you look at the *Sunrise Tai Chi* book (page 67) and DVD, you will see that you can also stretch this muscle through the mind/body prescriptions called walk and kick back. If your knees are healthy and you do not feel the stretch even when your heel is touching the sitting bone, and if you are interested in the next step, you need to perform the next posture, which in Japanese is called seiza.

Seiza

Sitting in seiza regularly can help prevent knee problems and lower back injuries as well as ankle issues. Seiza is the posture of kneeling down on your knees while sitting on your toes. If you want to kneel down on your knees, you must make sure that your knees are healthy and strong and that you do not have any issues with them. If you have knee problems, added pressure from sitting in seiza on the floor may hurt them even more. Even if you do have healthy knees, I would recommend that you put a blanket under them or even two blankets to soften the pressure between the floor and the patella, which is the floating bone in the knee.

You should feel a comfortable stretch in your ankle as well as the front of your thighs rather than a pain in your knees. If you have any knee problems, do not do this floor stretch but do the quad stretch. The seiza stretch should be done carefully and you should progress gradually.

If your quads are really tight, you may not be able to kneel on your knees and sit all the way to your heels. Gradually work toward getting lower and lower in this stretch while using a pillow or block that is the right height for you. Usually I use the purple or the grey yoga blocks that allow me to practice at three different heights.

Place the block underneath your sitting bones. Use any block that reduces the pressure on your knees. As you become more flexible, you will be able to sit on the floor between your heels with no pain or strain in your knees or ankles.

Sit on the block and breathe deeply. Relax your weight into the block while lengthening through the spine. Relax your face and shoulders, coordinate the visualization of the baton with the empty/full moon abdominal movement, and put your mind high up in the heavens as well as deep down into the center of the earth.

Most people do not often stretch their quads. An excellent way of including this stretch in your life is to do it while doing other things; it can be done in front of the TV, you can eat your meals sitting in this posture, you can set up your laptop for this height. The way to achieve this posture is to just spend more time sitting in it. You can pretend that you are in Japan and you are sitting in that style.

The various blocks will give you ways to control the pressure in your knees. You do not want to have pressure on your knees. You want to feel the stretch in the tendons and in the quads, which run from the knee to the hip.

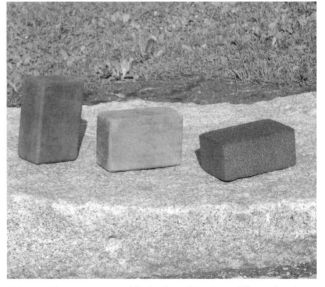

Use purple or grey yoga blocks that allow three different heights.

The ankles should be straight, the toes pointing straight backward, and the heels pointing up. Do not fold the ankles or the feet to the sides. Eventually, you will not need the block and you will be able to sit on the floor between the two heels. You should fit exactly between the two heels.

It is easier to sit in seiza, at first, with the knees apart. This allows a little more slack in the tendons, quads, and outer thighs. As you become more flexible, move your knees closer until they touch each other. The closer the legs, the more difficult it is to hold the posture because the femur bone is straighter and creates a longer distance between the knee and the hip.

Use the higher part of the block to start. When you feel comfortable, move to the second height of the block. Once you improve further, use the lowest part of the block.

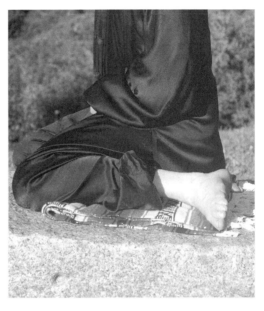

Do not fold ankles to the sides.

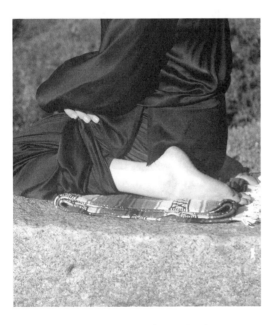

Fit exactly between the two heels, with the heels pointing up.

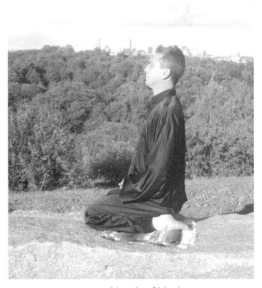

Second height of block.

When you are comfortable using the lowest part of the block, start moving toward the floor. You may need to use a book or a towel until you can sit on the ground.

You want to lengthen your spine all the way from the sitting bones up but at the same time drop the shoulders and relax the face. There are two forces that you want to pay attention to within this posture. The first sensation is a deep sinking heavy feeling from the belly button down to the floor, and the second sensation is a light rising from the belly button up through the spine and a suspension of your head. But you do not want to allow this light and up energy to influence the shoulders and the face. You want to drop through the shoulders, and relax and calm your face.

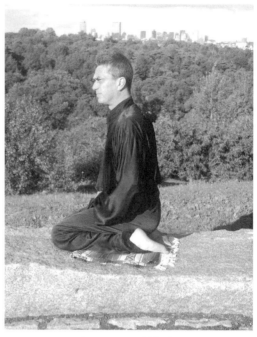

Lowest part of block.

In a Zen temple, seiza is the posture of meditation with a wooden block underneath the sitting bones, or without a block. If you do not use the block, the legs become numb from your weight. The weight pressing against your legs causes the legs to become slightly numb allowing the individual to experience only the trunk, which is one of the purposes of sitting meditation.

Facing the setting sun while sitting in seiza is a powerful experience. Try starting 10 minutes before the sun starts to set and keep going 10 minutes after it sets. Allow the setting sun to caress your entire body and melt, dissolve, and then pull away your impurities. When performing this exercise other times than during the setting sun, close your eyes and try imitating the sensation of the sun to the best you can. This experience means you are becoming more sensitive and aware of the natural energy around you and within you.

Once you feel a little bit of numbness in the legs, you may want to stand up and massage the legs: tap them, and allow the blood to circulate back into the legs. If your legs are numb, you may not be able to get up right away and you may need to sit on the floor and allow them to wake up. Tapping and massaging will always help. When coming out of the posture, be careful of moving sideways away from the posture; that is when you can injure your knees. The idea is to come out without twisting the knees. To come out of this posture, shift the weight onto your palms, into your arms, and then straighten the legs. Straighten them one at a time backward while your weight is on your arms. Sometimes you can hold this posture for two to five minutes. Then you can stand up.

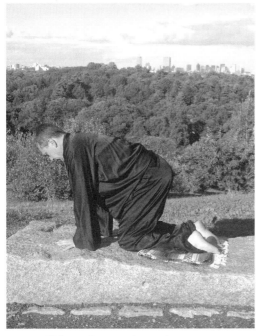

Shift weight into palms and into arms.

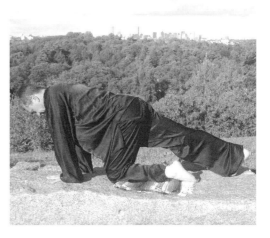

Straighten legs one at a time backward.

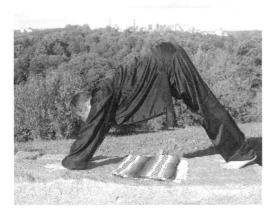

Sometimes hold posture for three minutes.

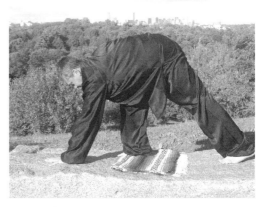

Bring one leg forward, and then stand up.

Over time, you will be able to decrease the height of the block underneath your sitting bones, and then once you are able to sit on the floor and you do not feel the stretch in the quads anymore, your next goal is to lie backward until you are able to lie flat on the ground. Remember, do NOT force this posture. It can injure your knees as well as your lower back very easily. Use caution at all times and recognize at which level you are. You can start by leaning backward against a chair and then gradually work your way down to the floor.

Sit-Ups

This abdominal strengthening exercise should be done carefully. If you have any lower back problems, you should first resolve them before you put any strain on your back. Begin by establishing your personal number of sit-ups, the number you can do comfortably without being too sore or injured the next day. My experience is that most of the people who do some sports can do about 10 and the ones that do not do much with the abdominal muscles can do about five. If you can do 20 to 30 sit-ups, I would consider you to be at an intermediate level and if you can do 30 to 50, and you are not sore the next day, you are in the advanced stage. As your stomach becomes stronger, your number of sit-ups and your level will increase.

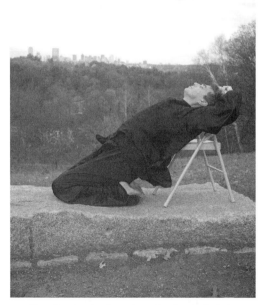

Start leaning backward against back of chair.

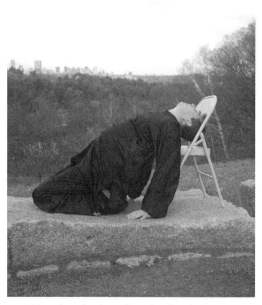

Next, lean backward against the chair seat.

If you are doing sit-ups with your legs under a sofa or having somebody hold your legs, you are defeating the purpose of the exercise. You are not isolating the abdominal muscles purely.

It is not wrong, but you need to understand that you are also strengthening your leg muscles because the fixed point is now at the ankles, which adds the leg muscles to the action of lifting the trunk off the ground. Some individuals will feel pain in the back when doing this kind of sit-up without the legs. In that case, you should stop and not do the sit-ups in this way. Many times, people use their back muscles to lift the trunk and the head. You should learn to use the abdominal muscles and let go of the back ones when moving the trunk off the floor. The minute you sense you are using your back muscles you should stop. It will take longer to achieve the fullest strength in the abdominal muscles if the leg muscles are involved. Both ways are fine as long as you can perform both sets of sit-ups without pain in the lower back.

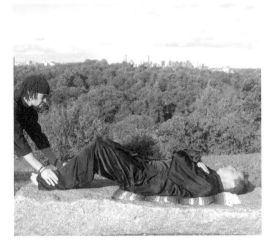

Someone holds legs thus defeating purpose.

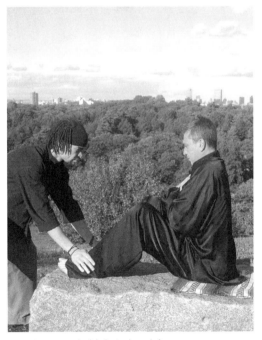

Someone holds legs thus defeating purpose.

Level 1: Lie on your back on top of a blanket with your knees bent. Stretch your arms straight behind you so you can use them to help you do your sit-ups. Relax for a few seconds and breathe deeply. On an inhalation, get ready and as you exhale, swing the arms forward toward the legs and sit up, and bring your chest to your knees. Keep going up and down slowly until you reach your number. If you sense that you are starting to use your back muscles, you have reached your limit and you should stop. Build up the number of sit-ups you do gradually as well as keep stretching this area to avoid injuries.

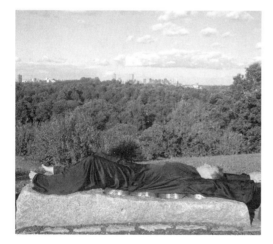

Beginners. Stretch arms straight behind you.

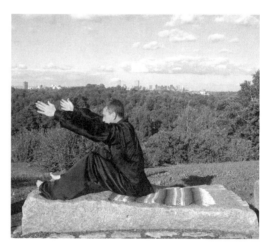

Beginners. Sit-ups using arms.

Level 2: Lie on your back on top of a blanket. Bend your knees. Place your arms in an X on your chest, relax for a few seconds, and breathe deeply. On your next inhalation get ready, and as you exhale, sit up and bring your chest to your knees.

Keep going up and down slowly until you reach whatever number of reps is best for you. If you sense that you are starting to use your back muscles, you did too many and you should stop. Build up the number of sit-ups you do, gradually, and keep stretching this area to avoid injuries.

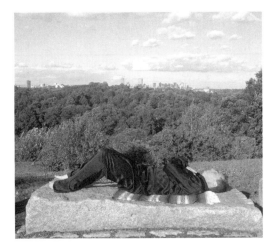

Intermediate. Bend knees and place arms in an X on your chest.

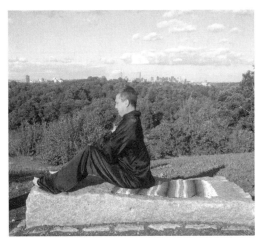

Intermediate. Exhale and sit up bringing chest to knees.

Level 3: Lie on your back on top of a blanket, place your legs on a chair or any other object that will hold your knees in a 90% angle, and place your arms in an X on your chest. Relax for a few seconds and breathe deeply; on your next inhalation get ready and as you exhale, sit up and bring your chest to your knees.

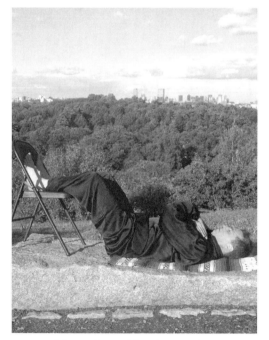

Advanced sit-up. Place legs on chair.

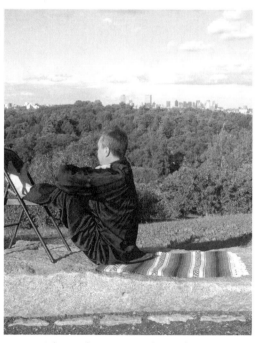

Advanced sit-up. Bring chest to knees.

Keep going up and down slowly until you reach your number. If you need help to start this posture, use the trick of starting with your arms behind your head and using them to help lift your trunk. After just a short period of time, you will not need your arms any more.

If you sense that you are starting to use your back muscles, you did too many and you should stop. Practice at whatever level is best for you. Work toward the goal of practicing sit-ups with the feet elevated. This may take weeks or months of regular practice. Set a goal for yourself, balance with serious stretching, and progress gradually to avoid injuries

The setting sun is used to expel impurities from the body. When you come up, you exhale and that is when you send your impurities toward the horizon, toward the setting sun. The power of the setting sun will dissolve, pull, and take your impurities away quickly and efficiently. That means that when you are inhaling and moving back and down, you also need to scan the body, collect your impurities, and bring them to the solar plexus area. When you come up and forward, exhale and send the impurities toward the setting sun.

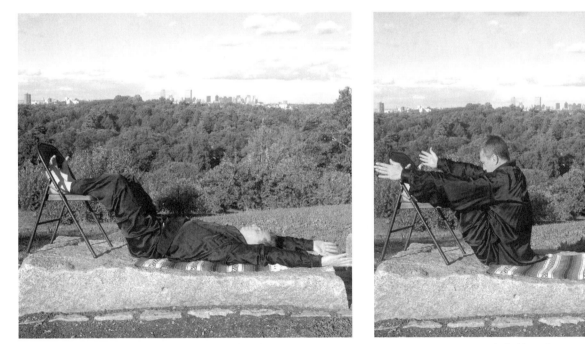

Arms behind your head.   Use arms to help lift trunk.

SIT AND REACH FORWARD STRETCH

Sit and reach is a stretch that helps balance the neck, upper back, lower and middle back, and the back of the legs. When you are able to just 'fold in half' or reach your toes with your palms, you will experience the most enjoyable transparency through most of the back of the body. It gives you the unique sensation of being loose and free that may have a positive effect on negative moods for some people. There are studies documenting that losing physical independence leads to depression. This stretch, because it involves a big part of the body, is extremely effective in preventing loss of physical capabilities. To start this stretch, you may want to sit on a block or something that will give you an angle down from your sitting bones toward your toes.

Of course, if you had a board set at an angle that will be the optimal tool for the beginner's stage.

Sit on the floor, or the board, and straighten your legs. Flex the toes toward you and flex the heel forward. Bend forward and reach toward your toes. Keep the knees as straight as you can without hyper-extending them. If you cannot reach the toes, place a belt around the balls of your feet and use the belt as an extension of your arms.

Remember to use 80% effort. Relax and let the lower back and hamstrings gradually stretch. Breathe deeply into the back of your lungs and, as you exhale, soften the muscles. Lengthen through the spine upward instead of thinking downward. You want

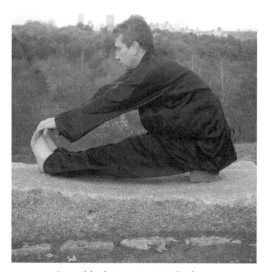

Sit on block to give an angle down
from sitting bones toward toes.

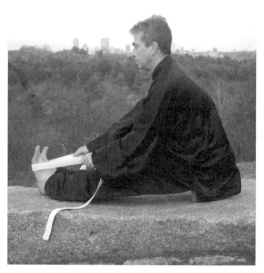

Place belt around balls of feet
and use it as extension of arms.

to keep your spine straight and do not break the alignment. At the beginning level, you should be able to achieve a 45-degree angle with your spine.

Over time, the muscles will stretch and you will be able to move to the next level in this stretch.

The next goal with sit and reach is to move the trunk lower and to try grabbing the toes with your hands without the belt. Stretch forward and reach your toes with your fingers, grasp the toes gently, and lengthen through the spine. Keep moving the thoracic spine in and up to prevent the spine from collapsing. The sensation in the spine should be like an airplane taking off. Start from the sacrum and take off along your spine all the way to the top of the head.

This level will open your lower back and stimulate the kidneys. Gradually work toward getting lower; your arms and hands will help adjust the height to be right for you. Lengthen your back, so that you have a straight sensation through the spine rather than a curved sensation. Relax your face, neck, and shoulders while breathing deeply into the back of your lungs.

Over time, you will be able to fold in half, which means that you have freed yourself from being a prisoner of a major portion of your soft tissues.

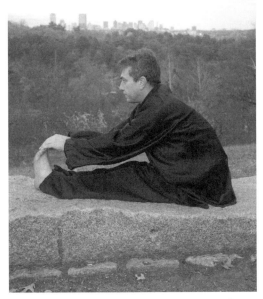 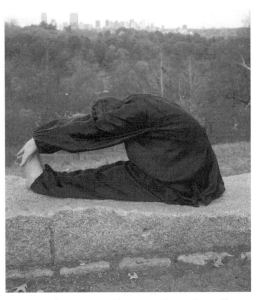

Sensation in spine like an airplane taking off.

Start from sacrum like an airplane taking off along spine all the way to top of head.

When you use the belt or the fingers to pull the trunk toward the toes, you are actively performing this stretch, pulling with a bit more force. There is yet another way to do this stretch that is more passive.

The idea is that you can use both styles. Some days we need to be aggressive and other days we need to balance with being passive. Sometimes you can start aggressively doing the stretch and finish passively, and vice versa.

First, you want to put some pillows on top of your thighs right around the knee area; any pillow will do: a bolster or yoga pillow. Yoga blocks on a chair work well. Then lean just your forehead on the pillow while your legs are straight and the feet are relaxed, not flexed as they are when doing the stretch actively. Make sure you leave room for breathing. Your nose and mouth should be unobstructed. That means that only your forehead is leaning, gently, on the objects in front of you.

Relax and drop the weight of your trunk into the pillow or whatever is supporting your head. In this posture, the spine is relaxed. You are allowed to have some slack in the legs and a mild collapsed sensation through the spine because you are being passive. Breathe deeply and stay calm.

Over time, you will be able to straighten and lengthen the spine and you will be able to fold in half within the passive posture. That is the goal. Different people will feel the stretch in different areas. Some will sense their neck and upper back being stretched,

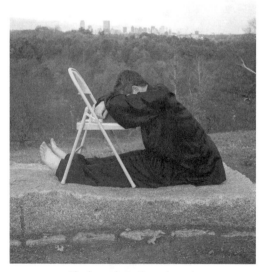

Block on chair. Sit and reach
with the legs relaxed (passive).

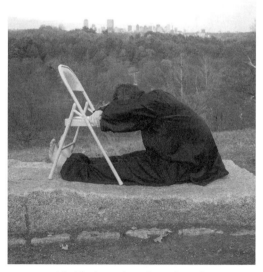

No block on chair. Sit and reach
with legs relaxed (passive).

and others may sense the calves, the hamstrings, or lower back. Over time, you will loosen the tight muscles that restrict your freedom of motion. This is why this is a great stretch; it stretches you all the way from the heels along the calf, hamstring, lower back, upper back, and neck.

Pull yourself slightly back and do not try to reach as far as you do in the active stretch. Make sure your spine is straight. You are moving your trunk down from your hips so you should be able maintain a straight spine. Also, the object in front of your chest should help you maintain a straight spine. Eventually, you will be able to move all the way down while your spine is straight. Using a yoga block or some books under your sitting bones creates a little bit of an angle between the sitting bones and the heels. This angle will make a huge difference; it restricts the legs from bending at the knees and it gives you a bit of an advantage because gravity is now on your side.

Doing this posture at sunset or at night is special because it strengthens the visualization of draining the energetic baton. You move the trunk and the spine up and forward while the mind is moving from the upper energy center down to the lower one. When your mind can reside in the lower energy center and your upper energy center is cool and calm, you will experience your bubble more strongly as well as in a unique way because this posture is not one that occurs very often.

The ability to fully do this stretch reflects a flexible individual because the stretch involves so many groups of muscles. Many people think that children are flexible. From my experience, I have noticed that if you do not have them do the stretch sit and reach, you will realize how stiff children are. If they do not train, they are not flexible at all. They just seem to be flexible. They do not have as much strength in their muscles, which means less resistance, not more flexibility, and their flexibility is at the joint areas. Sitting on the floor requires much joint flexibility, and children's ability to sit comfortably on the floor makes them look like they are flexible. Ask any child to do this stretch. Kids who are seven or eight years old, toddlers, babies, and especially teens will not be able to grip their toes while keeping their legs and knees straight.

The general population is stiff because of lifestyle, not natural ability. Many of our muscles are tight and stiff simply from the lack of use.

The good news is that it does not matter what age you are. With the correct information and practice, you will be able to free your skeleton from being a prisoner of your soft tissue, and you will be able to sit and reach all the way down to your toes.

The setting sun will help with the sinking of the trunk toward the legs. Remember, although you do not only sink, you also have a lengthening through the spine, which is represented in the moving of the sun. Sink and lengthen especially if you have the opportunity to do this exercise while the sun is setting. Use the setting sun to encourage these forces, sinking and lengthening, when stretching aggressively or passively. Use the setting sun to cleanse the entire body when you are in this stretch.

Sit and Reach on Two Chairs

This stretch can be also done between two chairs. Sit on one all the way back and have the heels on the other. The same rule that we talked about when doing the posture on the floor applies to when doing it on two chairs. Just make sure your chairs are strong and stable.

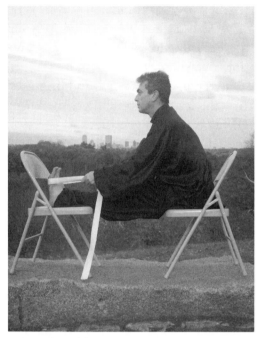

Sit and reach between two chairs with yoga belt.

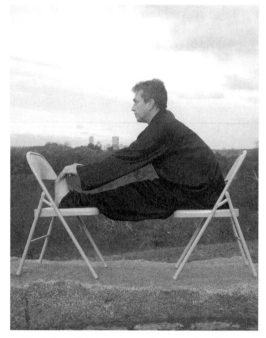

Sit and reach between two chairs, and grab toes.

BALANCING THE LOWER BACK

The Three Musketeers or Vitamin 'L'—Lower Back

Balance is a big word and achieving this with your lower back requires constant practice between stretching and strengthening while knowing when to take a break. It also means to keep the lower back warm if you live in a cold climate or close the window at night. One of the reasons I called the next set of stretches Vitamin L is that over the years I have witnessed how disciplined many individuals are with their vitamins and other pills. I would wish that they would be as disciplined with the various principles of the Eastern arts. I thought that if I called it Vitamin L, people would treat this stretch as a pill and consistently take it or use it the same way they are consistent with their other pills. I analyzed the lower back structure and found out that, between the vertebrae, there are three major small groups of muscles that create the various movements we can perform with our back: forward, rotation, and lateral. This is the reason for the second name for this mind/body prescription, the Three Musketeers. The names attempt to motivate individuals to stick with the routines of the mind/body prescriptions.

The three musketeers are the three different postures that you are doing while sitting on the floor or a chair. The first is straight: forward and down. The second is left: forward and down, and the third musketeer is moving forward and down to the right. You can use the setting sun to cleanse the body from stress and tension that we built throughout the day, but we also use the setting sun to imitate the setting of the trunk to the different directions.

Our lifestyle contributes to tight and stiff lower backs, especially in men. Before we know it, we are waking up in the morning with a stiff lower back and it takes hours before we feel we can function again. By the time men are 35, most cannot touch their fingers to the ground while keeping their legs straight. Some of the problem is the hamstrings but another big part is the lower back. Parents cannot play with their kids on the floor and lifting them becomes harder. If you let this tension build for too long, you may develop sciatica nerve problems, bulging discs, or, even worse, ruptured discs. This situation can be prevented, and much agony, pain can be prevented. All you need to do is to make this stretch part of your day-to-day routine, and you will enjoy a strong open back that will lead to a positive chain reaction in the rest of your life.

This stretch is one of the most effective ways to release the lower back muscles, as well as to prevent lower back injuries. Many individuals only stretch straight forward, which is only one of the three musketeers that stretch the muscles on both sides of the lower back. Yet they do not spend the time to stretch the muscles on each side of the spine separately.

Stretching the lower back and stimulating the kidneys are very important exercises in all Eastern arts because on our middle back around the kidney area, we have a small gate, which is considered as the life doors of our energetic system. This gate acts like the valve in a pressure cooker. This valve regulates our energetic system when too much fire energy is filling our bodies. If the area is not open, loose, or flexible, this valve will not function to its potential resulting in an unbalanced energetic system.

Another important reason for this posture is that when breathing deeply, the lung cells in different parts of your lungs are stimulated. While in this posture, the gentle tension in the front directs the breath into the back parts of your lungs. While in this forward-bending posture, try moving the skin on your back with your breathing and regain control over those muscles.

This stretch, like several others, can be practiced at a basic, intermediate, or more advanced level. Practice whichever one is appropriate for you. Start while sitting with your legs crossed, or as my kids call it 'criss cross apple sauce.'

Some of you may be stuck on this posture for a while until your knees are touching the floor. If you start moving forward toward the groin and your knees are not fully down, you will hurt your knees or your lower back. To release the knees down, you need to spend more time in the posture. For example, do it while watching TV or when reading a book. I recommend placing a pillow(s) under each knee that is not resting on the ground.

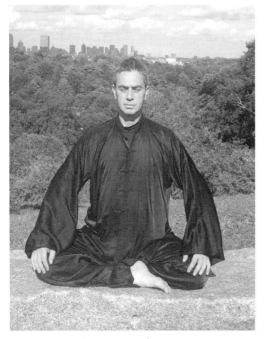

Criss cross apple sauce.

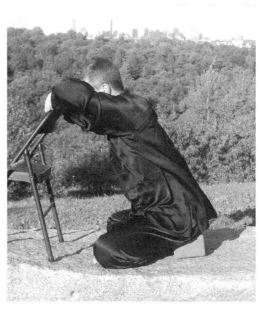

Beginners. Straight forward with yoga block.

When putting the support under your knees, you are first preventing injuries to the joints, the knees, or hips, and second, you are tricking the mind to let go and release the entire leg. You will achieve more in this stretch by backing away through using the support. For the knees to touch the floor, you need both your groin and your hips to be open. These areas are part of the pelvic floor, an area that is very dense with soft tissue. It may take some time to achieve this posture. Until you reach the time that your knees are touching the ground in the crossed leg posture, you can achieve the benefits of the three musketeers, forward, right, and left, to your lower and middle back, the neck as well as the energetic benefits, through doing the stretch using two chairs, or a chair and a table. (Sit on the edge of one chair and lean toward another chair or a table.) Keep sitting on the floor to create the flexibility in the groin and outer hips. Once your knees are touching the ground, you are ready to move to the floor and enjoy the full benefits of the complete postures.

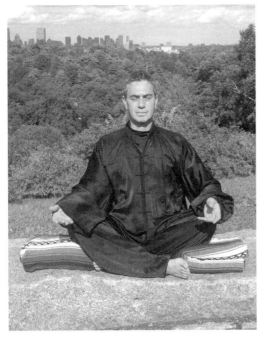

Placing pillows or blankets under each knee.

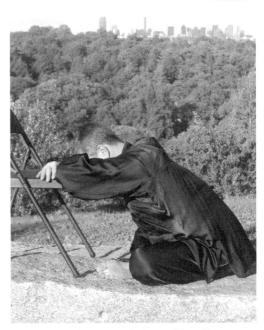

Intermediate. Straight forward from floor.

First Musketeer: Straight Down and Forward: 12 O'clock

Sit with your legs crossed. Relax for a few moments, and breathe deeply and quietly. Use the inhalation to move the spine upward and the exhalation to relax your shoulders and face. On your next inhalation, move downward from your hips. Imagine two handles at the outer hips and by turning them forward, your entire trunk moves forward. Your spine should stay straight when you lean your forehead on the support or the floor.

Place your elbows over your head while your forehead is leaning on the support. Leave space for your eyes and nose so you can breathe comfortably.

Stay in this stretch for two to three minutes. Lengthen through the spine and sink through the legs and pelvis. Breathe deeply and perform empty-full moon, drain the energetic baton, and build your energetic bubble. Over time, you will be able to move through the different heights while keeping your spine straight. Notice the sensation around both kidneys when you are down and then again when coming up. The tension when going down slows the energy flow through the life doors, mingmen, and when coming up and releasing the lower back muscles, the life door gate will open and you may sense the energy moving out.

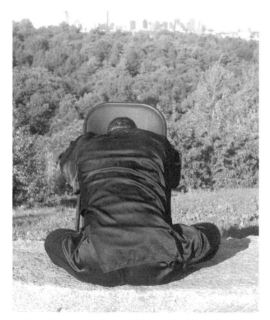

First Musketeer. Forward from hips (12 o'clock).

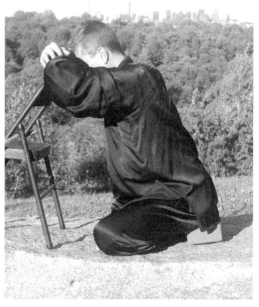

Elbows over head with forehead leaning and leaving space for eyes and nose.

Second Musketeer: To the Left Down and Forward

After you finish moving to the center, you can either come up first and then turn a notch to the left, and move down to your left. The other option is to swing your body to the left from your forward position. Different individuals experience the two options differently. Experiment and see for yourself what is best for you. I like to come back up and then go down again. When ending in the stretched posture, there is a tendency to move to the left slightly farther than needed. Move in the direction of 11 o'clock and not 10:00 o'clock. If you angle too far left, you will break the alignment in both the spine and the ribs, and you will lose the pure stretch.

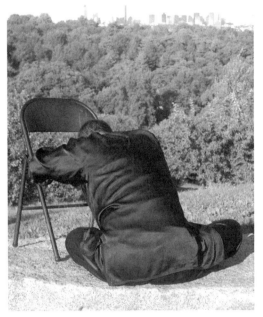

Second Musketeer. Left down and forward (11 o'clock).

People sometimes have a tendency to twist a bit to the side in this stretch. Try to keep your chest parallel to the floor during the stretch. The body will find whatever way it can to achieve the tasks we give it, but sometimes this option comes at the expense of correct alignment. Use your chin and forehead as indicators to make sure that your trunk is straight. Choose two spots on your forehead, one on the left and the other on the right, as indicators. If you are going down to the right, there will be a tendency to touch the object in front with the right part of your forehead. It is easier for the body to get down this way. Balance this tendency by tilting from the trunk, not the neck. Create an even, gentle pressure on both spots of your forehead.

You can do the same with the chin. Choose two spots on your chin, one on the outer left and the other one on the outer right. When going down, make sure both spots touch the object you are using as a prop, gently and evenly. If you want to find the middle, just use the forehead and the chin as indicators. Turn your trunk slightly to the right and then to the left and then you will find your center. This is a tai chi key point: "Look to the left, be aware of the right, then you will have a center." Once you have identified and understand the use of the two spots as indicators, do the same when going to the sides.

Third Musketeer: To the Right, Down, and Forward

After you spend two to three minutes on the left, come back up and turn slightly to the right; then stretch down to the right while keeping your spine straight. Place your forehead or your chin on the object in front and use the two spots on the chin or the forehead to make sure your trunk is straight. Breathe deeply—elbows over your head.

Notice the sensation in the lower back area in relationship to the center. You will find that when moving to the right or left, one side of your back will more tense than the other. These three stretches create various positions in which the tensing and relaxing of different groups of muscles also performs a gentle massage to your internal organs, especially the kidneys.

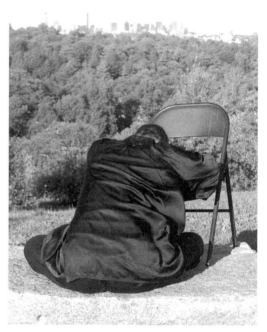

Third Musketeer. Right down and forward (1 o'clock).

Remember to change your leg position from day to day. Have the right leg in front on some days and the left one on others. If you do not do this, you will create an imbalance in the groin and the hips, which can lead to problems in the lower back. Changing the leg position allows you to stretch evenly in all directions.

Gradually work toward getting lower, using the various props and blocks to adjust the height to be appropriate for the condition of your body. Lengthen your back, so that you have a straight sensation through the spine, rather than a curved sensation. Relax your face, neck, and shoulders while breathing deeply into the back of your lungs. Mix in all your visualizations and you will enjoy this stretch tremendously. The 12 o'clock stretch is another one of the stretches besides the passive sit and reach stretch during which I can fall asleep doing. When having neck problems, this stretch is a tremendous help. Placing your forehead on a support gives the neck a rest. If you touch your neck while in this position, you can feel how loose it is.

Lower Back Stretch on a Chair

If you cannot sit on the floor with your knees flat, do this variation of the stretch first. You can stretch using two chairs to achieve the important stretching of your back and the regulating of your life doors.

Sit on the edge of a chair and place another chair in front of you. First, place the chair with the back rest toward you, and put your elbows over your head.

Then when you do not feel the stretch anymore, turn the chair around and put a yoga block on top of the seat. The next step is to stretch from one seat to the other.

The same rules apply to this stretch as doing it on the floor. Do all three postures or angles while breathing deeply and trying to move the skin on your upper back through the deep breathing. Integrate the visualizations and our other skills. I stretch from a chair every now and then even though I can do it on the floor. Pulling yourself back to the basic version of any exercise while practicing is a good habit. It gives you an opportunity to experience various aspects of the five building blocks differently.

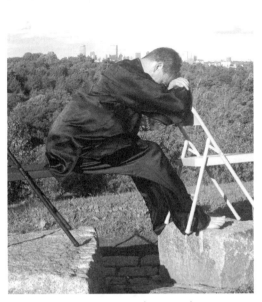

Beginners. From a chair to a chair.

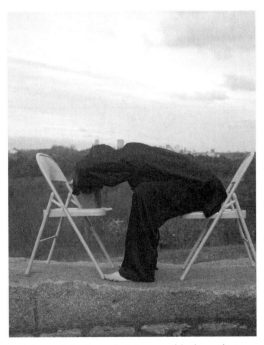

Intermediate. From chair to yoga block on chair.

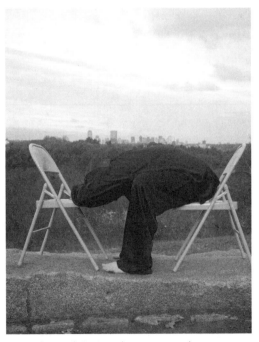

Advanced. From a chair seat to a chair seat.

HAMSTRING STRETCHES

Because the hamstrings are the most stubborn muscles in our body, we need to constantly stretch them. If you think about it, the hamstrings are one of the muscles that do not have any strengthening exercises. The reason is that the function of the muscle puts them in a special category. They are constantly working and working hard. This is why you can find stretching exercises for hamstrings but not much when it comes to strengthening.

The hamstring is connected to the sitting bones at the top and to the back of the knee at the bottom. The hamstring's job is to hold the whole trunk upright when standing and while sitting (Figure 47).

THE HAMSTRING MUSCLES
The most stubborn muscle in the body, made up of three parts

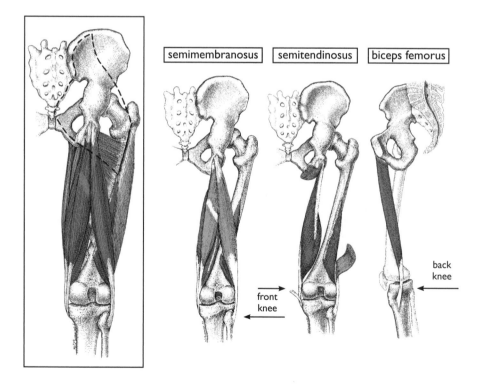

Figure 47. The Hamstring is in charge of bending the knee and holding the trunk muscles upright.
LifeART image copyright 2010. Wolters Kluwer Health, Inc. – Lippincott Williams & Wilkins. All rights reserved.

This task puts tremendous stress on the hamstrings and if not stretched properly, it also puts stress on the lower back as well as the knees. Another symptom that is a byproduct of tight hamstrings is pain from the sciatic nerves. When your lower back and your hamstrings reach a certain tight point, the fiber puts pressure on the sciatic nerves. It is often painful and debilitating.

It is very important to stretch the hamstrings so I am including several ways to stretch them. In this way, you can include stretching into your life and you will have different options to achieve the goal of keeping the hamstring flexible at all times. One leg up is one way to stretch the hamstrings. Another is Vitamin H, an exercise from the *Sunrise Tai Chi* book (page 57). Another way is by putting one of your legs up on the wall while the other is straight on the floor.

Having the hamstrings flexible at all times is a martial arts concept. After all, the hamstrings are the muscles that help perform kicks. Imagine a martial artist stumbling into a fight and telling his or her opponent that today is not a good day for him to fight because his hamstrings are too tight. No, that is not even an option. As a martial artist, my leg should always be able touch my opponent's face, but that takes constant stretching of my legs, not my face.

The variety of the stretches will give you the opportunity to incorporate hamstring stretches into your life. When you are outside waiting for the trolley, subway, or the bus, you can put your leg up on a fence, a bench, or a wall. You can bend over when in the shower, or when waking up or after work you can lie on your back and stretch more passively.

The bottom line is you need to stretch the hamstrings a few times a day and not for short one minute stretches. Stretch for three to four minutes at a time. If you do reach a stage of having flexible and strong hamstrings, you will enjoy higher performance in your legs as well as have a sense of lightness and speed. But most importantly, you will prevent injuries in two major areas: the lower back and your knees. By preventing injury, you will save yourself pain and agony while having an excellent quality of physical functioning no matter what your age.

Hamstring Stretch–One Leg Up

Stand with your feet straight and take a few breaths. Place one leg straight forward into a chair, or any other surface, that is the right height for you.

Breathe deeply, with long, calm, quiet, peaceful inhalations. Some days, hold on to the wall or another chair to eliminate any issues with balance that can inhibit your ability to relax and stretch properly. On other days, perform the stretch without support to experience performing the stretch while challenging your balance.

To create a good stretch in the calf, you will need to flex the ankle of the leg that is up. The toes move toward you while the heel pushes out and away. Allow your hamstrings and calf muscles to stretch gradually over two to three minutes.

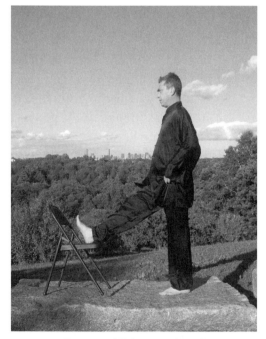

Beginners. Left foot straight and right leg/heel on chair.

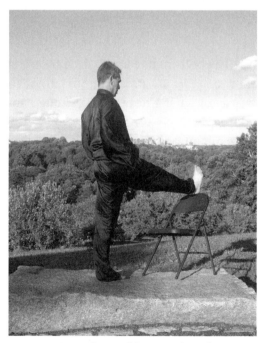

Intermediate. Left foot straight and right leg/heel top of chair.

The leg muscles of the standing leg should be active. Raise up the kneecaps with your thigh muscles while pushing gently against the floor with your heels. Do not lock the knees. The spine should be relaxed. Distribute your weight between the ball of the foot and the heel and make sure the inner arch of the standing leg is not collapsed. The toes of the standing leg should eventually face forward, but to control the 80% effort in this stretch, you may find that by angling the toes slightly to the outside you can lift your leg higher as well as control the stretch through the standing leg's quads. Yes, some individuals feel the stretch in more than one place. To be able to do the stretch with the toes of the standing leg facing forward will demand more stretching if you are tight. It is important in all your stretches to take your time and gradually work toward the final posture.

The next area that often needs work to do this stretch properly is the pelvis. In order to lift the leg up, the body will compensate by tilting the pelvis. This tilt of the pelvis is not correct alignment.

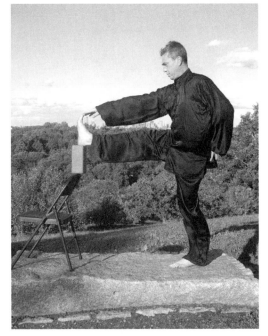

Advanced. Left foot straight and right
leg/heel on yoga block on chair.

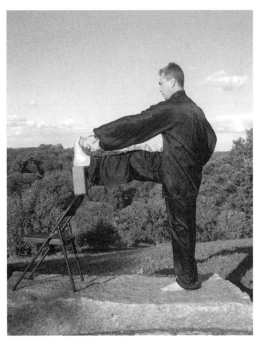

One leg up, final posture.

This tilt of the pelvis occurs more in the martial art world where the goal is to kick someone and it does not matter if the hip is tilted or not. In fact, by tilting the hip, you can generate more power to your kick. Because we are not kicking anyone, we need to have correct alignment. You may find that by lowering the height of the stretched leg, you will be able to drop through the hip of the leg that is up and lift through the hip of the standing leg. This movement through the hip will align the pelvis. When looking from the back, you should see a straight line through the pelvis and sitting bones.

Many individuals, when performing this stretch, bend down with their spine to reach the toes of the leg that is up. Doing so increases the sensation in the hamstring of the leg that is up but again, you are breaking alignment in your spine, your lungs are collapsed, and the rest of your internal organs are compressed.

Straighten your spine, drop your shoulders, suspend the head, and relax your face.

Next, you would want to start rotating toward the leg that is up. Rotate your trunk to the left if your left leg is up. Keep the hip evenly open as well as the standing leg's toes facing forward. Over time, when your leg can reach higher to about solar plexus height, you will be able to touch the toes of the leg that is up without collapsing the trunk but while actually lengthening through the spine while reaching your toes with your palm.

Once your leg is up around the solar plexus height, if the left leg is up, reach with the left hand and touch the toes of your left foot.

Perform the stretch for 2 to 3 minutes. After a few weeks, try reaching your toes with the opposite palm/arm.

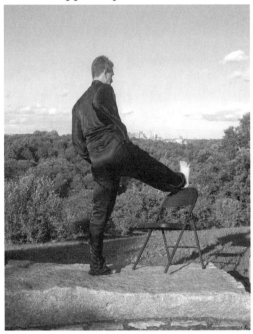

This tilt of pelvis is not correct alignment.

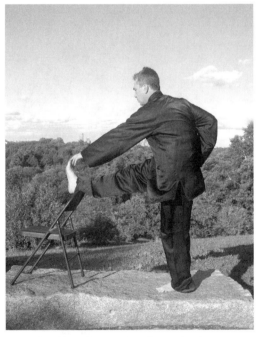

Breaking alignment in spine so that lungs are collapsed and organs are compressed.

Once you are done stretching the left leg, switch legs and now lift the right leg and place it on a chair or any other surface. Flex through the right ankle to stretch the calf. Raise the kneecap of the left leg while pushing down into the floor with the sole of your foot, and then lengthen the spine and drop the right sitting bones while lifting through the left hip joint. As you become more flexible, you will be able to close your eyes as well as to put your leg higher and higher while keeping correct alignment.

When stretching, remember to use your mind to sense deeper and deeper into the layers of soft tissue. Also, use the setting sun to cleanse the entire physical as well as energetic body. Allow the setting sun to caress your face and dissolve any tension or stress. This skill will improve over time.

Hamstring Stretch–While Sitting on a Chair

This stretch can be done using two chairs on days you cannot stand or when you do not feel like standing. Sit on the edge of one chair and place your left leg on the other. Use a belt to pull on the ball of the foot of the left leg. Keep your spine and trunk relaxed and open.

When you do not feel the stretch any more, lift the leg higher, maybe onto a table or the back part of the chair. At this point, you are not going to need the belt unless you are very tight in the lower back, in which case you should not lift your leg to a higher height.

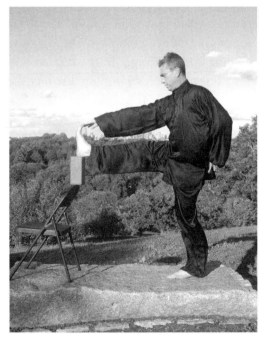

Right leg at solar plexus height
while right hand touches toes.

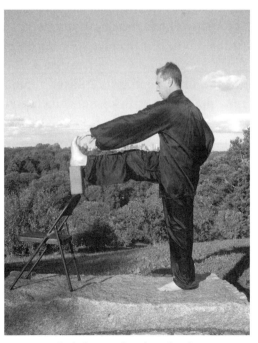

Right leg at solar plexus height
while left hand touches toes.

SUNSET MEDITATION

This meditation can be practiced indoors or out. For best results, face the West. At the end of the day, our bodies are often stiff and sore. For many of us, our minds are still at work. It is very important to make time to wind down and let go of this stress that accumulates and is held in the body. We all know the typical sayings and sensations of how difficult this change could be: "It is hard for me to let go," or "I cannot wind down." This meditation is designed to help you dissolve this tension as well as rejuvenate the body and evoke spirituality. By adding this meditation at the end of the mind/body practice as well as at the end of every day, you will not only release tension and impurities, but you will also increase your own energy while experiencing the natural forces around you.

The sunset meditation is an ancient traditional method of allowing the power of the setting sun to pull away the tension and stress that has built up through your day and is stored in the physical and energetic body. It is an essential method to achieve balance. If your winters are cold and you want to be outside when performing this meditation, wrap yourself with a blanket.

Sit on the edge of the chair or stand with your feet shoulder-width apart. Face the setting sun, close your eyes, breathe calmly, and sense the warmth of the sun on your face and the entire body. Relax your entire body. Drop your shoulders, keep your head suspended, drop your tailbone, lengthen the thoracic spine, slightly bend your knees, and have the tongue touch the roof of your mouth.

After you have been standing for a few minutes, add some visualizations. Allow the setting sun to first dissolve your impurities. Then visualize the setting sun pulling away all the tension and impurities that have built in your body throughout the day. As you become more familiar with this meditation, bring your mind down into the earth at the same time you are dissolving and emptying out all your impurities.

One of our biggest problems is that many of us do not know how to wind down or change phases when we come home. We do not know how to change the racing mind that was needed at work. Activating higher brain waves to achieve success at work is essential and changing that when coming home is very difficult. Over time and with practice, you will be able to let go more easily and quickly. The Sunset Tai Chi mind/body program is very effective in helping you make this transition.

For example, if you are home from work at five or six o'clock, you could finish a set of the Sunset Tai Chi program by seven o'clock, which will allow you four to five hours of being in a relaxed state before bedtime. But if you do not let go and you still carry that stressful stuff with you and at eleven o'clock at night you are still thinking of work, you have a problem. You go to bed but you cannot sleep because your brain needs time to wind down. When you do fall asleep, you will not get deep, restful sleep. It is all about the positive chain reaction versus the negative chain reaction. By doing that little step right in between coming from work and starting your evening at home or whatever you do after work, you allow a very strong, efficient transition that will allow you to enjoy the rest of the night as well prepare you to enjoy the next day.

Sunset meditation can be done either sitting or standing. You can start by standing and then sit as well. Stand and open the palms sideways, almost like putting yourself in a vulnerable energetic position, as if you are exposed and open.

Close your eyes and look toward the sun. Relax the entire body; relax, but do not collapse. Breathe deeply through the nose and sigh to relax the lungs. Lengthen through the spine, drop the shoulders, and relax your face. Scan the body—you will notice that if you put your mind just a millimeter away from the muscles, you can feel your skin. Scan the entire skin from the top of the head down to your toes. Just sense the skin of your body. Once you scan from the top down, move a little deeper and feel the fascia, the thin membrane between the skin and the muscles. Sense and notice the fascia in a continuous web throughout your body. Keep breathing deeply through the nose while the tongue touches the roof of the mouth. Then move your mind a little further inward and sense the muscles. You

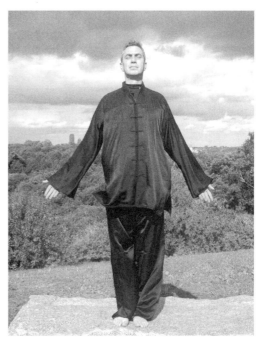

Sunset meditation. Open palms with legs together (standing).

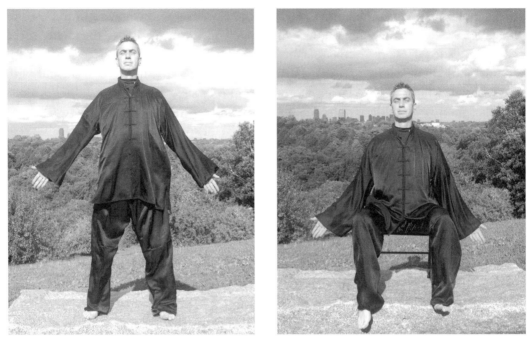

Sunset meditation. Open palms
with legs apart (standing).

Sunset meditation. Open palms (sitting).

may notice that the muscles feel a little warmer because the blood flows through them while the skin does not have as much circulation. Move your mind deeper within the body and sense the bones and the bone marrow. You may notice that they have a cooler sensation than the muscles.

When you scan the various soft tissues, you may find that within the various soft tissue there are little pockets of stagnation, stress, or areas that feel tight or tense. This feeling is associated with dark colors or a cold feeling for some people. You may feel tingling or numbness in those areas. You may know of an area in your body that is holding stress. We refer to these pockets of stress as impurities. On an inhalation, scan the various soft tissues for those impurities. We tend to store and hold much stress in the physical body but also in the energetic body. *Remember, you may also scan the energetic body, which is an energy field a fist away from our skin.* You will be surprised; you may find some impurities actually residing within the energetic body.

Once you identify the impurities, use the mind and the warmth of the setting sun to help dissolve those impurities. Work with these images: ice to water and water to gas, or solid to liquid and liquid to gas. Our mind is very powerful and is able to dissolve some of those pockets and impurities. Utilizing the sun will provide an even stronger and much more powerful effect.

After you spend some time and allow the impurities to be dissolved by your mind and the setting sun, allow the energy of the setting sun to draw out all those melted impurities, as well as the ones that you did not melt, and release them far into the horizon. The more you relax and not collapse, the easier it will be for the sun to draw those impurities away from your body. Lengthening gently through the spine, dropping the shoulders, and keeping the lungs relaxed, the head suspended, and the face relaxed, will allow the impurities to leave your body more easily.

Even after years of training, the first few minutes of dissolving the impurities are important. The extra help you get from the setting sun is worth making time for. I feel the impurities leaving my body one by one in maybe five to ten second intervals. I wait another 10-15-20 seconds and maybe another one will leave and disappear or dissolve. As I continue the visualization, the impurities leave my body more quickly and more easily. It is like making popcorn; at first, you hear a few pops and soon you hear more and more. That is very similar to my experience of dissolving the impurities using the setting sun.

When holding the arms to the sides, palms facing forward, some individuals may experience fatigue throughout the arms and the shoulders. The more you lengthen through the spine and drop the shoulders, the less fatigue you will feel. If the arms do get tired and you want to switch, you can lay your arms on top of your knees if sitting, or on the front of your legs if standing. The palms still face forward.

Breathe deeply, close your eyes, keep the palms a fist away from the body, face toward the sun, and the tongue touching the roof of the mouth. Lift the head slightly toward the heavens. You do not need to perform any of the other skills; just scan for impurities, dissolve, and allow the sun to take them away. This is a more passive process than other mind/body prescriptions. Your only task is to try maintaining alignment through the body. Do not collapse or stress any joint soft tissue or muscles. You achieve the alignment by suspending the head and dropping the shoulders.

Once you find the alignment, start to breathe deeply to supply as much oxygen as possible to your body, but in a very relaxed way. You do not want to breathe in such an intense way that it will steal your mind

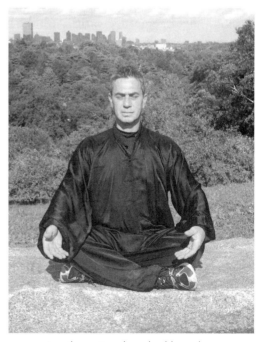

Lengthen spine, drop shoulders, place arms on knees with palms forward.

away from dissolving and releasing the impurities. Use your mind and move into the various soft tissue, skin, fascia, muscles, organs, and bones. Scan for impurities, and then start dissolving them using this visualization: from ice to water, water to gas. At the same time, ask the sun politely to help you with dissolving the impurities. Now you are using two forces: one internal, your brain, and one external, the sun.

I have a theory about why qigong has proven to be so effective in the cancer studies that I have been involved with. Cancer cells start about pinhead size. If you have both forces dissolving and releasing the impurities, the brain and the sun, you have an effective method of dealing with the pinhead impurity. Remember, dissolving and releasing the impurities takes time; it is slow. While they are leaving, you are also relaxing more and more throughout the layers and that allows the impurities to free themselves from being captured by the soft tissue.

The best time to do the sunset meditation is, of course, when the sun is setting. Watching the sunset and being outdoors will provide the strongest experience. When you do not have that luxury, then you can do it at a later time and still benefit from the pulling down energy of the setting sun. You can also use the moon energy to draw the impurities away because the moon is yin and we are yang. Some practitioners of the internal arts will practice meditations at midnight instead of with the setting sun, to dissolve and release their impurities.

In general, 20 minutes is the minimum time needed for an effective meditation session. The time needed varies with the individual. If you are able to immediately calm your brain waves to the state between awake and asleep, then the dissolving will happen sooner. If you sit only five or ten minutes, you still enjoy some benefit. The goal should be to work up to 20 to 30 minutes. If you spend 30 minutes, you can catch the sun setting 15 minutes before it sets and then 15 minutes after. In the first 15 minutes, locate the impurities, and then dissolve and release them as the sun sets until you have a clear and light feeling throughout the body.

CHAPTER 4
Tai Chi Movements

The tai chi movements are organized in small steps from the basics principles and stances to the more complex parts of the drills and tai chi forms. First, learn and practice the stances, stationary and moving, while maintaining correct alignment, and then move to the drills. Again practice both the stationary and the moving ones. Do not forget to also practice on the edge of a chair when you tackle the drills and the tai chi form. The mind/body program prepares you to perform all physical and mental skills described in the tai chi sections of the book. You will need to learn the movements and finally put them all together. Practicing with a different partner regularly is highly recommended. Although this arrangement is very important, most of the practice is done on your own. At some point, teaching will contribute tremendously to your learning. Once you are ready to share your understanding and knowledge with others, start teaching, but when you do, remember two important principles: staying humble, and developing your patience and empathy. Your final goal is to perform or teach all aspects of the tai chi while integrating the five building blocks—body, breath, mind, energy, and spirit—with every move or posture. Achieving that is easier said than done, but with practice and more practice, you will be able one day to become one with tai chi versus just practicing it. When doing the tai chi form, use the setting sun to help with some of your visualizations as much as you can.

The Complete Sunset Tai Chi Form

To the Left ⟶

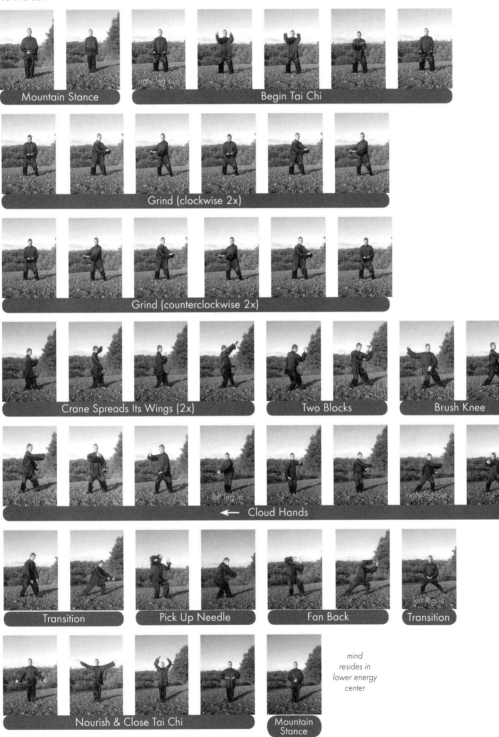

Mountain Stance

Begin Tai Chi

Grind (clockwise 2x)

Grind (counterclockwise 2x)

Crane Spreads Its Wings (2x)

Two Blocks

Brush Knee

⟵ Cloud Hands

Transition

Pick Up Needle

Fan Back

Transition

Nourish & Close Tai Chi

Mountain Stance

mind resides in lower energy center

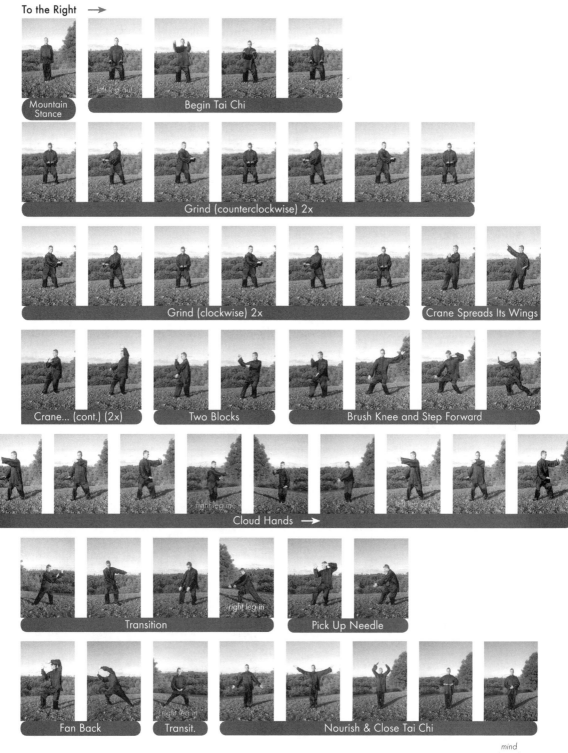

To the Right →

Mountain Stance

left leg out

Begin Tai Chi

Grind (counterclockwise) 2x

Grind (clockwise) 2x

Crane Spreads Its Wings

Crane... (cont.) (2x)

Two Blocks

Brush Knee and Step Forward

right leg in

left leg out

Cloud Hands →

Transition

right leg in

Pick Up Needle

Fan Back

Transit.

right leg in

Nourish & Close Tai Chi

mind resides in lower energy center

SACRUM DROPPED

If you want to achieve the maximum benefits from the mind/body program in this book and if you are interested in better health and the ability to generate more strength with minimum effort, alignment of the sacrum is essential. Because the sacrum is at the base of the spine, working on the sacrum will give you a starting point in achieving a larger goal, which is alignment of the spine as well as the entire skeletal system. Through correct alignment, we become directly connected physically and energetically to the earth and heaven. This is the fundamental first step on the path of achieving abundant energy through our bodies. At first, you will need to be more active muscularly, using your abdominal and hip muscles to tuck in your sacrum. This will cause tension. Over time, however, as you become more flexible, you will be able to just drop the sacrum, using less force and generating less unwanted tension.

HEAD SUSPENDED, SHOULDERS DROPPED

We often allow our head to hang, and allow the neck to be compressed. We also have a tendency to have floating shoulders, and we hold tension in them and in the upper back. For these reasons, many individuals suffer from headaches, migraines, and neck issues. In many instances, the shoulders are a major part of the problem, as well as the solution. The positions we sleep in for hours each night have a major influence on

our neck and shoulders. Each one of us needs to find the best way to sleep, without compressing the shoulders or creating torque in the neck.

The first step is to maintain awareness of correct alignment in the neck and shoulders at all times. Second are the mind/body prescriptions that give you tools to increase flexibility and strength in the upper body from the solar plexus up.

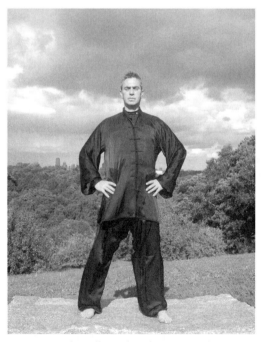

Drop the tailbone, lengthen spine, relax shoulders, and suspend head.

In the East, head problems are not only addressed through the neck and the skull areas, but treatment includes the shoulders, as well as the chest and upper back. It is understood that there are thick, complex, and intertwined layers of soft tissue from the solar plexus area all the way up to the face. Therefore, the first step is learning the sensation of keeping the chin parallel to the floor. We tend to slouch and drop the head down, which puts it in misalignment. Some of us tend to tilt the head somewhat to the left or right, which again throws the alignment off.

Our shoulders are often misused. There are three common problems: We tend to have one shoulder higher than the other. We tend to carry one or both shoulders slightly forward, which throws it out of correct alignment. Lastly, we tend to crunch or shrink the shoulders inward toward the neck, which can be associated with mentally holding tension in this area.

Sometimes these behaviors happen because we do not use our shoulders much. If you do not use them correctly and regularly, you may lose their optimum alignment. Often we suddenly abuse them or demand more than they can take while engaging in sports and other physically demanding hobbies. In addition, we do this after a sedentary period during which the shoulders have become weak and distorted.

Balance between strength and flexibility and an understanding of alignment are the keys to having healthy shoulders, and a pain-free neck and head. Some of the instructions that you hear again and again when learning Chinese tai chi, for health or martial arts, are tuck your tailbone in, keep your chin parallel to the floor, lengthen the spine, drop your shoulders, and keep your head suspended.

EMPTY MOON/FULL MOON

The abdominal and the back muscles should move and be coordinated with every breath you take. When they move out, it is a full moon. When they are drawn in, it is an empty moon.

ELBOWS DROPPED AND SUNK

In order to have a strong flow of energy through the limbs, we should keep them slightly bent and sunk while performing all of the internal practices. Hold the elbows near the body, about the distance of one fist away from the ribs, when doing the tai chi drills or the tai chi form. The hands stay at the height of the navel. Do not let your hands and elbows float around randomly.

WEIGHT THROUGH THE KNEES AND NOT INTO THE KNEES

We tend to misuse our knees, putting our entire body weight into the knees. Because the ligaments in the knees are not designed for that purpose, the pressure that accumulates in those ligaments is like a negative bank account. In this situation, many different problems can occur; some people gradually develop knee problems, such as persistent pain, and others end up with torn cartilage (meniscus), hyper-extended ligaments, and eventually many develop various types of arthritis. Our modern lifestyle does not include walking, climbing, proper leg exercises, and activities that provide weight-resistance through the legs. However, the biggest reason for so many knee problems is a lack of knowledge and attention toward correct alignment and not enough practice in the correct body mechanics during regular physical tasks. The knees are delicate. You need to master the skill of directing power through the knees and not into the knees. You must always pay attention to them and be careful with them.

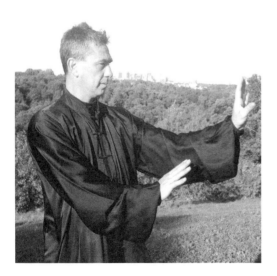

Elbows are near body, one fist away from ribs.

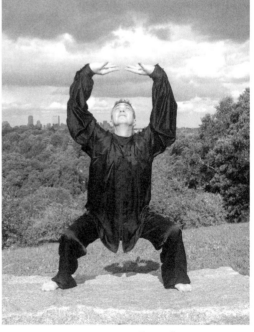

For strong energy flow, elbows
are always slightly bent.

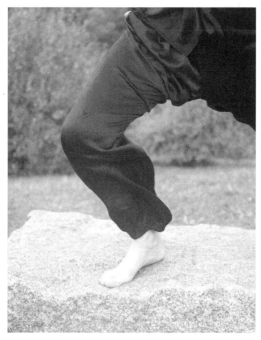

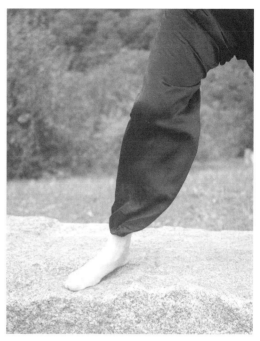

Misuse of knees; putting body weight into knees.

Misuse of knees; putting body weight into knees.

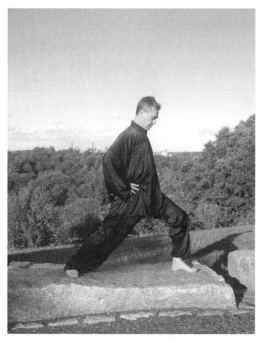

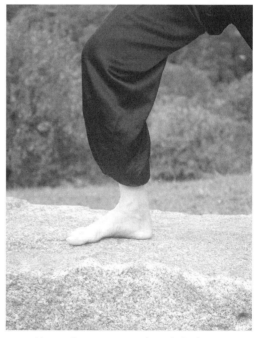

Master directing power through the knees.

Master directing power through the knees.

Turn and Lift Using the Heels

There are four simple rules regarding the feet: when lifting and placing the soles of the feet up and down, and when turning.

First, when putting the leg down, start from the ball of the foot or the heel. Second, when lifting the foot up, peel it off the ground from the heel to the ball of the foot or from the ball of the foot to the heel. Third, lift the legs and do not drag them. There is a tendency to collapse the inner arches. Make sure that you maintain alignment through the inner arches.

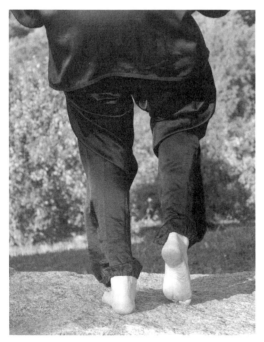

Leg down while rolling from ball of foot to heel.

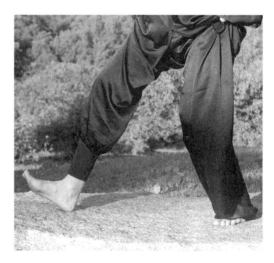

Leg down while rolling from heel to ball of foot.

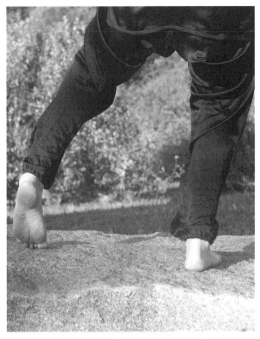

Leg up and peel from heel to ball of foot.

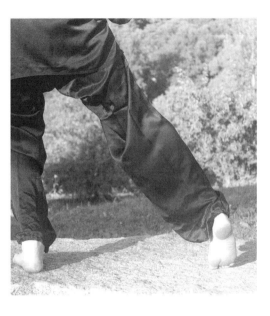

Lift and place leg down and roll
from ball of foot to heel.

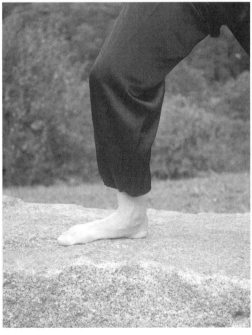

No alignment because inner arches are collapsed.

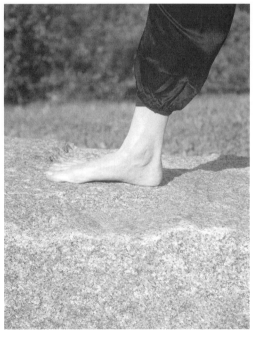

Maintain alignment through inner arches.

Lastly, when the foot is turning, it should have no weight on it, and you should turn on the heel.

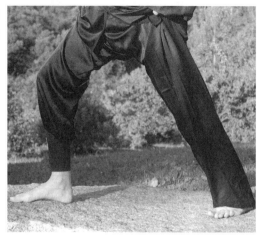

Front stance getting ready to turn right foot.

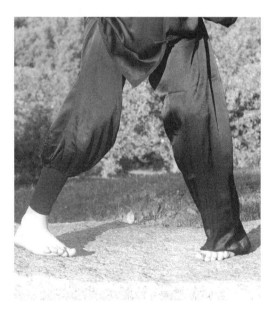

Right foot turning. Turn on the heel bearing no weight.

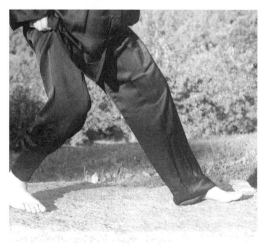

Back stance, right foot at 45 degrees.

TAI CHI HAND FORM

At this time, you should learn the Yang-style Tai Chi Hand form. Hold your hands in front of you, palms out. Starting with your left hand, slightly push the pinky sideways toward the left and the thumb sideways toward the right. The middle finger moves gently forward and up. On the right hand, the pinky moves to the right and the thumb toward the left while the middle fingers move gently up and forward. If you hold a ball between your palms, the middle fingers presses more on the ball than the pinky fingers and the thumbs that move away from the ball. The finger movements also create a cup-like shape with your palms. The tension in the fingers slows down the flow of energy to the fingers and leads the energy flow to the centers of the palms.

The reason that we hold our fingers in this manner is to create tension in the palm. The tension creates a small dam that slows down the energy flowing into the fingers and allows energy to accumulate in the center of the palm.

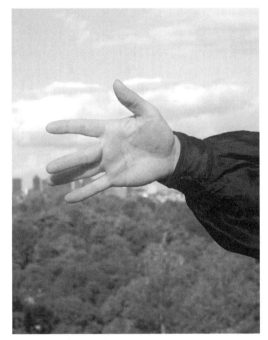

Yang-style Tai Chi Hand form.

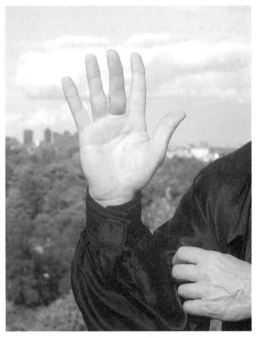

Yang-style Tai Chi Hand form.

THE SETTING SUN AND TAI CHI DRILLS

Remember, if you have an opportunity, perform the tai chi drills as well as the tai chi form in the setting sun. Relax, but do not collapse your entire body and surrender physically and mentally to the gentle warmth and to the powerful drawing and cleansing energy of the setting sun. Of course, second best would be indoors while the sun is setting. You can still use and sense the drawing setting sun energy to achieve the cleansing but will need to imagine the feeling of the gentle warmth of the setting sun.

STANCES

Stances are the bases of the tai chi form. You have to understand the stances, leg positions, and movements before you can perform a tai chi form. You have to focus on maintaining correct, healthy alignment in your entire body and remain aware of your body weight as it gently shifts from side to side in each stance.

Start in a high stance at first, and then over time lower your stance and practice longer. Train the stances before you work on the upper body movements. Later, you can also train only the upper part of the tai chi movements by, for instance, doing the form while seated on the edge of a chair. This helps you to fine-tune the movements, and your tai chi will be improved when you put them back together. Remember, as we begin to move into the tai chi postures and forms, to maintain the skills and principles, both physical and mental that we trained earlier.

Key Points about the Stances

Each stance should be trained in a stationary position, and then you should train moving from one stance to the other. Remain relaxed, with a little bit of slack throughout the body, which allows the energy and blood to flow and nourish the body. Connect energetically to the ground. If there is too much tension in the muscles, the blood and the energy is stagnant and sealed, and your tai chi is not an internal art anymore; it is only an external form.

When you turn the body, be sure to turn the hips and face them forward in the direction of the feet. Push off the heel of the back leg whenever you move forward. When you lift your foot at any time during the form, slowly 'peel' it off the ground by rolling and lifting it from the heel to the ball of the foot or from the ball of the foot to the heels. When placing the foot down, 'smear' it from the ball of the foot to the heel or from the heels to the ball of the foot. Sense your body weight as it shifts from one leg to the other. Look for other differences throughout the entire body as well.

Experience the substantial and insubstantial, which is the difference in levels of tension and relaxation, weight and lightness, in your legs, throughout your torso, and the rest of your body. This internal sensing will raise your total body awareness. It is said in the *Tai Chi Classics*: "Substantial and insubstantial must be differentiated, not only in the legs, but in the entire body."

Mountain Stance

Stand with both feet together, hands beside the body with the middle finger touching the middle of the outer thigh.

Try to sense a connection to earth and heaven. Align the spine, drop the shoulders, breathe deeply, and put your mind in your center of gravity energy center. This stance can also be trained with your hands on your belly to reinforce the sensation of the lower energy center. When standing, repeat this thought: "I am a great mountain." You should be calm, quiet, and centered.

Horse Stance

Stand with the legs about shoulder-width apart, feet pointing straight ahead, and slightly bend the knees, but not too much. The weight is evenly distributed, 50% in each leg. Keep the head suspended. Breathe deeply through the nose. The tongue touches the roof of the mouth. During exhalation, emphasize the sensation of the mind going out into the four gates, and on inhalation, back into your lower energy center.

Horse stance is very common in all Chinese martial arts. In horse stance, your squat can be as low as bringing the thighs parallel with the floor. In this tai chi form, you will not be asked to squat that low, but that can be an excellent additional training method for the thighs and entire body. You will experience horse stance throughout the Sunset Tai Chi form at various times, as you transition between the postures.

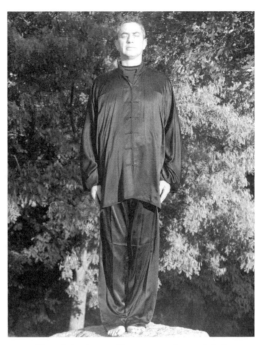

Mountain stance. "I am a great mountain."

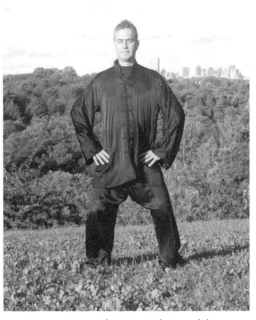

Horse stance with 50% weight in each leg.

Empty Stance

There are two empty stances. In the first empty stance, the feet are close to one another.

In the second empty stance, one leg is out in front of you, ready to kick or step.

In both empty stances, 90% of your weight is on the back leg and 10% of your weight on the front leg. The front leg gently touches the ground with the ball of the foot and is turned inward 45 degrees. It is important to distribute the weight of the back leg through the knee, down to the floor, and mentally, you may go down even deeper into the ground, into your roots (30 inches deep). This stance is also called cat stance, which reflects the spirit that needs to be felt when holding this stance.

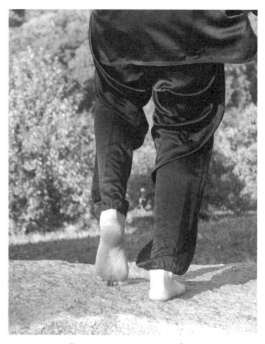

Empty stance. Legs together.

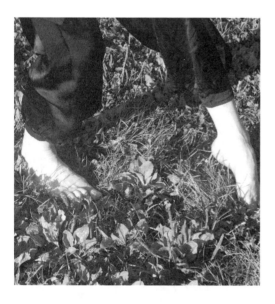

Empty stance. Weight 90% on back leg and 10% on front.

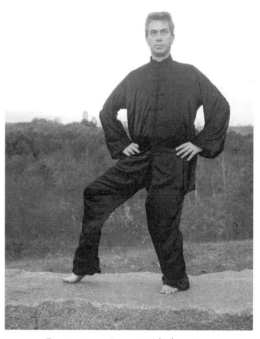

Empty stance. Leg out to kick or step.

First, start this stance standing high and as your legs become stronger, drop the stance lower and lower while holding it for longer periods of time: three to five minutes on each leg. To make sure you do not injure your knees, develop a balance between strength and flexibility in your legs before you require them to perform difficult tasks, such as low stances.

Your waist can be in one of two positions. At first, turn the waist away from the front leg, the leg with no weight. Then when you can keep your weight moving down through the back leg, which holds the stance, you can move the waist toward the front leg, which has no weight. You will see that the second waist position in this stance is more difficult, both on the knee of the back leg, as well as on the lower back.

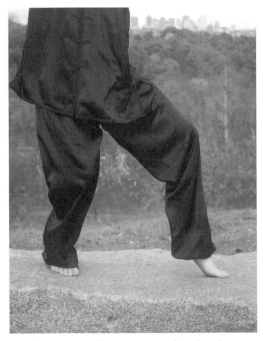

Empty stance. Turn waist away from front leg.

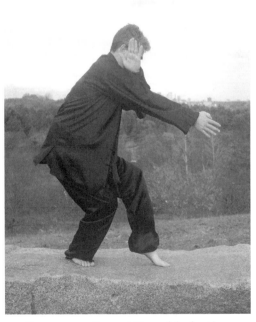

Empty stance. Turn waist toward the front leg.

Forward Stance

Forward stance has 70% of the body weight on the front foot and 30% on the back foot. The back leg is slightly bent. Do not bring your weight farther forward than the toes. Your knee should not be farther forward than the toes. The best indicator is the sensation that the weight is moving through the knee rather than into the knee. Direct your body weight through proper alignment of the leg into the ground. The toes should be turned so that there is a 45-degree angle in the feet and about one to two inches from an imaginary line drawn between the toes of the front leg and the heels of the back leg. Make sure your legs are always at least shoulder-width apart. In traditional tai chi chuan, this stance is called mountain climbing stance or bow and arrow stance.

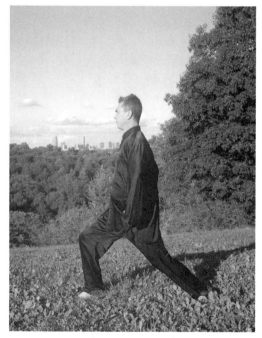

Forward stance. 70% on front leg
and 30% on back leg.

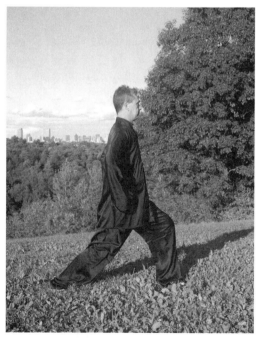

Forward stance. Back leg slightly bent.

Back Stance

Back stance has 60% of the body weight on the back leg, 40% on the front. The principles are the same as forward stance. When you sink into the back leg, be sure to tuck the tailbone slightly in. Distribute the weight right into the floor, not your knee. You should maintain a solid connection to the ground with the soles of the feet.

Tiger Stance

Stand in horse stance with your feet parallel, sacrum tucked in, head suspended, and shoulders dropped. Put the center of your palms on your waist. On the next inhalation, focus your mind in the lower energy center and on the sensation of 50% of your weight on each leg. Then, to begin shifting your weight from left to right, close your eyes and try to move as if you were pouring your body weight like sand, moving from the left leg to the right, slowly, paying attention to the sensation of pouring the sand, grain by grain.

On the next exhalation, continue to shift your weight from the left leg to the right leg, ending with 80% of your weight on the right leg.

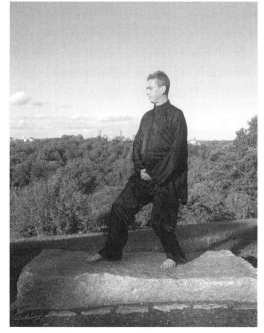

Back stance. 60% on back leg and 40% on front leg.

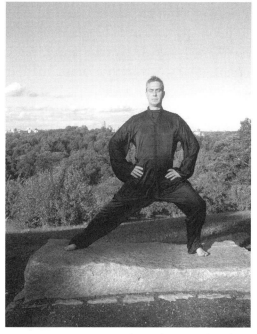

Tiger stance. 80% on one leg and 20% on the other.

Emphasize your weight moving down through the right knee into the floor and not into the knee. The left leg, which has 20% of your weight on it, is still parallel to the right leg. The inner soles of the feet are parallel to one another. You also want to keep both inner arches 'alive' and engaged, especially on the left, because the action of shifting into the right leg tends to collapse the arch of the left foot, and vice versa.

When a tiger attacks, the warrior waits until the last moment to respond. When the tiger jumps to attack, the warrior shifts his weight to the left side to evade the attack while his right arm sticks a knife in the tiger's left temple (do not try at home!). Try to recreate the spirit of the warrior when performing this stance. Shift your weight from side to side 20 to 30 times. Over time, you will be able to perform lower and longer stances. There are other traditional stances commonly used in longer tai chi chuan forms, but these are the stances you will be learning for the Sunset Tai Chi form.

MOVING STANCES

Once you understand the stances and can perform them without thinking, you should start mixing them and move from one to the other while maintaining the internal visualizations you have learned in this book as well as in *Sunrise Tai Chi*. To make the visualizations easier to perform, keep your eyes closed at first, and as your physical skills and mental skills improve, you can open your eyes. Make sure you understand the concept of 'leading' weight through the knees, rather than into the knees. Remember that in order to prevent injuries and obtain the most out of the information presented in this book, the entire program needs to be practiced and used in a balanced way.

When practicing your stances, especially the moving ones, you have an excellent opportunity to experience substantial versus insubstantial in your legs. Substantial and insubstantial are also known as yang and yin, respectively. When the weight is in the leg, it is substantial physically, but due to the increased muscular tension, it is insubstantial energetically. Tension creates energetic stagnation.

Observe these differences during your stances and as you shift your weight from one side to the other. An expert in the understanding of qigong can go through at least ten levels of yin and yang when analyzing a posture or movement.

From Mountain Stance to Begin Tai Chi Stance

Stand in mountain stance, the center of your palms two inches below your navel over the lower energy center, or with the middle fingers on the center of the sides of your legs in a straight line down from the hipbones. Breathe deeply when inhaling, focusing your mind in your center of gravity energy center, and upon exhalation, lead your mind down from your energy center through your legs, thirty inches below the soles of your feet.

On the next inhalation, draw your mind up from the floor through your left leg to your lower energy center; shift your weight to your right leg, slightly sinking into that leg. On the next exhalation, move your left leg to the left, parallel to the right, and smear the sole of the foot gently on the ground, from the ball of the foot to the heel, without dragging the weight of the leg. The sole of your left foot is about eight to twelve inches away from the right foot, or shoulder-width apart.

Leading with your mind, move your weight onto the left leg until your weight is distributed evenly on both legs with your sacrum tucked in. Your mind is equally strong through both legs and into the earth below both of your feet. While you move your left leg, move your arms as well, with the palms facing down toward the floor, to the area two inches below your navel and with the elbows one fist away from the hipbones. Close your eyes and practice four gates breathing, and if you can, add the baton and bubble visualization as well. When your eyes are open, show strong, intense eyes to raise the spirit.

On the next inhalation, shift your weight to the left leg and draw your mind up through it. Pull the right foot, starting from the heel, and gently bring that foot back to mountain stance. Bring your arms back to your lower energy center or beside your legs.

Keep moving from one foot to the other, first in a straight line from side to side and then in any direction you desire. You should always finish mountain stance with your feet parallel and palms gently on the sides of your legs. When you finish the 'begin tai chi stance,' your sacrum should be tucked in and the feet should be parallel to one another, knees slightly bent, elbows one fist away from the trunk, and with the palms facing down, two inches below your belly button. There is a tendency to have one foot turned to the outside, which is not the neutral position of your femur bone. The neutral position of your femur bone will line up correctly when the feet are parallel to one another.

From Horse Stance to Empty Stance

Stand in horse stance, with 50% of your weight on each leg, and put your palms on your waist. Close your eyes and visualize four gates breathing as well as the baton and bubble breathing. Shift your weight to the left without showing it externally, just enough that you can turn your right foot inward to 45 degrees. On the next inhalation, draw your mind from the floor through the left leg and shift the weight to the right leg, slightly bending the right knee and sinking your weight into it. Lift but do not drag the left leg. Place the ball of your left foot gently on the ground without weight. Your weight should be 90% on your right foot and 10% on the left foot. Try to hold this stance for 30 seconds. As you progress, you will be able to crouch lower and turn the waist more toward the left leg. Shift your weight back to the left foot and return to horse stance.

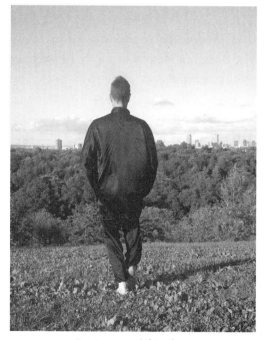

Empty stance shifting from
empty stance to horse stance.

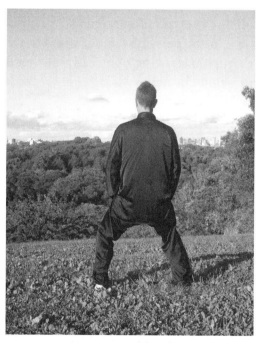

Horse stance shifting from
horse stance to empty stance.

Keep changing from horse stance to empty stance either to your left or right side. When your skill with these stances improves, you can turn and face any direction you desire, while keeping the weight down through the knees, head at the same height, hips straight forward, a 45-degree angle in the feet, and about one to two inches from the imaginary line drawn between the toes of the front leg and the heels of the back leg. Remember when you are in horse stance to keep your feet parallel, shoulder-width apart; also, drop your sacrum down, lengthen the spine, and maintain the internal visualizations.

When in empty stance, keep both feet at 45 degrees, with the sacrum tucked in and the weight distributed through the knees into the floor. The exercise 'up like smoke, down like a feather' in *Sunrise Tai Chi,* page 69, will help create the needed strength for these stances. To gain flexibility, work on the lower body stretches described in this program. To properly perform the tai chi form you will learn in this book, you will need to develop all these skills.

Forward Stance to Back Stance

Stand in forward stance (mountain climbing stance) with 70% of your weight on your right leg and 30% on the back left leg, with your feet set to 45 degrees. Turn your hips, pointing them straight ahead like the headlights of a car, toward the right. The back knee is slightly bent. You do not want to have your weight going into the front knee but rather through the properly aligned front knee into the ground. Place your hands on your waist or the center of your palms on your lower energy center. The tongue touches the roof of the mouth.

Close your eyes as you visualize four gates breathing as well as your baton and bubble visualization. When you are ready to move, inhale and gradually shift your weight to the rear (left) leg, and draw your mind up from the floor through the right leg into your lower energy center and then down into the left leg as 70% of your weight settles into it, turning your waist toward the left leg.

Stay in back stance for 30 seconds. Tuck the tailbone in, lengthen the spine, suspend the head, relax the face, and drop the shoulders. Continue breathing deeply. Coordinate the movement of the abdominal and back muscles with your breathing. Remember, when the muscles are drawn in, we refer to it as empty moon, and when they are out, full moon. Maintain your internal visualizations. Push the outer edge of your left foot gently down against the floor. There is a tendency to collapse the inner

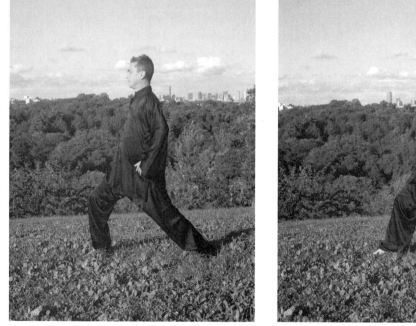

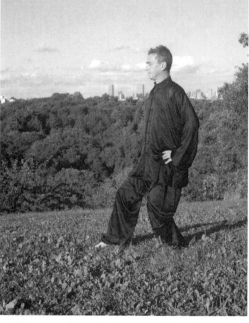

Forward stance. From forward stance to back stance.   Back stance. From back stance to forward stance.

arches of the weighted leg, such as when we are in back stance. The weight goes into the knees rather than the floor and that pulls on the inner arch, causing it to collapse.

We also tend to collapse the inner arches of the back leg when we are in forward stance. Some of this is caused by lack of flexibility and some of it is just awareness. On your next inhalation, focus your mind in your lower energy center, and on an exhalation shift your weight back to the right leg and lead your mind down through that leg all the way to the floor and beyond. Turn your waist toward the right leg so the hip bones are set straight forward.

Practice moving to and from back stance and forward stance. Train for three to five minutes with one leg forward, and then switch and train for another three to five minutes. The sacrum should be tucked in, the head suspended, and the shoulders dropped. Over time, as your flexibility and strength improves, you can perform these stances lower and longer.

From Horse Stance to Tame the Tiger Stance to Empty Stance

Moving from horse stance with your hands on your waist or two inches below your belly button in front of your lower energy enter. Shift your weight to your left leg, until you are in tame the tiger stance on the left leg. Move slowly, close your eyes, and experience a strong sensation of the kua, or the dome-like, powerful foundation of your legs. Once your weight is on your left leg, peel your right foot off the ground, starting with your heel. Then lift, not drag, the right leg and place it next to the left foot. You are now in empty stance with 90% of the weight on your left leg. Roll the right foot down, starting from the ball of the foot, and shift your weight to the right leg while emptying the left leg. You are now in empty stance with 90% of your weight on your right leg.

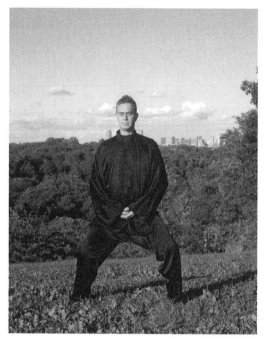

Horse stance. From horse stance to tiger stance to empty stance.

Now, lift the left leg and place it a few feet to your left away from the right leg; roll the soles of the left foot from the ball of the foot to the heel. Now you are in tame the tiger stance with 80% of your weight on the right leg. Shift your weight slowly again to the left and stop when you are in horse stance. Move about 10 times to the right and then 10 times to the left. Sometimes, you want to pause in between each stance for 30 to 60 seconds. During this time, close your eyes and visualize four gates breathing, as well as your baton/bubble visualization. This kind of training builds a strong experience of each stance and will improve these stances and postures and make it easier to perform the tai chi form.

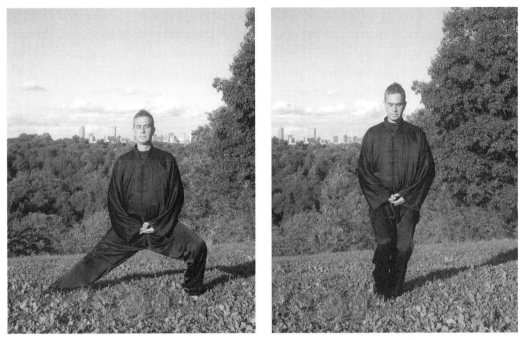

Tiger stance. From horse stance to
tiger stance to empty stance.

Empty stance. From horse stance
to tiger stance to empty stance.

Forward Stance to Forward Stance

This time we will perform forward stance from side to side. Start in forward stance with the right leg forward and your hands on your waist, left leg back and the knee slightly bent. Push from the outer sole of the rear (left) foot and lead the weight through the right leg into the floor. Maintain your internal visualizations. The rule is that you can turn the foot only when there is no weight on it.

Start by facing to the right. You will need to turn the right leg and foot 45 degrees inward. Because you have 70% of your weight on that leg, you need to empty this leg so you can turn the right foot on the heel. As soon as you empty the ball of your right foot, turn it inward so it is at a 45-degree angle. Then, pushing from the right foot, lift the left leg, continue the turning of the entire body to face the left, and then place the left leg down, slightly to the left of where it started, ball of the foot first. Repeat this change from side to side for three to five minutes.

You should always push off the back foot as you move into forward stance, maintaining the connection of the body from the toes to the fingertips. Maintain proper alignment, posture, and distance between the feet. Keep practicing the mental skills.

At first, you should empty the front leg completely and after turning the foot, fill it up again completely in order to experience the substantial and insubstantial through the body and especially in the legs. If you were to look at yourself from the side, you would look as if you are bobbing from side to side, left to right. This is acceptable because this is only an exercise, but eventually you should refine the movement so that the weight shifting is not externally visible. In tai chi and qigong practice, it is traditionally more proper for the movement to be smooth and continuous.

This exercise helps you to experience your body mass and to understand the substantial and the insubstantial aspects of the legs and the entire body. Through repeated practice, you can learn to smooth out the corners and stop bobbing from side to side. Experiencing the substantial and insubstantial in your legs is much easier than in the rest of the body. This is why we start from the legs using big movements, such as, in this case, bobbing. As your sensitivity and awareness improves, smooth out the corners and move in a straight line from left to right without bobbing.

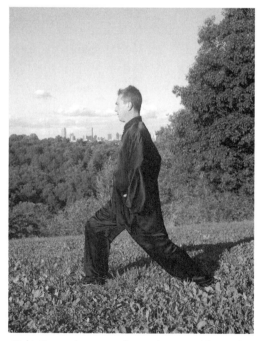 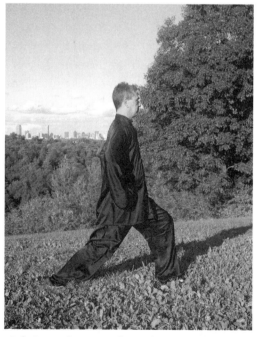

Right. Forward stance to forward stance, side to side.   Left. Forward stance to forward stance, side to side.

From Back Stance to Back Stance

Stand in a back stance with 60% of your weight on your back (left leg) and 40% on the front leg. Place your palms on your waist or on the lower energy center. Make sure you distribute your weight through the knees into the floor, especially the back leg. Keep your head suspended, tailbone dropped, breathe deeply, and use empty/full moon breathing, coordinating the abdominal and back muscles with your breath. Maintain your internal visualizations.

Your front (right) leg is already lighter because there is only 40% of your weight on it. Just turn the foot of the right leg inward to 45 degrees, and then shift the weight to that leg while lifting the left leg outward and placing it down from the heel to the ball of the foot. Keep your waist at 45 degrees. Practice moving from side to side for three to five minutes. As you become stronger and more flexible, you will be able to move in a lower stance and perform the stance for longer periods of time.

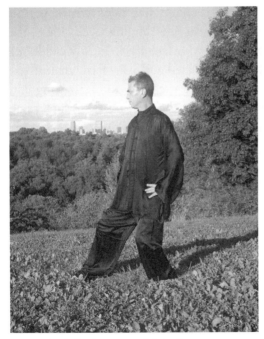

Right back stance to left back stance.

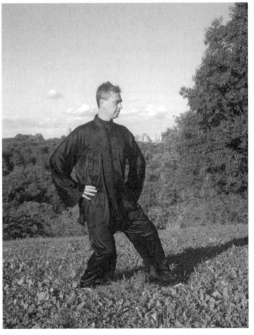

Left back stance to right back stance.

STATIONARY TAI CHI DRILLS

The tai chi stationary drills are designed not only for better health, but also to prepare you for the tai chi form. The stationary movements give you the opportunity to emphasize and experience the physical and mental skills more strongly. The drills also give you the opportunity to figure out how to put together the physical and the mental visualizations with movements from Yang-style Tai Chi. Each one of the tai chi movements you learn and perform have a martial application as well as specific benefits toward better health, longevity, and a higher quality of life.

The first part of each drill is stationary and the second part includes moving. Your body must be connected from the feet to the fingertips. To accomplish this sensation of the body moving as one connected unit takes time and practice. Remember that when you are pushing or striking forward, you must also be mindful of your rear foot and its connection to the ground. This is your root. A strong root allows you to manifest maximum power through your hands. Your power is generated from your, feet directed by the waist, and manifested through the palms and fingers.

Begin Tai Chi

Stand with your feet parallel, shoulder-width apart, and slightly bend the knees. The palms face downward, at belly button height. Your elbows should be one fist away from your ribs. Inhale, and turn the palms to face each other, while stretching the bows. Lift the arms to shoulder height, while visualizing an energy ball between the palms. Then, exhale and turn the palms to face downward. Release the bows, and lower the arms to their original position. Keep the inner arch of your feet alive. Tuck the tailbone in and keep your head suspended. Your shoulders are relaxed and your face is calm. You can practice the begin tai chi movement by moving only the arms and stretching and releasing the bows, and you can also practice by bending the knees and sinking when the hands reach the navel. The main goal of this movement is to sink your mind to the lower energy center.

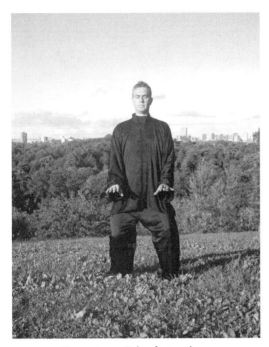

Horse stance. Palms facing down
and mind is in lower energy center.

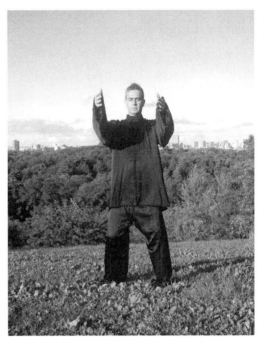

Turn arms with palms facing each
other and lift up to head height.

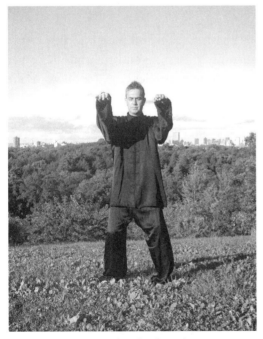

Turn arms with palms face down,
mind in lower energy center.

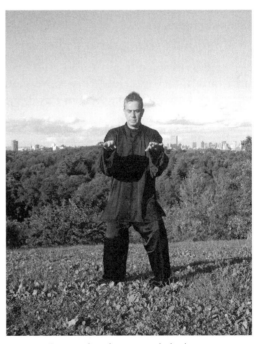

Drop palms down, stretch the bows.

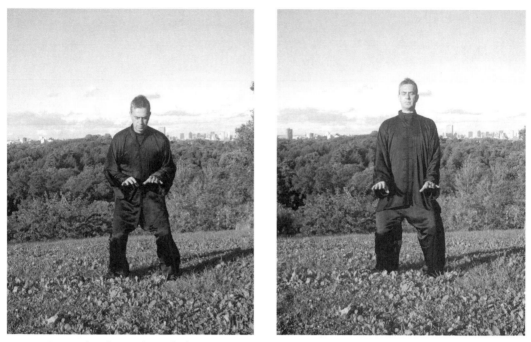

Drop palms down, release the bows.   Back to original position, mind in lower energy center.

Crane Spreads Its Wings

Inhale and cross your arms in front of your chest. Exhale and raise one arm to the side, rotating the arm outward, while simultaneously dropping and rotating the other arm outward. Try to lead this movement by stretching and releasing the bows. Make sure your wrists are relaxed and shoulders stay down.

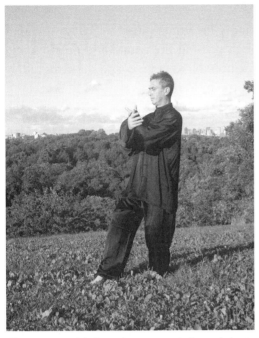

Empty stance. Inhale and cross arms in front of chest.

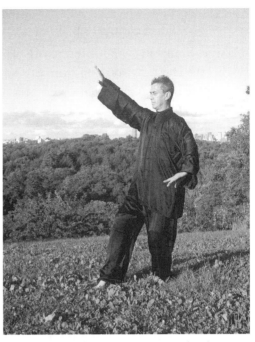

Raise right arm rotating outward and drop left arm down rotating outward.

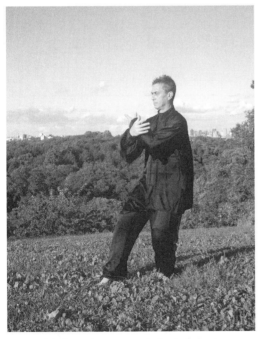

Inhale and cross arms in front of chest; reside in lower energy center.

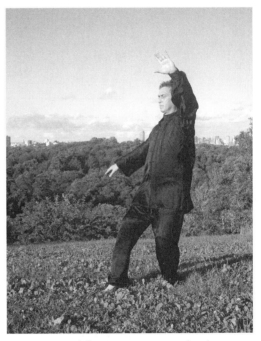

Raise left arm rotating outward and drop right arm down rotating outward.

Two Blocks

This exercise simulates blocking two imaginary incoming punches. The movement massages your lungs and internal organs through turning the trunk, and opening and closing the chest. By rotating from the waist, the upper body moves and the arms follow in order to block. Coordinate your breath with the movement.

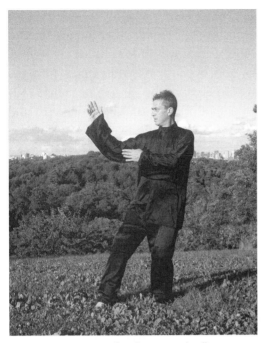

Empty stance. Left palm near right elbow.

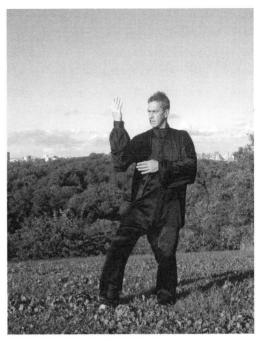

Block with right arm. Left near right elbow; turn trunk.

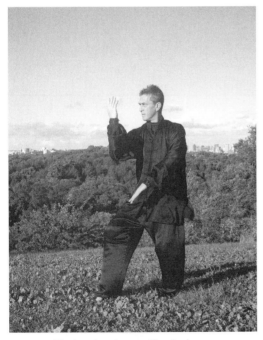

Block with right arm. Use the bows;
mind in lower energy center.

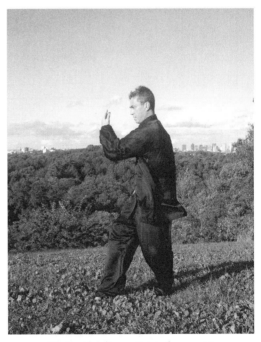

Block with left arm. Rotate from waist;
maintain alignments in legs.

Brush Knee

As you inhale, lift one arm to the blocking position while the other hand points to your elbow. Then the waist turns, and the blocking arm moves in toward the centerline. At the same time, the other hand moves back and upward. As you exhale, turn the waist, brush your knee, and push forward from the height of the ear. Do not tense your shoulders. The wrists are loose and relaxed. At the end of the push, settle the wrist and keep your elbows slightly bent.

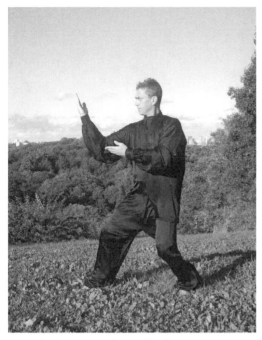

Back stance. Right arm blocking position;
other hand points to elbow.

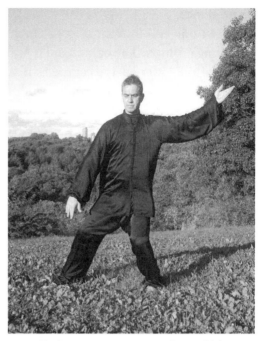

Blocking arm moves to centerline and left
arm moves back and upward.

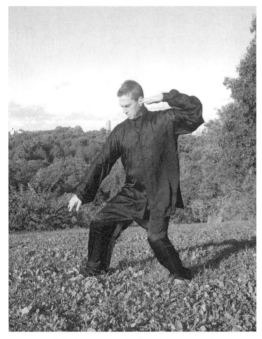

Exhale. Turn waist, brush knee, and
push forward from ear height.

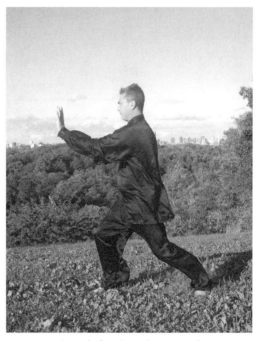

At end of push, settle wrist, and
keep elbows slightly bent.

Cloud Hands

Raise one arm in front of your chest in a hugging position. The other hand is at the height of the lower energy center, as if you were petting a big, tall dog. As you inhale, turn the waist and rotate your body in the direction of the raised arm. Exhale as you switch arms and repeat to the other side. Relax your neck and shoulders. While you are turning, it is important to keep your inner arches alive. Do not allow your knees to move inward.

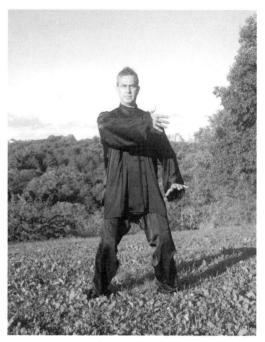

Horse stance. Right hand in front of chest and left hand at height of lower energy center.

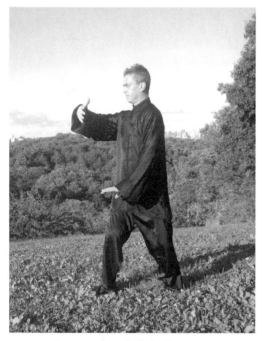

Turn to right and inhale. Turn waist in direction of raised arm.

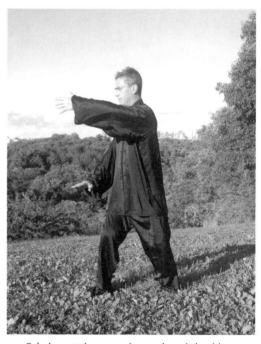

Exhale, switch arms, relax neck and shoulders.

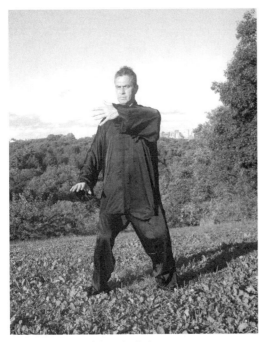

Turn to left and inhale. Turn waist,
rotate body in direction of raised arm.

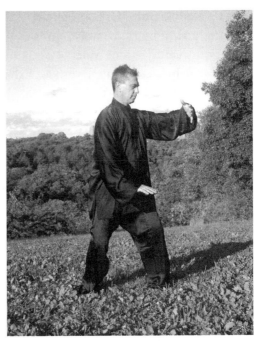

Keep turning and maintain alignments in legs.

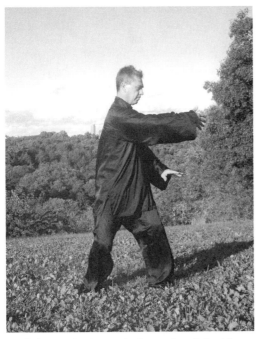

Exhale, switch arms, and relax neck and shoulders.

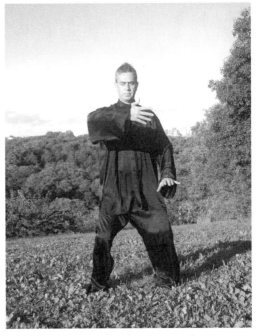

Back in original position; reside
in lower energy center.

Pick Up Needle from the Sea Bottom

While turning your waist, inhale and raise both hands to one side of your face with the palms facing each other. Exhale and strike forward with the rear hand, and sting downward toward an imaginary opponent's lower energy center. At the same time, the other hand blocks and protects your face. Inhale, and draw the hands back to the other side. Exhale and repeat the sting with your hand.

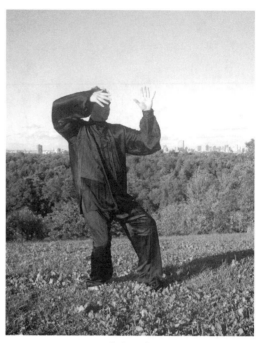

Empty stance. Inhale and pull arms up to ear height with both palms facing forward.

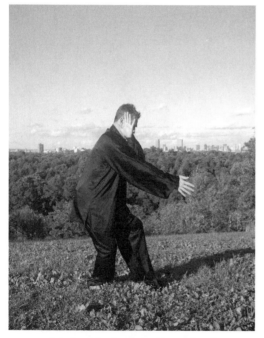

Exhale, strike forward with rear hand while other hand blocks face.

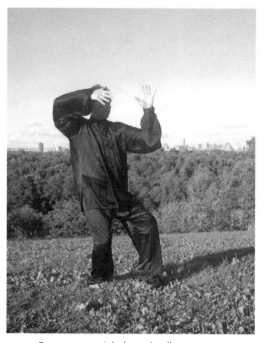

Empty stance. Inhale and pull arms up to ear height with both palms facing forward.

Fan Back

Inhale and pull your arms up to ear height with both palms facing forward, with the legs in empty stance. As you move forward to front stance, exhale, and both hands push at face height.

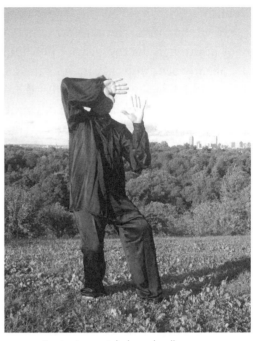

Empty stance. Inhale and pull arms up to ear height with both palms facing forward.

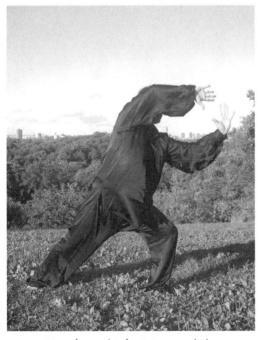

Move forward to front stance, exhale, both hands push at face height.

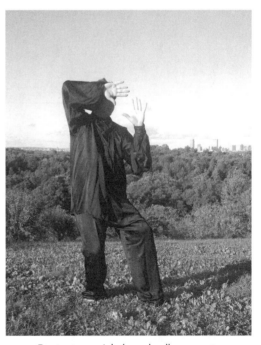

Empty stance. Inhale and pull arms up to ear height with both palms facing forward.

Nourish

Inhale and draw clean, healthy energy from your surroundings. Allow the energy to pour in through the top of your head, filling the body from the ground upward.

Slightly bend your knees. Tuck the tailbone in. Suspend the head. Drop your shoulders. Breathe deeply so you can feel the ribs expanding. Visualize your body's energetic circulation. Feel the relationship of your body to the earth. Feel the relationship of your body to the heavens. Draw earth energy into your fingers. Draw in energy from the trees. Draw in mountain energy. Draw in ocean energy. Lead this energy inward to nourish your entire body.

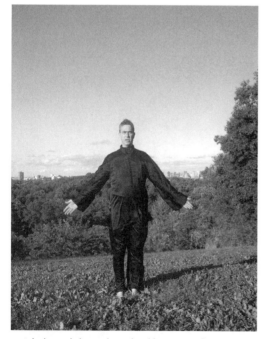

Inhale and draw clean, healthy energy from your surroundings (earth, oceans, trees).

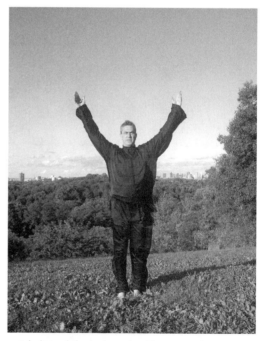

Inhale and draw clean, healthy energy from your surroundings (mountains, sky, stars).

Close Tai Chi

As you finish, return the palms to the front of the body, placing the center of the palms over the lower energy center and keeping them there for a few minutes, or as long as you like. Stand in mountain stance and allow the energy created to return to your lower energy center. The *Tai Chi Classics* says, "When standing still in your mountain stance, stand as still as a mountain. Look for the motion in the stillness."

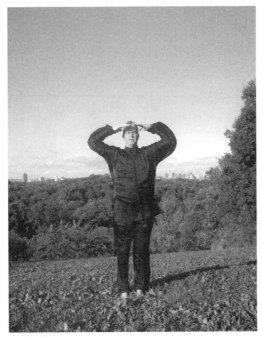

Allow positive energy to pour in through top of head.

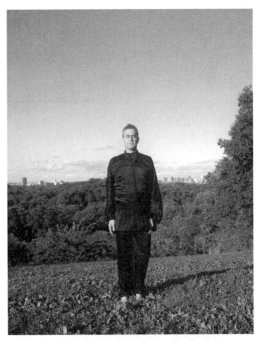

Filling body, from the ground up, and nourish entire body.

MOVING TAI CHI DRILLS

Now that you have learned the basic movements, practicing moving drills will allow you to refine each movement separately before you string them together into the Sunset Tai Chi form. The moving drills below are practiced from side to side, so that you may train even in a small space. You may also drill each movement while walking in a straight line, or free form, out in the park or at your home. Only when you have drilled each movement to the point that you feel you understand the subtle points of the movement and the sensation and spirit of each movement should you move on to the complete form.

Below is a selection of moving drills for some of the movements. You may make your own combined drills, such as crane spreads wings, into two blocks and back again.

Begin Tai Chi

In this drill, start by standing in mountain stance, with your arms at your sides, fingers pointing downward. Then, step so your feet are parallel, shoulder-width apart, and the knees are slightly bent. This is a high horse stance. The palms face downward, at belly button height. Your elbows should be one fist away from your ribs.

Inhale, and turn the palms to face each other, while stretching the bows.

Lift the arms to shoulder height, while visualizing an energy ball between the palms.

Now, exhale and turn the palms to face downward. Release the bows and lower the arms to their original position. The head is suspended. Your shoulders are relaxed, and face is calm. Continue practicing this transition along a straight line to the left and right.

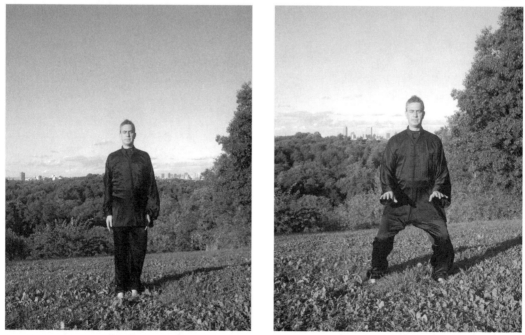

Mountain stance. Arms at your sides with fingers pointing downward.

High horse stance. Palms face downward and elbows are one fist away from ribs.

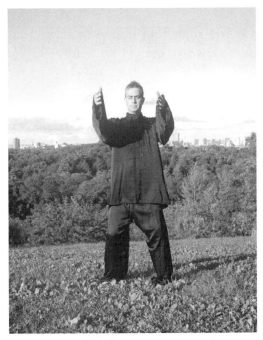

Lift arms to shoulder height while visualizing energy ball between palms.

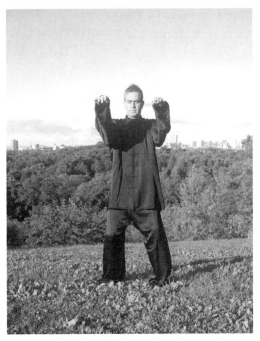

Exhale and turn palms to face downward.

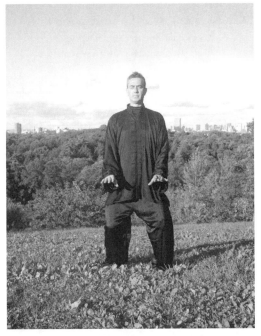

Release bows and lower arms to original position.

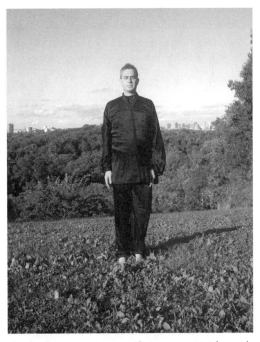

Back to mountain stance with arms at your sides and fingers pointing downward. Your mind resides in the lower energy center.

Crane Spreads Its Wings

Repeat from side to side. Make sure that as you shift from side to side that your weight goes through the knee, rather than into the knee, to prevent knee injuries.

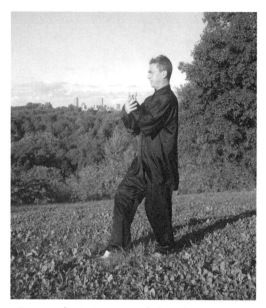

Turn to right empty stance, inhale and cross arms in front of chest; reside in lower energy center.

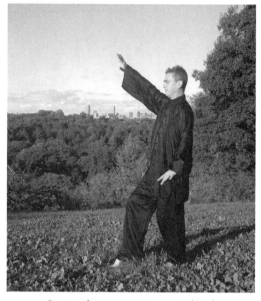

Raise right arm rotating outward and drop left arm down rotating outward.

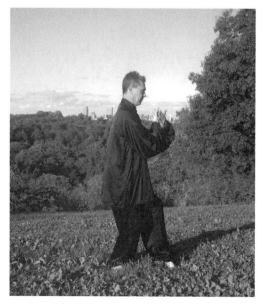

Turn to left empty stance and inhale while crossing arms in front of chest; reside in lower energy center.

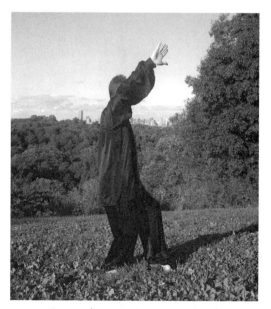

Raise right arm rotating outward and drop left arm down rotating outward.

Two Blocks

Step into empty stance and practice your blocking. Shift the empty stance from side to side. By rotating from the waist, the upper body moves and the arms follow in order to block. Coordinate your breath with the movement. Be careful to protect your knees. Your weight should go into the floor, rather than into your knee.

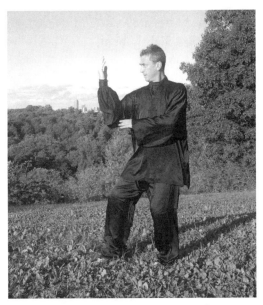

Turn to right into empty stance with
left palm near right elbow.

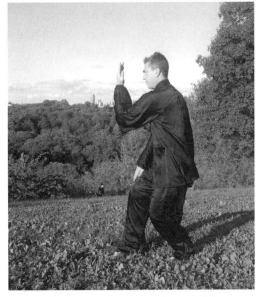

Block with right arm and then with left
arm, while turning from waist.

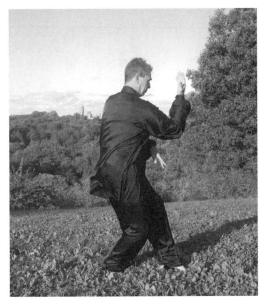

Turn to other side into empty stance
and block with right arm.

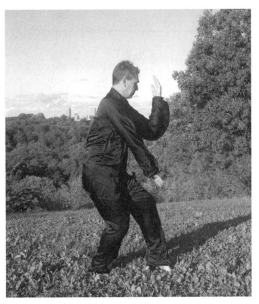

Block with left arm while rotating from
waist, and maintain alignments in legs.

Brush Knee and Step

Start in back stance. As you inhale, lift one arm to the blocking position while the other hand moves back and upward. As the waist turns, start to shift your weight forward. Exhale, brush your knee, and push into front stance.

When you complete the push into front stance, make sure your hips are facing square forward. To prevent damaging torque in the knee, make sure your feet stay shoulder-width apart. Do not tense your shoulders. The wrists are loose and relaxed. At the end of the push, settle the wrist and keep your elbows slightly bent.

Repeat from side to side.

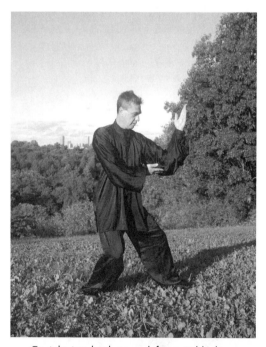

To right, into back stance left arm in blocking position while other hand points to elbow.

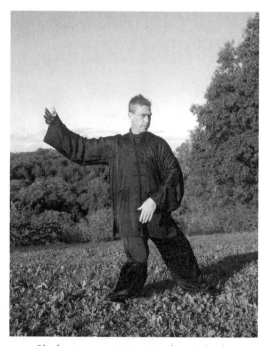

Blocking arm moves to centerline and right arm moves back and upward.

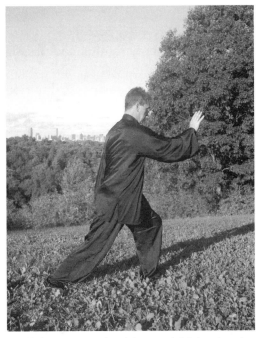

Exhale. Turn waist, brush knee with left hand, and push forward, with right, from ear height.

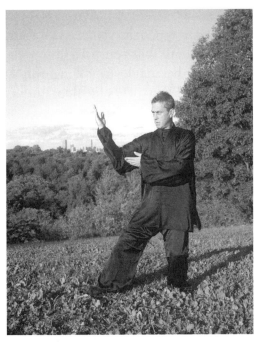

To left; turn to other side into back stance and block with right.

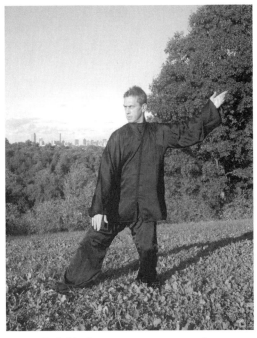

Right blocking arm moves to centerline while left arm moves back and upward.

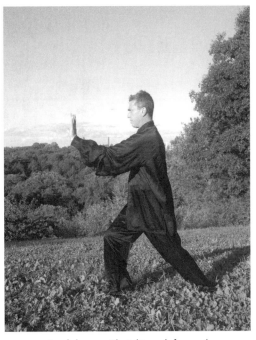

Brush knee, with right, push forward with left; from ear height.

Cloud Hands

Stand in mountain stance, with your palms on your lower energy center.

Inhale, and shift your weight into one leg, picking the empty foot up and placing it down to the side slowly, rolling from the ball of the foot to the heel.

As your heel touches the floor, turn the waist and rotate your body in the direction you are stepping.

Exhale as you switch arms and repeat from side to side.

Relax your shoulders. Do not allow your knees to move inward. Experience a light and airy sensation in your upper body as you turn the waist softly. Your lower body remains grounded and rooted. Imagine that you are a cloud gently moving through the sky.

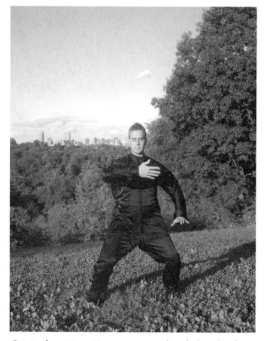

Original position. Horse stance with right hand in front of chest and left at height of lower energy center.

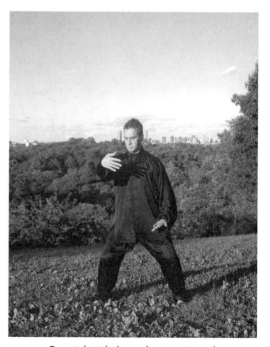

Turn right, inhale, and turn waist and arm in direction of raised arm.

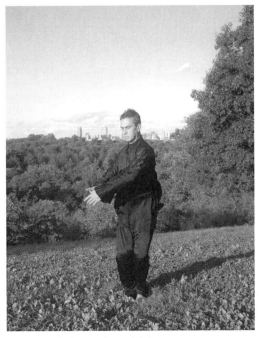

Exhale. First bring left leg into empty
stance, then turn to your left.

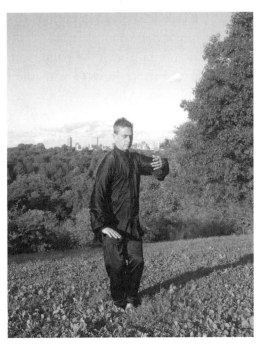

Continue to exhale. Maintain your empty stance
and get ready to switch the arms.

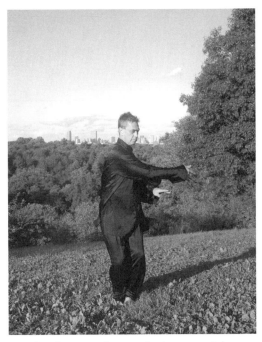

Switch arms and turn and twist to your right.

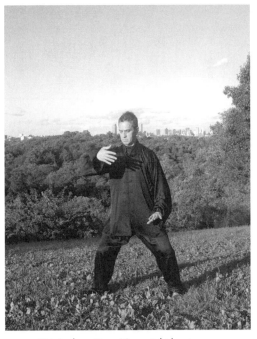

Original position. Move right leg to your
side, horse stance keep turning left.

Pick Up Needle from the Sea Bottom

Step into empty stance. While turning your waist, inhale and raise both hands to one side of your face with the palms facing each other.

Exhale and strike forward with the rear hand, and sting downward. At the same time, the other hand blocks and protects your face.

Inhale, draw the hands back to the other side, and switch into empty stance on the other side and strike again with one arm while protecting with the other.

Exhale, and repeat the sting strike from side to side.

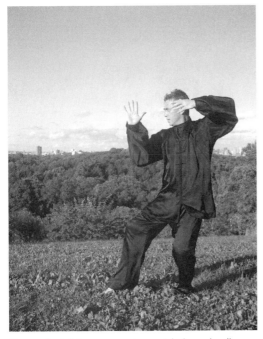

Turn to the left into empty stance. Inhale and pull arms
up to ear height with both palms facing forward.

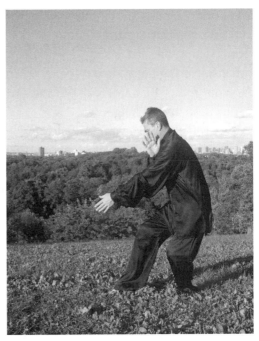

Exhale, strike forward with rear hand
while other hand blocks face.

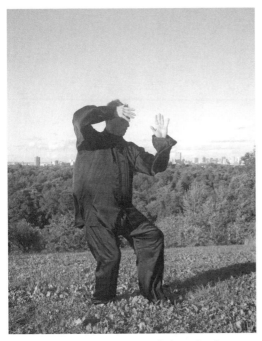

Turn right into empty stance. Inhale and pull arms
up to ear height with both palms facing forward.

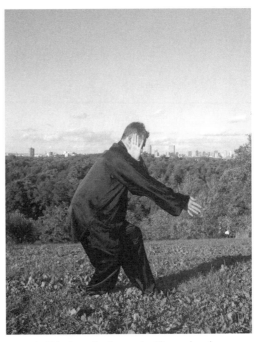

Exhale, strike forward with rear hand
while other hand blocks face.

Fan Back

Shift your weight from empty stance to front stance on one side. Repeat on the other side using horse stance as a transition. As you move forward, exhale and both hands push at face height.

As you shift backward, inhale, and circle both hands down toward your waist and then raise them on the other side.

Repeat on both sides until you can perform it smoothly with the internal skills.

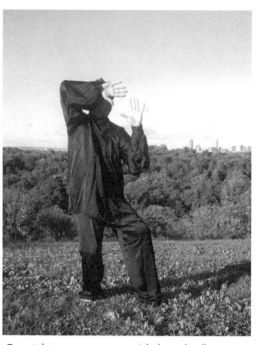

Turn right into empty stance. Inhale and pull arms up to ear height with both palms facing forward.

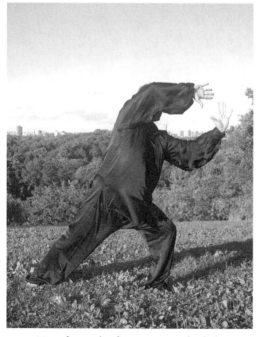

Move forward to front stance, and exhale with both hands pushing at face height.

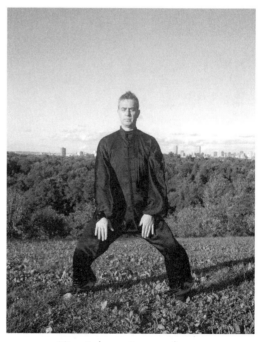

Move to horse stance and move arms down with palms facing in.

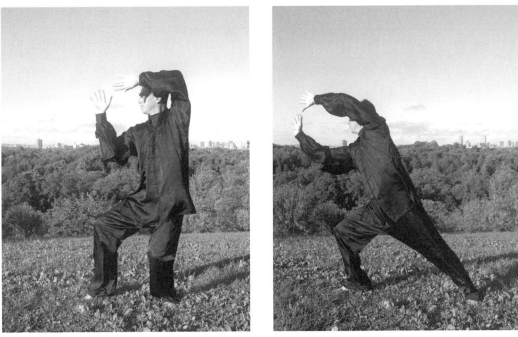

Turn left into empty stance. Inhale, and pull arms
up to ear height with both palms facing forward.

Move forward to front stance, exhale,
both hands push at face height.

Remember to eventually integrate all of the internal skills within each tai chi drill
and within the tai chi form.

CHAPTER 5

Sunset Tai Chi Form

Tai chi is beautiful. The form is soft and agile and flowing. The practitioner appears to be at peace. This Sunset Tai Chi form is a short sequence of traditional movements common to almost all tai chi styles. Regular practice of this form will allow you to fine-tune your tai chi skills and bring your awareness into the present moment, so you may make the most of your downtime at home, alone or with family.

On a physical level, the tai chi postures engage the whole body. The stances we have just learned utilize strength and flexibility, while maintaining or increasing the range of movement in the joints. The stances, especially when performed low, will increase muscle mass and bone density, which is important for health, as well as martial arts. The pulsing and pumping of the joints and ligaments boosts our energetic circulatory system, the same system that we work on when we go to an acupuncturist.

Relaxing and tensing various groups of muscles creates a cycle of holding and releasing blood, oxygen, and energy into the veins and capillaries, as well as into the energy pathways, known as channels, vessels, and meridians. This works to open up and nourish the body's trillions of cells on the deepest level, and all the way to the extremities. You will enjoy stimulation of your acupuncture points and experience a deep tissue massage at the same time.

When we practice tai chi slowly and mindfully for the purpose of improving our health, it is considered a qigong practice. Qigong and tai chi are sometimes thought of as doing acupuncture on yourself, without the needles. The breath is used as a tool to quiet the mind and to lead energy in and out of the body. For martial applications, in general, when inhaling we block, and when exhaling, we strike. For health purposes, inhaling and exhaling is used for moving/leading energy to a desired area. This deep breathing brings more oxygen in and more toxins, like carbon dioxide, out, thus upgrading the functioning of every cell in your body and giving you abundant energy.

The Complete Sunset Tai Chi Form

To the Left ⟶

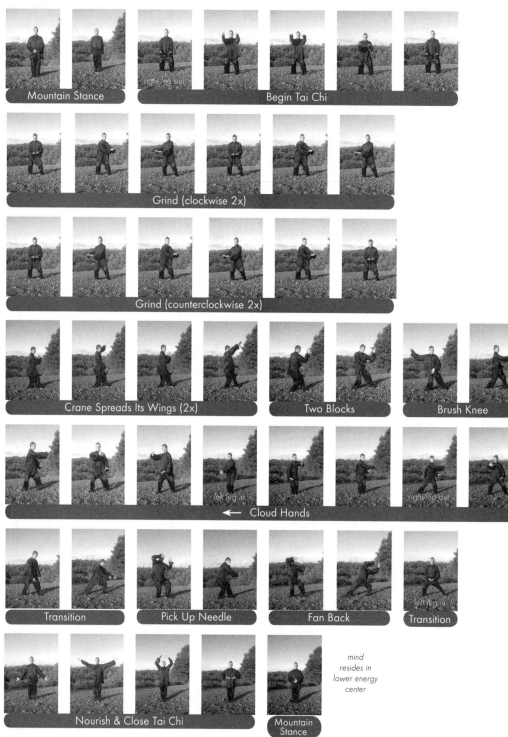

Mountain Stance

Begin Tai Chi

Grind (clockwise 2x)

Grind (counterclockwise 2x)

Crane Spreads Its Wings (2x)

Two Blocks

Brush Knee

⟵ Cloud Hands

Transition

Pick Up Needle

Fan Back

Transition

Nourish & Close Tai Chi

Mountain Stance

mind resides in lower energy center

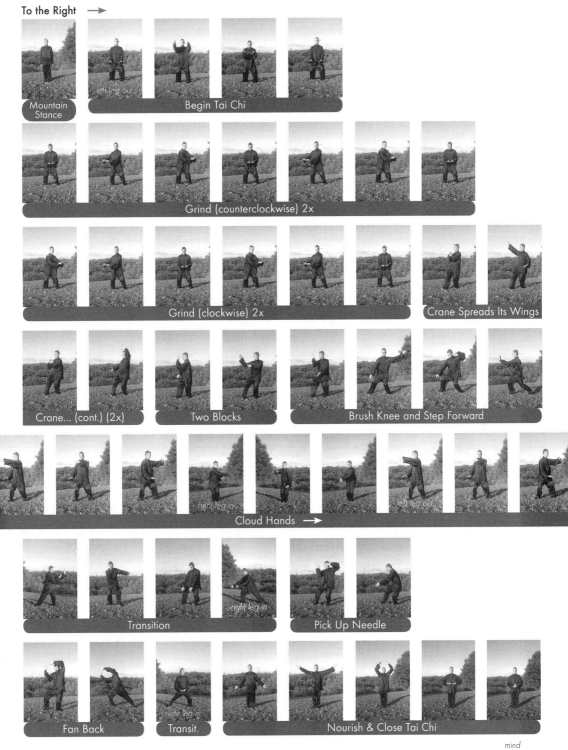

To the Right →

Mountain Stance

Begin Tai Chi

Grind (counterclockwise) 2x

Grind (clockwise) 2x

Crane Spreads Its Wings

Crane... (cont.) (2x)

Two Blocks

Brush Knee and Step Forward

Cloud Hands →

Transition

Pick Up Needle

Fan Back

Transit.

Nourish & Close Tai Chi

*mind
resides in lower
energy center*

ELEMENTS OF THE SUNSET TAI CHI FORM

You have already learned the movements. Now they will be strung together into the Sunset Tai Chi form, and we will show the details of each transition from movement to movement so that you can learn this form thoroughly and begin practicing today. These movements are performed as a slow, continuous sequence with an emphasis on relaxation, correct posture, and balance. Eventually, the practitioner may speed up the tai chi form, but increase the speed of your movements gradually, while keeping the postures correct. The goal is to reach the point where the movement is able to generate or emit power, as if you were involved in combat.

At this point, we are focusing on the beginning stage of practice, moving slowly, with an emphasis on the healing benefits of tai chi. This leads to increased awareness and vitality, and helps you to eliminate tension, regain your health, and experience the natural energy within your body and surrounding you. This tai chi form will help you transit from one stage to another and will transform you to a new and refreshed person.

The entire body should always move as one connected unit. While doing the postures, be sure that your arms are moving in conjunction with your torso and that your torso is pushed by the legs. Your arms should not move unless the rest of your body is in motion. Remember to always line up the knees in the direction of the toes, and do not extend the knees past the toes.

As you exhale, the energy goes out through the four gates—the center of your palms and the center of the soles of your feet. Keep your hands in the tai chi hand form—relaxed, and slightly cupped, with the middle fingers downward slightly and the pinky fingers extended. By holding this hand form, you cause some of the energy to stagnate slightly inside the palms, making the energy there stronger. Do not move the arms from the shoulder joints only, but instead through the stretching and releasing of the spine and chest bows.

Once you can perform the form standing or sitting on the edge of the chair with all the external and internal skills taught in this book, use the setting sun to help your entire body to relax, and start using the setting sun and your mind to dissolve and melt the tension and stress through your physical and energetic bodies. Recognize your impurities and allow the mind and the sun to dissolve and cleanse them. The short tai chi form and the powerful energy of the setting sun, over time and practice, will allow you to experience a unique connection between you, the heavens, and the earth.

MOUNTAIN STANCE

Sunset Tai Chi Form's First Move

Stand with both feet together, palms placed two inches below your navel. Breathe deeply and close your eyes until you are calm and centered.

When standing still, bring to mind the big mountains and when moving, flow like the great rivers. On an inhalation, open your eyes and move your arms beside your body. You are still a great mountain.

You have awakened, yet you are relaxed. Your brain waves are between the states of being awake and asleep. Sense the earth beneath you and the heavens above. You are a part of the universe.

Key Points. Hold your hands beside the body, the middle finger touching the middle of the outer thigh. Try to sense a greater spirit, a connection to the earth and heavens. Align the spine, drop the shoulders, and use deep center of gravity breathing. This stance can also be trained without removing your hands from your belly (two inches below the navel), to reinforce the sensation of the lower energy center. "You are a great mountain." You should be calm, quiet, and centered. You can stay in mountain stance for 20 seconds or 20 minutes, until you are ready to proceed to the next movement: begin tai chi.

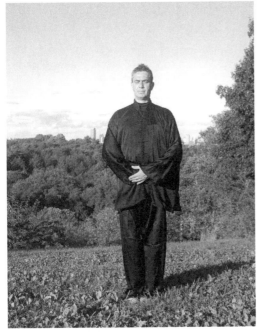

Put feet together and palms below navel.

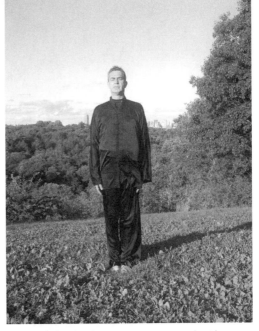

Inhalation. Open eyes, move arms beside body. You are a great mountain.

BEGIN TAI CHI

Sunset Tai Chi Form

From mountain stance, shift your weight to the left leg.

Peel up the right foot, from the heel to the ball of the foot.

Place the right foot down a shoulder's width away from the left foot.

Smear the sole of the foot from the ball of the foot to the heel.

Stand with your feet parallel, shoulder-width apart, and slightly bend the knees. The palms face downward, at belly button height. Your elbows should be one fist away from your ribs.

Inhale, and turn the palms to face each other, while stretching the bows. Lift the arms to shoulder height, while visualizing an energy ball between the palms.

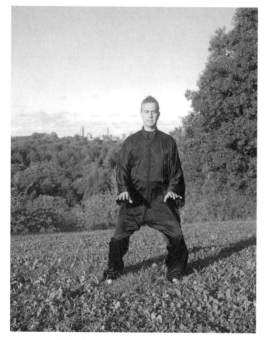

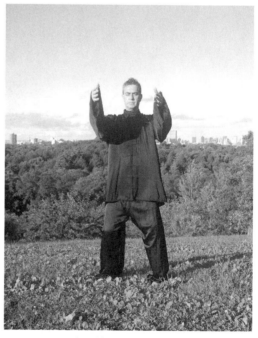

Feet parallel, shoulder-width apart; bend knees with palms facing downward at belly button height.

Turn palms, lift arm to shoulder height.

Now, exhale and turn the palms to face downward.

Release the bows and lower the arms to their original position.

Key Points. Keep the inner arch of your feet alive. Tuck the tailbone in. Your head is suspended. Your shoulders are relaxed and your face is calm. The main goal of this movement is to sink your mind to the lower energy center.

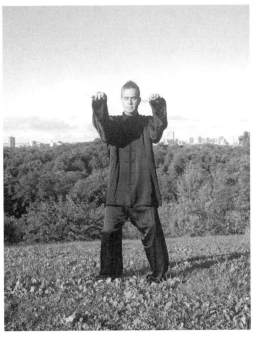

Exhale, turn the palms to face downward.

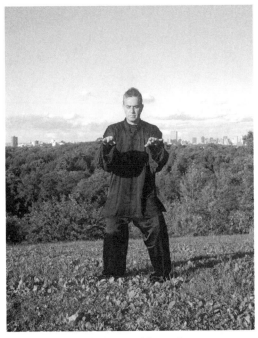

Release the bow and lower the arm.

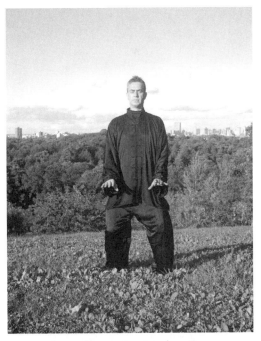

Lower the arms to original position.

Martial Arts Application of Begin Tai Chi

One martial art application of this posture can be used when you are facing an opponent who has his hands on top of yours or is grabbing your wrists.

Raise your arms and coil your hands around and over the outside of your opponent's hands or arms, and then push the arms downward, gaining an advantageous position for punching or kicking.

If you are interested in a take down, you can use your leg to also drop him to the ground.

If you choose to control your opponent, you can lock him so he cannot move anymore.

Begin tai chi trains us to do two things that are essential for both health as well as martial arts. The first action we do when performing this move is to sink the mind

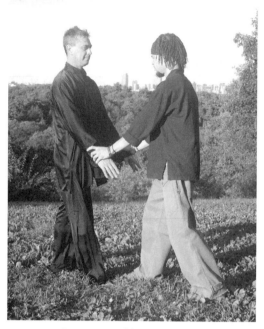

Opponent grabbing your wrists.

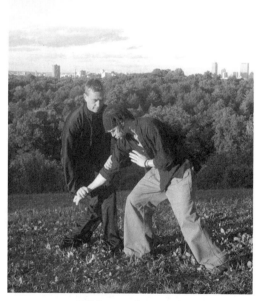

Pull the arm downward.

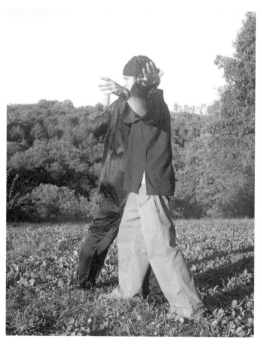

A take down.

into the center of gravity energy center. This visualization will lead and focus the scattered energy through the body right down to the center where it can be ready for any martial art need or use. It is a stage of being prepared; calmness is an essential principle of being ready for a fight and for preventing illness. The second part of this move is being still. It is written in the *Tai Chi Classics*: "When being still, be as still as a great mountain." This stillness is the key to seeing and reacting more efficiently to any energy that may come at you. It is much easier to react effectively to a punch from a still position than when hopping and jumping around. When you are still and calm, your ability to see or sense the punch or kick coming at you improves with practice, and you can even reach a point where you can sense the punch before it is launched.

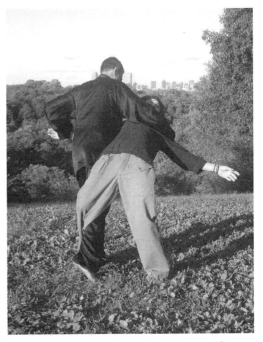

Use your leg to drop opponent to ground.

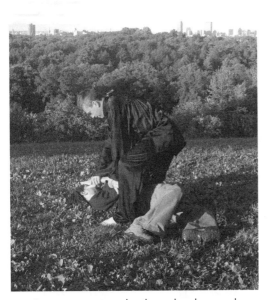

Raise your arms, and coil your hands around and over the outside opponent's arms.

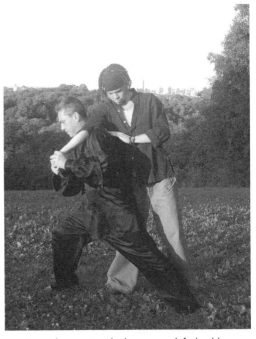

Control opponent; lock arm over left shoulder.

Looking and Sensing–Moving or Standing Still

Find a partner. At first, both of you will jump around like boxers. Your partner's task is to touch your chest using three different speeds, slow, medium, and fast, and your task is to block the attacks. Your partner will jump and hop around you and will try to touch your chest by surprise. Your job while also jumping is to try to block his touch to your chest.

The second time, have your partner jump around like the boxer but you just stand still. Ask your partner to approach you with three different speeds: first, slow touches, then medium ones, and last, fast ones. Take a few minutes' break to breathe deeply and become calm, and then stand still. Focus on your partner's chest area while he or she is hopping and jumping. Stay as still, relaxed, and focused as you can.

Next, your partner will try the three-speed touch: slow, medium, and fast. You block the touches or just avoid them by moving your body out of the way. What was your experience?

Most probably, your reactions are much faster when you are starting from a still position than when you are jumping and moving around. This part of martial arts training is called Yi Chuan, which means 'standing still meditation.' It is a part of every traditional Chinese martial arts training. It is one of the most important stepping stones of training internal martial arts. The reason for that is that all motion starts from stillness. You have a better chance of detecting movement if you are still, rather than jumping and moving around.

Standing Meditation (Yi Chuan)

Different internal styles have different standing meditation postures. The two standing meditations chosen for this book are from yoga and from Yang style Tai Chi.

The first meditation comes from the yoga tradition. Stand in the mountain stance posture.

Empty the mind, and then gather and focus your entire energy at your lower energy center while connecting to the three forces: heaven, human, and earth.

This standing meditation should be practiced on its own until you can stand for 30 minutes.

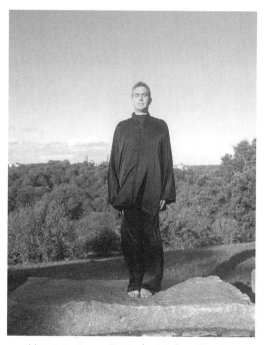

Mountain stance. Empty the mind, and gather and focus energy at lower energy center.

The second standing meditation comes from tai chi, four gates breathing.

It is challenging in a more physical way, especially for the arms and legs. Train with the mind on the four gates visualization as well as the bubble. On an inhalation, move your mind to the lower energy center from the four gates and the bubble and on exhalation, back to the four gates as well as the bubble.

If you are interested in more standing meditation (Yi Chuan) training, you can take the eleven moves from the tai chi form and make each one into a standing meditation. Also, I recommend, for your collection of books, the two-volume *Warriors of Stillness* by Jan Diepersloot. It is difficult to find this book but is worth the effort. The author teaches the art of standing Chinese meditation in a very traditional way. It is full of pictures of world-renowned masters of the various internal styles.

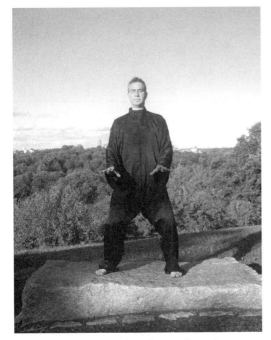

High. Four gates breathing with mind in four gates and energetic bubble.

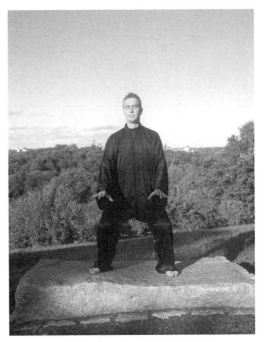

Low. Four gates breathing with mind in four gates and energetic bubble.

GRIND

Sunset Tai Chi Form

From the horse stance at the end of begin tai chi, start grinding counterclockwise two times and then clockwise two times. When grinding, keep your stance at the same height and your hands two inches below the navel. Have a sensation of the grinding not only at the hands and palms but also at the bottom of the soles of your feet. Use the grinding motion to lead more of the energy from the upper energy center to the lower energy center, and to lead the energy down the energetic baton in a spiral.

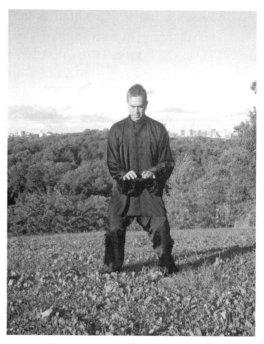

Horse stance; mind in 4 gates, lower energy center and bubble.

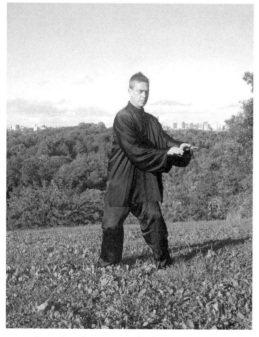

First. Grinding counterclockwise two times.

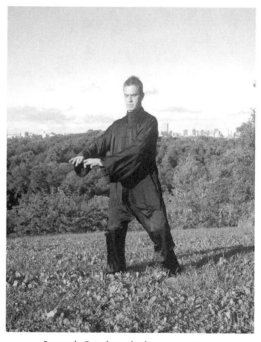

Second. Grinding clockwise two times.

Tai Chi Ball

Use the tai chi ball to strengthen the tai chi movement.

The tai chi ball is a traditional training tool used to strengthen the muscles, joints, and bones on a physical level. It is also an important tool that helps with strengthening the visualizations of the lower and upper energy centers as well as the small circulation that gives us physical feedback. This projection that is done with the external ball in our hands can be done when the ball is stationary, when working on just the centers and moving, and when focusing on the small circulation. The tai chi ball is usually made out of natural wood to allow the energy to pass through. If you are lucky, it is made from one piece of wood such as mahogany, oak, cherry, or walnut. You may use any kind of ball, such as a medicine ball, a round object, or a rock.

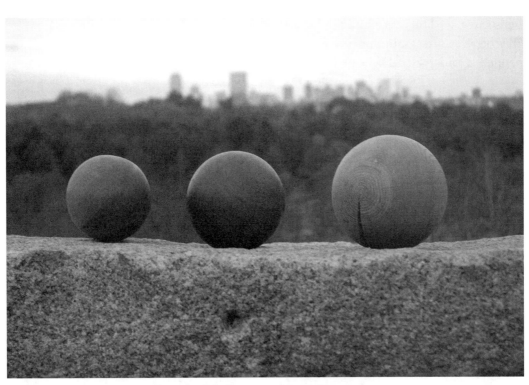

Using tai chi balls to strengthen tai chi movement.

Stand with the feet parallel and the weight distributed evenly between the ball of your foot and your heel in both feet.

Alternatively, you could sit comfortably on the edge of a chair.

Maintain a healthy alignment: tailbone dropped, head suspended, face and shoulders relaxed, and knees slightly bent. Visualize that there is an internal energetic circulation in your body that follows the outer movements of the ball in your hands.

Start moving the ball in a circle from left to right, parallel to the floor at dan tian height. Start with small circles, and as you become stronger in your legs and are able to hold the knees and inner arches of your feet still, while the pelvis is turning, you can make the circle bigger and squat lower. Change and circle in the opposite direction for an equal number of repetitions.

When you are comfortable performing this physical exercise, add the mental visualization of circling the mind in the direction that the ball is turning along the belt energy vessel around your waist.

Visualize the energy getting bigger and bigger until it extends past your waist and circles about one foot around your body.

Maintain alignment throughout the legs. The knees should point roughly over the middle toe, and the feet should be parallel, inner arches alive, and the huiyin cavity (the area between the groin and the anus) pointing down. Keep the top of the head suspended. Hold the ball two inches below the navel. Concentrate on the lower energy

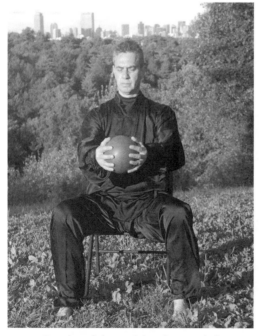

On edge of chair with head suspended, and face and shoulders relaxed.

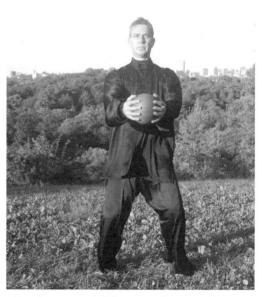

Visualize energy belt becoming bigger and bigger, extending past waist and circling around body.

center. Then imagine the lower energy center is like the sun and imagine the ball as the earth. Rotate the ball or earth around the center or sun. Start going toward the right, counterclockwise, and make a flat circle and bring it back to the center. Try to keep your circles symmetrical. When you turn to your right, do not let the left knee and the inner arch of the left foot collapse. When you turn to your left, do not let the right knee and the inner arch of the right foot collapse. The knees and the inner arches need to stay aligned. Do not let the waist and the tai chi ball pull on the legs and break that alignment. To achieve that, start by doing a small circle. When you feel comfortable and are able to maintain the correct alignment in your legs, gradually increase the size of your circle.

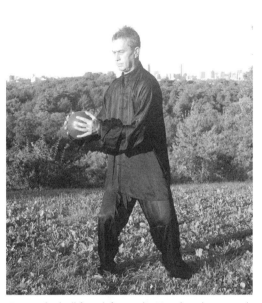

Rotate the ball from left to right. Visualize the internal energetic circulation that follows outer movements of ball in hands.

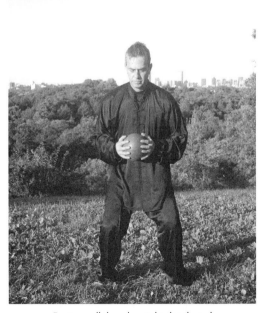

Feet parallel and weight distributed between ball of foot and heel.

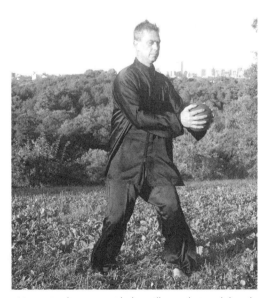

Maintain alignment with the tailbone dropped, head suspended, face and shoulders relaxed.

Make sure that the groin area is opening and closing, and is not just still. When you move to your left, the inner groin on the left is closed and the inner groin on the right is open and when you move toward the right, the groin on the right closes and the one on the left opens.

Often beginners and sometimes even advanced practitioners make the mistake of moving their arms without moving the pelvis because it is easier to maintain alignment since there is no pull on the legs from the pelvis. Be aware of this tendency and avoid it.

Eventually, after you are comfortable maintaining the physical alignment, you will want the ball that rotates outside to correspond to the energy that rotates around the lower energy center in the belt vessel. Remember that holding the ball is just a way to help the mind transform or project this circle into the belt vessel that is around the lower energy center.

Try integrating the skills of stretching and relaxing the bow with the movement of the waist and ball. This can be done in two ways. You can start by holding the ball at the lower energy center with the stretch the bow posture.

As you rotate the ball away from your body, you release the bow. You stretch the bow when the ball is close to the body and you release the bow when the ball moves away from the body at the furthest point: that is the switching point.

To finish the circle pull the tai chi ball back in to your energy center and release the bow.

Circle an equal number of times in each direction.

Key Points about the Tai Chi Ball. Your palms should be soft and your wrists should be relaxed when you hold the tai chi ball. You should be like an octopus. Imagine every part of your fingers and palms have suction cups and when you touch the ball, you feel or sense every millimeter in your palms.

Your wrists should be soft. Your shoulders should drop, relax, and sink. There is a tendency to raise the shoulders when working with the ball. Coordinate the movement with the breathing. For example, you can inhale during half the circle and exhale during the other half, or you can inhale during a whole circle and exhale during the next one, or you can inhale for three circles and exhale on the next three circles.

Breathing is a tool, it is a strategy, and you can utilize it in whatever means you want or for whatever purposes you need. If you are training for the reason of learning martial arts, most of the time the inhalation goes with the movement inward and exhalation goes with the movement outward. When looking at the empty full moon as well as the long and the cross bows that we learned, most of the time inhalation will go with the empty moon and stretch the bow, and exhalation will go with full moon, release the bow. But if you are doing the tai chi ball for health purposes, you can change the order of the breath and bow skills.

Remember, the spirit of this motion with the tai chi ball is grinding as in grinding rice.

If you use a pestle or any other hand tool to grind, you will find that you need to push down as well as circle around to achieve good results. When real grinding was done, the downward pressure was created by using a heavy stone. You need to create that down feeling or sensation when you circle the tai chi ball. There is a sense of sinking through the tai chi ball, through the elbows, through the energetic baton, and eventually sinking through the belly button and all the way through the legs deep into the earth.

When the tai chi ball is the farthest from your belly button, this is when you want to sink the most. It is not that you rise along the other parts of the circle; it is just that you want to counter the tendency to be pulled up when the ball is at the farthest point from the body. There is a heavy sinking through the legs and there is a heavy sensation into the ball but there is a light feeling up through the spine, all the way to the top of the head. You want to sink throughout the whole movement.

You want to actually feel and sense the grinding or the 'moo' sensation in the bubbling well in the soles of the feet as if you were also grinding under the soles of your feet against the ground.

There is a little circle under the soles that does its own little grinding.

You could, for example, focus on the waist or the tai chi ball, or just focus on the soles of the feet, put your mind there and generate the whole motion of the circle from the soles of the feet.

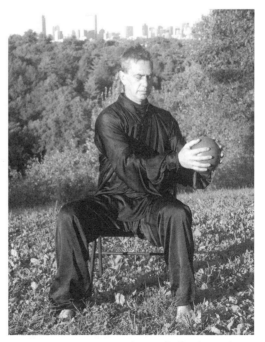

The tailbone, which is part of the long bow, should never stick out backward. It is either straight down or dropped in. When you stretch the bow, it is dropped in, and when you release the bow, it is straight down. If you stick the tailbone out, that will break the alignment. Make sure that your shoulders are relaxed. There is a tendency to raise the shoulder, so be aware of that. Keep the head suspended and be aware of the tendency to look down toward the ball. The eyes should look straight forward. Sometimes you can just close the eyes slightly and that will allow you to maintain a stronger internal visualization of the energy moving around the lower energy center and the belt vessel.

Lower energy center is the sun; ball is the earth; rotate ball/earth around center/sun.

There are many skills that you need to put together. It is useful to pull yourself back and practice each skill separately until it becomes comfortable and you can do it correctly. Once you are comfortable with each skill, you put them together. Eventually, you will be able to perform while standing in a low horse stance while rotating the pelvis without collapsing the inner arches or the knees, mixing the bows with the motion as well as the empty full moon, using the visualizations of draining the baton, the bubble, four gates breathing, and spiritual breathing. With practice, you can put them all together and will be ready to harmonize them with the three forces: earth, human, and heaven. Have patience and do not be hard on yourself. Practice, practice, and then practice some more.

Martial Applications of Grind

Grind to the left and right can be used for striking, controlling, or as a takedown move. The movements of the legs in the tai chi drills and tai chi form are not the movements you use for taking your opponent down. Not showing the leg application in the form or exercise was a very traditional principle. The form has layers and layers of applications, and except for the first layer, the individuals who came up with these forms tried to keep the applications secret. If you think about it, not long ago this was a necessary principle to win or lose a war. It was necessary to prevent your enemy from finding out the meaning of every move and then coming up with solutions that could lead to losing the fight and in turn the war.

Another application of the grind motion is to use the right arm to block by performing the grind clockwise and at the same time use the left arm to block through the counterclockwise circle. This application is an example of the ones hidden in the layers of the movement.

The first application is in the category of takedowns. The first half of the clockwise

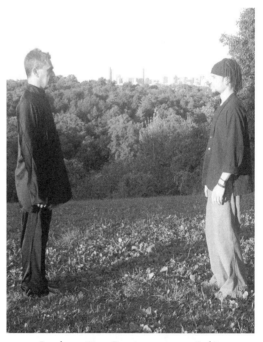

Ready position. Face opponent , mind in both lower energy centers and opponent.

circle of the grind is a block. Use your left arm to block your opponent's punch.

The second half, along with the proper use of the leg, is the takedown. Place your leg behind your opponent and circle the right hand/arm toward your opponent's neck.

The second circle could be used to break the opponent's neck once he or she is down.

Another application to this move is under the category of controlling your opponent. The first circle is used to block and stick.

The second circle can be used to control, or pop and break.

The last application is from the category of kicking and punching. The first circle is the block and a grip.

The second half of the circle is to knee your opponent in the ribs, or strike with your arm to his neck or face.

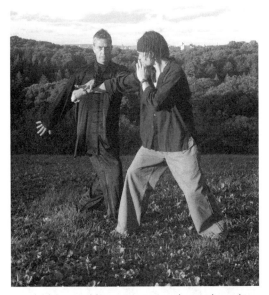

Takedown. Yield to opponent's right punch, circle to the left, use your left arm to block punch.

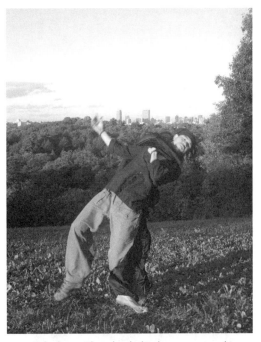

Takedown. Place leg behind opponent and circle right hand and arm toward opponent.

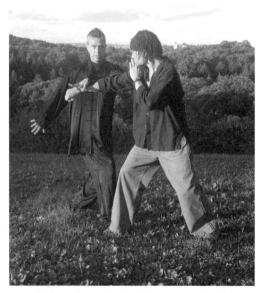

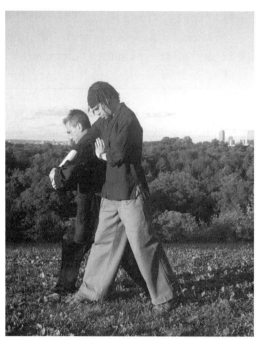

Controlling opponent. Yield to opponent's right punch. Circle to the left, use your left arm to block punch.

Controlling opponent. Stick and circle, control, pop, or break.

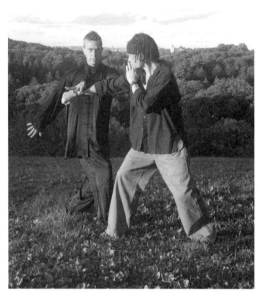

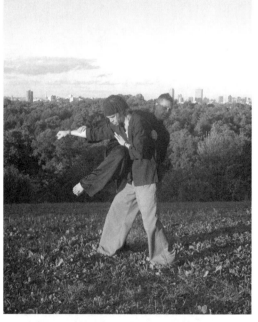

Kicking and punching. Yield to opponent's right punch. Circle to the left, use your left arm to block punch.

Kicking and punching. Circle knee opponent's ribs; or strike neck or face with arm.

CRANE SPREADS ITS WINGS

Sunset Tai Chi Form

Once you have finished grinding, from horse stance, shift your weight to the left leg and turn the right foot to 45 degrees.

Then shift your weight to the right leg. Lift the left foot and place it down gently, touching the floor with the ball of the foot. You are in empty stance to the left, your weight is on the right leg, you are facing the left, and your left foot just touches the floor, it has no weight on it.

While standing in empty stance, inhale and cross your arms in front of your chest.

Exhale and raise the left arm to the side, above your ear, rotating the arm and the palm outward, while simultaneously dropping down and rotating the other arm and palm outward.

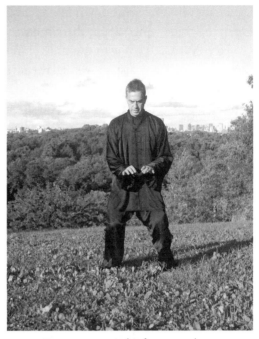

Horse stance; mind in four gates, lower energy center and bubble.

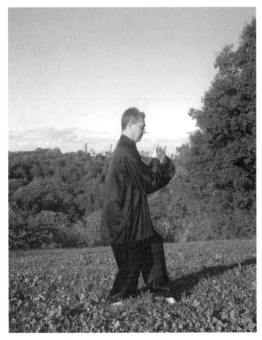

Empty stance to left. Inhale and cross arms in front of chest.

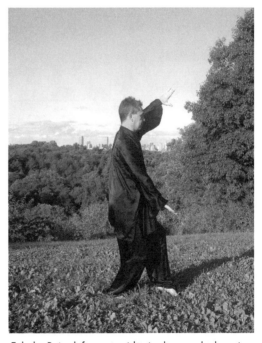

Exhale. Raise left arm to side simultaneously dropping right and rotate arms with palms facing outward.

Now bring the arms down and cross in front of your chest again, palms face inward. Open the crane wings again; this time you will end with the right arm and palm up high.

Key Points. Try not to use only your arms, but try to lead this movement from the movement of the waist as well as the stretching and releasing of the bows. Make sure your wrists are relaxed and shoulders stay down. When crossing the arms in front of your chest, inhale and exhale as you open the arms or when spreading your wings.

On an energetic level, when the arms/wings are crossed the long bow and the cross bow are stretched. Inhale and keep the mind on two visualizations at the same time. The first condenses the energy ball at your lower energy center (center of gravity energy center), and the second leads some of the energy from the lower energy center, upward through the governing vessel to the area between the shoulder blades.

When exhaling, lead the energy from the shoulder area to the palms and at the same time lead the energy from your lower energy center to a few inches below your feet.

When the waist and the bows are active while performing the movement, the internal organs are being massaged. This move is especially good for your liver and spleen in the front and the kidneys in the back.

Once you feel comfortable with one side, practice the movements on the other side. Your goal is to be able to move through different stances as well as from side to side while performing crane spreads its wings. When you are doing the Sunset Tai Chi form,

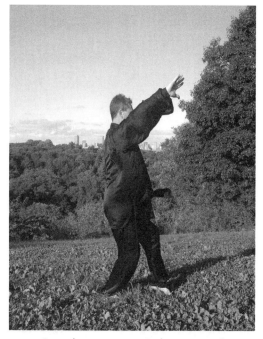

Open the crane wings. Right arm up and left down, and use tai chi hand form.

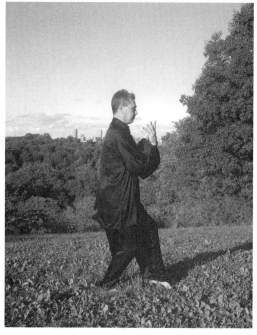

Bring arms down and cross them in front of chest.

you perform crane spread its wings to one side only. You need to isolate this move, as well as the other moves, which are done to one side only, and practice it to both sides.

It is important to practice while sitting on a chair. This regular practice will give you the opportunity to learn some of the skills in a way that does not happen when standing up. It also gives you an opportunity to practice on days that your legs are sore or injured. Finally, in order to really experience this move to its fullest, you want to not only perform the movement of the crane's wings but you want to be the crane. Try to become a crane, opening your wings to ward off your enemies or to protect your young. The eyes condense when inhaling and become 'fiery eyes' when exhaling. At this point you have integrated into the move the five building blocks: body, breath, mind, energy, and spirit. At this point in time, your tai chi is no longer just a dance with no internal skills.

Martial Arts Applications of Crane Spreads Its Wings

One of the applications is a kicking and punching application and involves both the upper body as well as the lower one. You can see that one leg is empty while the other is fully weighted. The empty leg is there to kick after blocking a punch or a grab.

When a punch comes at you or someone is grabbing your shirt, move to the left and repel their grip or punch with the left arm as it moves up into crane spreads its wings.

Next, move that hand downward, leading your opponent's arm down as you do.

You can see the form crane spreads its wings in the application. You block up and

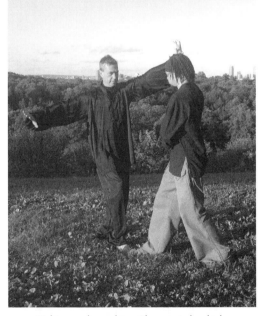

Kicking and punching. The empty leg kicks
after blocking a punch or a grab.

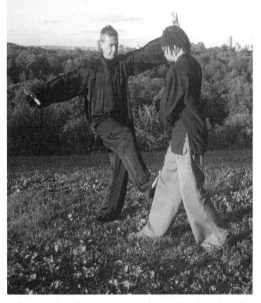

Block and Kick. Crane Spreads Its Wing. Block with
left arm, kick the knee or the patella with right foot.

continue the move downward to neutralize your opponent. At the same time your other arm, the right one, will strike your opponent in the face. There are many death points in the face. There are approximately 70 points or cavities that you can use to neutralize your opponent for a short or long time. There are 36 points that can knock him out totally or kill him.

At the same time your leg is ready to kick the patella, a floating bone in the knee, or you can kick the groin.

If your opponent decides to throw a second punch, or grasps you, apply the move again to his other arm. You can actually lock the two arms together, and then take him down.

To maintain the lock, you will take one arm, bring it down, and lock the elbow so

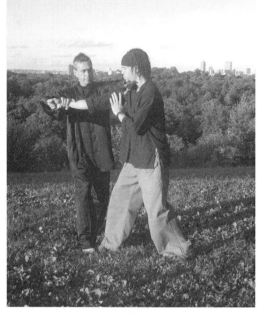

Kicking and punching. Circle to left, block with cross arms, and deflect sideways.

you can take him or her to the police. If you want to lock someone on the ground, you can entangle both arms, place your foot on him, locking him on the ground.

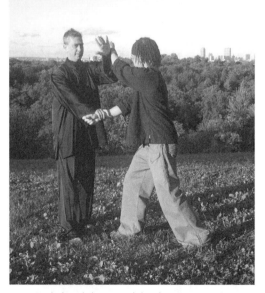

Right hand downward, leading opponent's arm down as you lead his other arm up.

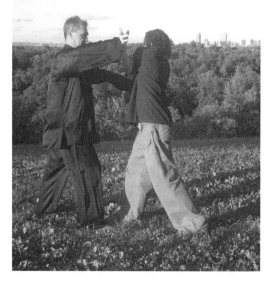

Block up and continue move downward to neutralize opponent.

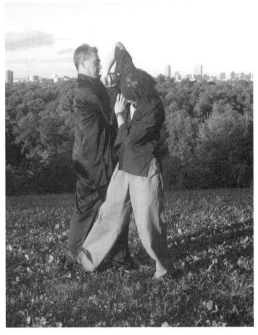

To maintain a lock, bring one arm down
and lock the wrist and elbow.

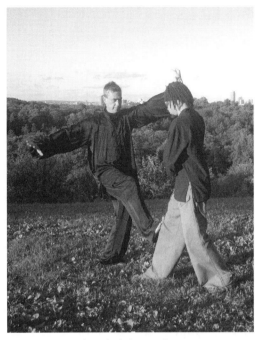

Leg ready to kick the patella or groin.

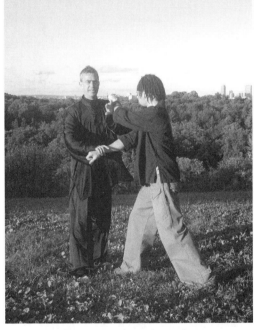

Opponent throws second punch. Apply move again
to other arm and lock his two arms together.

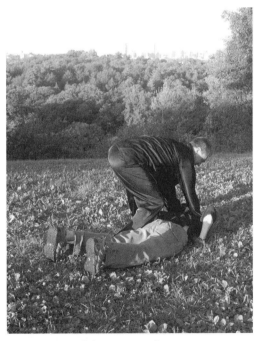

Take opponent down.

TWO BLOCKS

Sunset Tai Chi Form

Once you have finished your two crane spread its wings on the left side, you should have your right arm up while the left one is down.

From this posture, block with the right arm toward your left—first the chest and then the knees, while raising and blocking to your right with your left arm.

Key Points. This exercise or movement simulates blocking two imaginary incoming punches.

When performing this movement, the movements of your arms should come from the movements of the waist. Turn the waist from side to side and let the arms just follow. At the same time, stretch the bows on the first block and on the second one, stretch some more. Remember that at the end of the second block, you want to start releasing the bows that will prepare you for the next move. The bows close or stretch gradually from the first block to the second, but at the end of the second block you start to open or release them.

This movement of the waist from side to side as well as the movement of the bows and the empty-full moon around your center of gravity energy center massages all your internal organs through the trunk and especially massages your lungs and chest area. The breathing for this movement is a long inhalation through the two blocks. Inhale on the two blocks and when doing brush knee and step forward, exhale when stepping forward and pushing with your arm. When performing the two blocks, over time move slower and slower; that way you will bring more and more oxygen into your bloodstream as well as developing your lungs.

The mind should focus on the energetic visualizations. Move the energy of the imaginary two blocks first into your center, then take this energy as well as your own energy from the pituitary gland energy center and lead it all down to the lower energy center. Continue this visualization downward all the way to the floor. You are trying to dissolve all the energy from the two punches down into the earth. Your body structure and focus on downward movement will allow you to redirect any incoming force down and away.

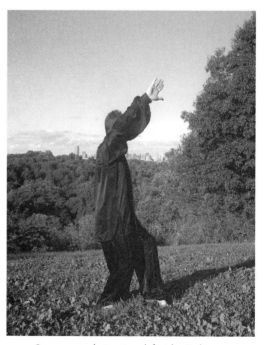

Crane spreads its wings left side. Right arm up, left arm down, and left leg forward.

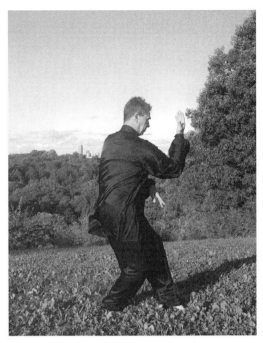 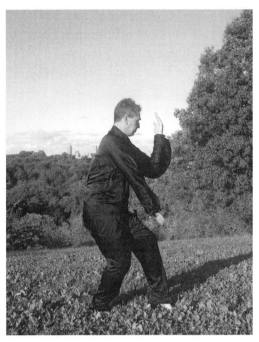

Block with right arm; chest. Block with left; knee.   Block with left arm; chest. Block with right arm; knee.

The head can do two things or take two different postures depending on the goal or purpose. For the martial artist, the head or the eyes face toward your enemy. For health purposes, you can move the head with the trunk, or if you are interested in stretching the neck, you can move the head farther to the left or the right. Just make sure it does not affect the integrity of the rest of your skills.

I encourage you to practice the two blocks on the edge of a chair, which will let you experience the upper body in a way that is not possible when standing. It will also increase the range of motion through your waist. The last element you want to evoke is your spirit. When performing the two blocks, you are like a whirlpool. Whatever stumbles into you will just get sucked down into the whirlpool.

Martial Arts Application of Two Blocks

A typical reaction from untrained individuals is to just meet a punch or a grab or, if having good instincts, step backwards.

As a martial artist, you train over the years not to stay with your body square forward when the energy comes at you but instead to move just enough that the opponent's arm slides beside your body.

Of course, this skill takes many years of practice but with the help of your arms, this becomes a skill easily learned.

Over time and with practice, not only can you move so your opponent's hands slide beside your body. You can become good enough so that you can grip his arm and with your ribs or stomach, you can control or pop out the elbow.

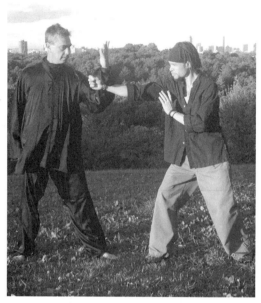

Turning right blocking with left.

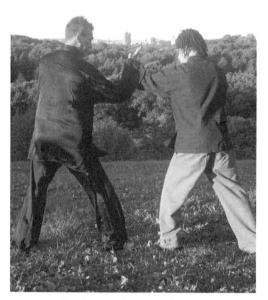

Turning left blocking with right.

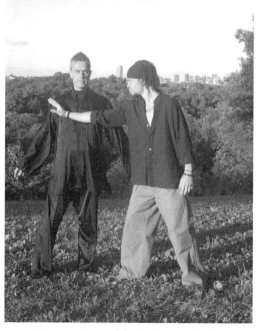

Opponent's arm slides beside your body.

If you want to do a takedown, just place your leg in the way of the opponent's movement that occurs as a result of the pain suffered in the elbow.

Usually if you use the two blocks, the second one is the strike and the first one will be the block.

If you are blocking from the inside then the second will strike the inner body.

If you are blocking from the outside, the strike will be to the back of your opponent's body, for example, the kidneys.

Challenge yourself and see how fast you can move your waist from side to side while holding your fists up by your head for one minute. Do it both standing and on a chair. Count left and right as one. If you can do 60 or more in 30 seconds, you are fairly fast.

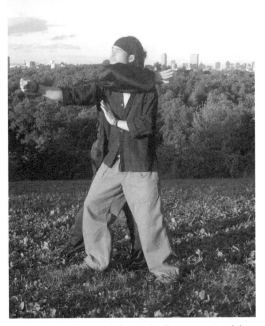

Takedown. Place right leg behind opponent's while wrapping right arm around opponent's neck.

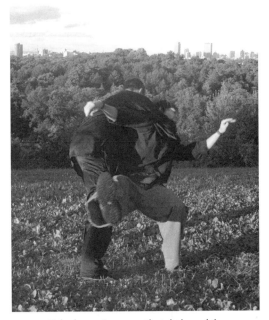

Takedown. Sweep with right leg while pushing down with right arm.

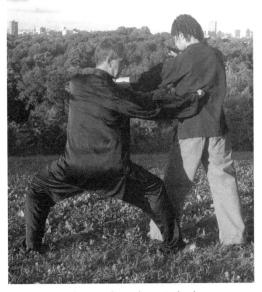

Kicking and punching. Strike the back of opponent's body: kidneys.

BRUSH KNEE

Sunset Tai Chi Form

You are in an empty stance, facing your left side, finishing your second block. As you inhale, lift your left arm to the blocking position while the other hand, the right, points to your elbow.

Then, the waist turns. The left, blocking arm moves from the waist, in toward the centerline. At the same time, the other hand, the right, moves back, through the waist, palm face up.

Continue moving the right arm back and upward, counterclockwise, over your head near your right ear.

While you lift the hand backward, your left leg moves forward, which will put you in a back stance.

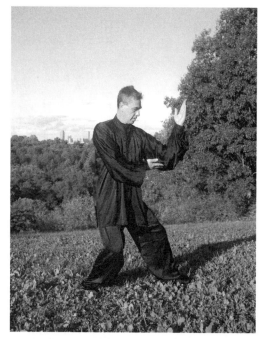

Back stance. Lift left arm to blocking position. Right hand points to elbow.

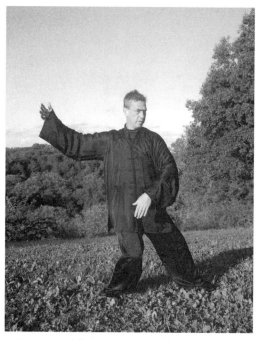

Waist turns, left arm moves toward centerline, and right arm moves back through waist.

Remember, from the beginning of the two blocks until this point, we are gradually stretching the two bows, the long bow and the cross bow. This is the most yin point of the physical movements.

Next you are going to move from a back stance to the forward one, the climb the mountain stance. As you exhale, turn the waist, brush your knee with the left arm, and push forward with the right arm, from the height of the ear. This is the most yang part of the physical posture.

Do not tense your shoulders. The wrists are loose and relaxed. At the end of the push, settle the wrist and keep your elbows slightly bent.

Key Points. Between the most yin point, back stance, with one arm backward at ear height and the other hand at a point right before brushing the knee and pushing forward, you should stretch the bows. As you finish the movements, or the push, or strike, release the bows.

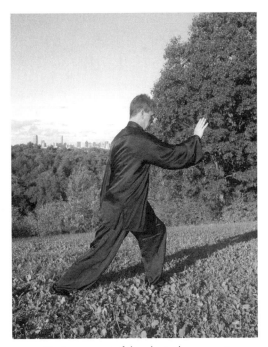

Most yang part of the physical movement
of brush knee and step forward.

When not doing the tai chi form, make sure you practice both sides as well as practicing while sitting on the edge of a chair. Another good way to practice is to practice the move beside a wall or tree. The wall or tree forces you to really use the bows as well as experience a strong sensation of energy between your trunk and the wall or the tree.

Some days when practicing brush knee and step forward near the wall or the tree, the sensation is like a great river, a strong stream of water running between you and the wall or tree. Other days, it could be just in your hand, or the sensation could be just a brook. When inhaling, the mind leads the energy from the lower energy center to the area between the shoulder blades while condensing in the lower energy center, and on exhalation, leads the energy to the center of your palms and at the same time a few inches below the soles of your feet. You can also, when inhaling, move your mind from the bubble, a fist away from your body, into your energetic baton and on the exhalation back into your energetic bubble. If you cannot do both the four gates breathing and the bubble visualization together, pull yourself back and do one. It takes time for the mind to be able to perform multiple visualizations while performing the physical moves. With lots of patience and mindful practice, you will get there.

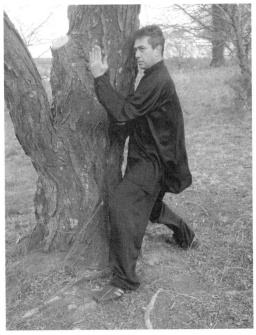

Left arm toward centerline and right; back,
through waist (release bows).

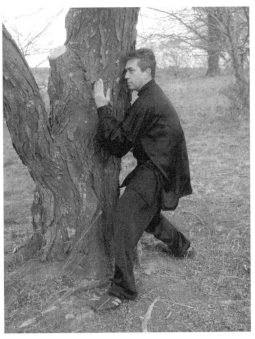

Left arm block. Right arm moves between
tree and hip (stretch bows).

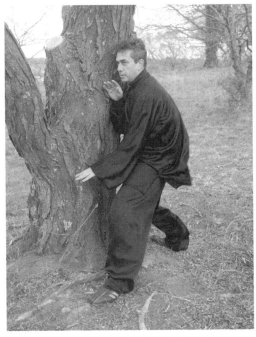

Left arm brushes left knee while right
arm pushes forward (start releasing bows).

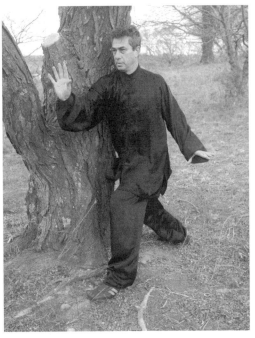

Forward stance with right arm pushing
forward and settle the wrist (release bows).

Martial Arts Applications of Brush Knee

Again the main principle in brush knee and step forward is to first listen, then yield, stick, and finally to adhere. When a punch or a grab is coming at you, first step back with your right leg and turn your body to the right while using your left arm to block.

To achieve the sensitivity, which allows you to know when to move your right leg back, takes practice. You can try facing your opponent and then have him slowly try to touch your chest.

As soon as you sense your opponent's movements, move your right or left leg back, while turning the body to the same direction.

This practice of listening is the way to develop better reaction time. It is a listening that is not done with your ears. It is a listening that is done with the eyes and the skin. For now, look at your opponent's chest. After you improve, look in his eyes. When you are being touched, you are listening from your skin and when you are being punched, you are listening from being still and looking at your opponent's chest or eyes. Also when you are neutralizing your opponent's energy while your weight is on the back leg, your front leg is ready to kick.

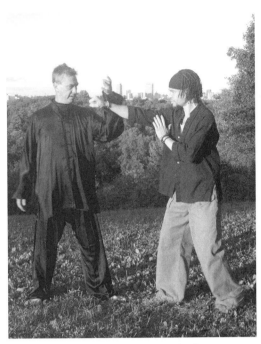

Right leg steps back, turn body
right, and use arm to block.

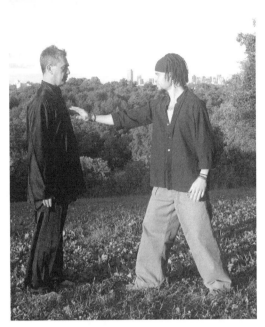

Listen, yield while facing opponent;
have him slowly try to touch your chest.

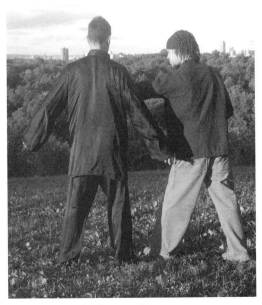

Stick and adhere, and sense movement.
Leg back turning body (back view).

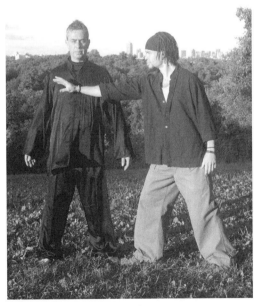

Stick and adhere, and sense movement.
Leg back turning body (front view).

Remember that the leg position in the tai chi form is not correct for applications. You will need to angle toward your opponent with your legs, and then kick.

You can also step forward and strike with your right arm if you blocked with your left and vice versa.

To do a takedown with 'brush knee and step forward,' lock the elbow of the arm you blocked and drag or drop your opponent down to the floor. Because his elbow is locked, he will follow you to the ground.

If you must, you can stick your left or right leg in your opponent's way to make the drop more harmful.

There are many ways to control your opponent with this move. I like the one that is called 'send the devil to the heaven.' As you block the punch, you grab the wrist of your opponent's hand and lift it up while holding his elbow. Your opponent will go up on his toes and will beg you to stop.

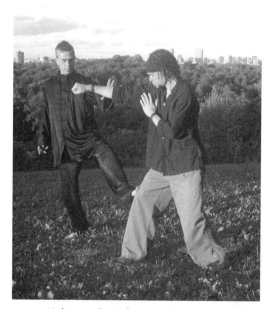

Kicking and punching. Angle opponent
with legs, and then kick.

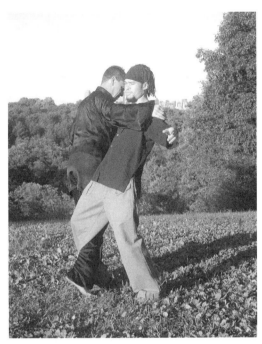

Takedown. Lock opponent's elbow of blocked
arm, and reach for neck with other arm.

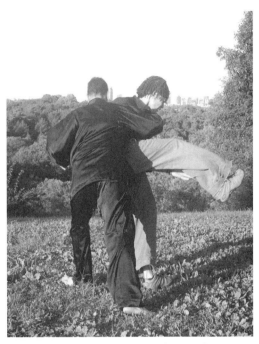

Takedown. Drop opponent down to floor.

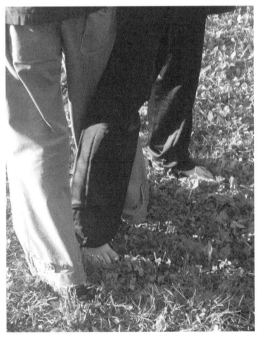

Takedown. Stick left or right leg in opponent's
way, and drop becomes more harmful.

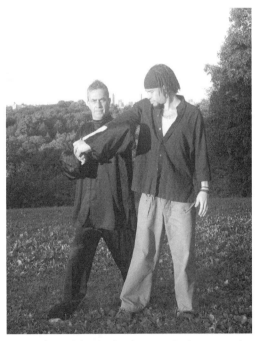

Control. Send the devil to heaven. Grab opponent's
hand and lift it up while holding his wrist and elbow.

CLOUD HANDS

Sunset Tai Chi Form

From a front stance to your left, move into a high horse stance by bringing the left leg in toward the right leg.

At the same time, the right arm is turned inward and brought in front of your chest as if you are hugging someone.

The left arm moves in front of you, palm facing down, as if you are petting a dog. The elbow is a fist away from your waist.

Now move to your right and do cloud hands three times. Your legs are already in position (horse stance) to do the first cloud hands to your right.

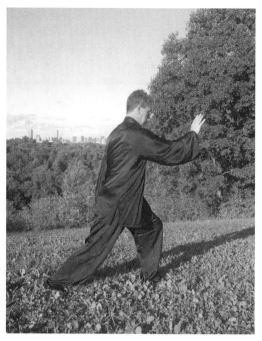

Brush knee and step forward standing in front stance to your left.

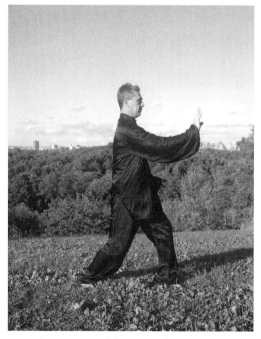

Front stance to left, move to horse stance.

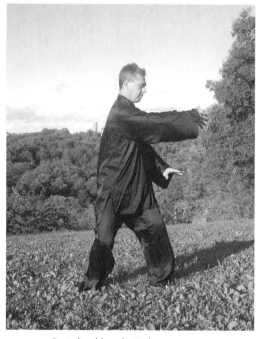

First cloud hands. Right arm moves turned inward in front of chest.

The second cloud hands moves left; bring your left leg near the right and shift your weight to the right leg.

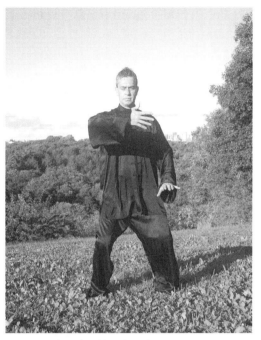

First cloud hands. Left arm moves with palm facing down.

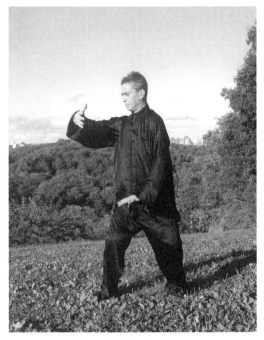

First cloud hands to right.

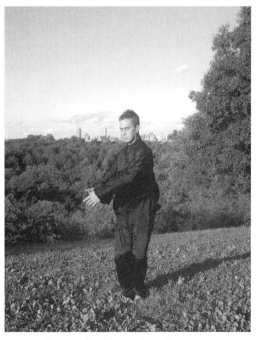

Second cloud hands. Bring left leg in, change the arms and move to your left.

For the third cloud hands, bring the right leg out and then as you move the waist and arms to the right.

Key Points. Changing the arms is a strong energetic experience. Keep pondering and practicing the up and down energies. While you are performing, imagine being a cloud moving through the blue sky. When the left arm moves up, the right moves down. When the palms rotate, they rotate as one. The fingers are in tai chi position and the wrists are totally relaxed. The legs are agile and the waist is alive. You are a powerful cloud in the sky.

Lengthen with a light sensation through the spine while creating a heavy sensation of sinking down through the legs. As you inhale, turn the waist and rotate your body in the direction of the raised arm.

Exhale as you switch arms. When you are moving to the right or the left, you are moving from the horse stance to the empty stance.

When standing in the horse stance, make sure you maintain the integrity of the inner arches of the soles of your feet, especially when the waist starts to turn.

When turning to the right, pay attention to the left inner arch. When turning to the left, pay attention to the right inner arch. After a while, you will learn the sensation

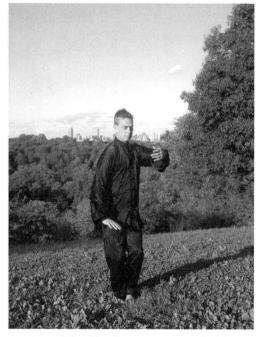

Second cloud hands. Keep turning to the left.

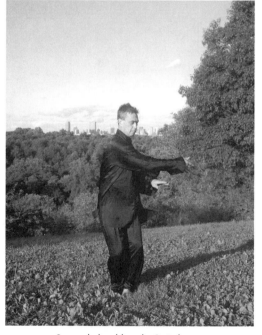

Second cloud hands. Switch arm position and turn to your right.

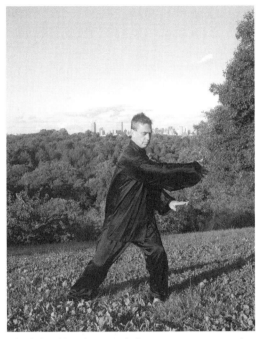

Third cloud hands. Put right leg out, turn to your right.

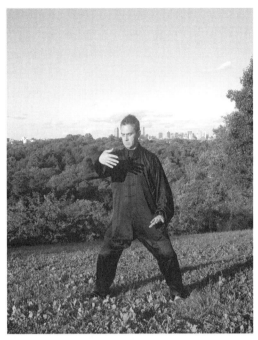

Third cloud hands. Keep turning,
do not break alignment.

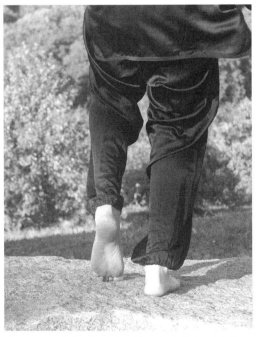

Getting ready for third cloud hands. Roll the right foot
down while rolling the left foot up.

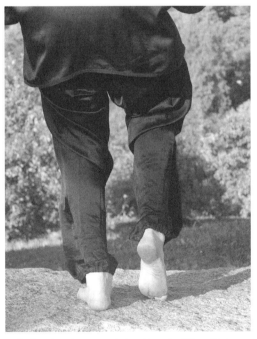

Performing the second cloud hands. Lift and bring
right leg in, roll from the ball of the foot to the heels.

and you will not need to pay attention any more. Do not allow your knees to move inward. Maintain the structure of the kua, which is the space that you create between your legs, through maintaining alignment through the legs.

When moving from the horse stance to the empty stance, if moving to the right, peel the left sole of the foot off the ground, and then gently place that foot right beside the right leg and smear it down gently to the floor.

When lifting the leg, lift with control until placing it down. Do not drag the foot on the floor. Once you are in the empty stance, the entire right sole of the foot should be touching the ground while just the ball of the left foot touches. If you want to change the feet so the right ball of the foot is touching and the left one is supporting your weight, do that through rolling the left down while peeling the right up. Now your right leg is ready to have the ball of the foot touch down and the left foot smears down while maintaining alignment through the knees as well as the inner arches.

Relax your face, neck, and shoulders. Your mind can focus on the energetic bubble. Maintain this visualization while moving to either side. The last element that you need to awaken is your spirit. When performing this movement, you want at first to imitate the clouds moving in the sky slowly over the earth. After a while, you will not only pretend to be a cloud but you will become one whenever you perform this movement.

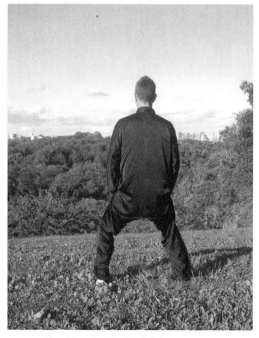

Cloud hands. Moving left horse stance.

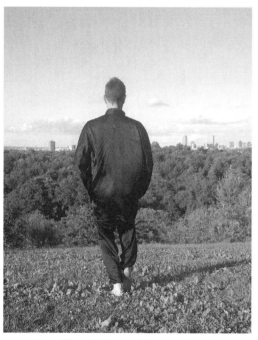

Cloud hands. Moving left empty stance.

Martial Arts Applications of Cloud Hands

When your opponent has his or her palms grabbing your elbow and wrist of your left arm, you can turn to the right and put the right arm under your left elbow to take away your opponent's grip.

Now you are grabbing your opponent's wrist.

Then your left arm moves over your opponent's held arm and you place it on your opponent's elbow. Now you have reversed the situation.

At this point, your opponent can do the same. This form is one of the basic double pushing hands practices. Pushing hands is the martial application training for tai chi. This can be done standing in a climb the mountain stance, or standing with your feet parallel, or even while sitting.

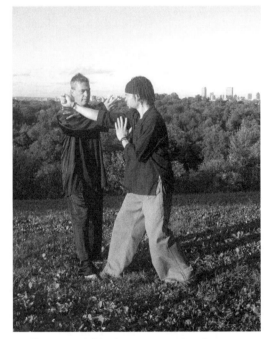

Turn left and put opponent's right arm under your left elbow.

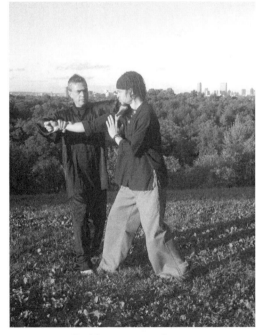

Grabbing opponent's wrist.

For striking and kicking, grab your opponent's wrist. Instead of grabbing the opponent's elbow with the free hand, strike the face with the side of the palm or the elbow.

You can also use the knee to strike the rib area while grabbing the head for better results.

To do a takedown, step behind your opponent with your right foot after the neutralization. With your right arm around your opponent's neck drop him or her to the ground.

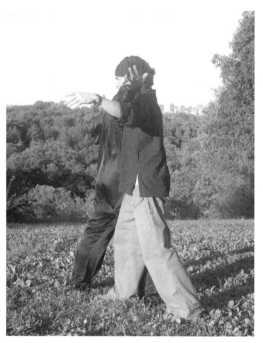

Striking and kicking. Strike face with side of palm or elbow.

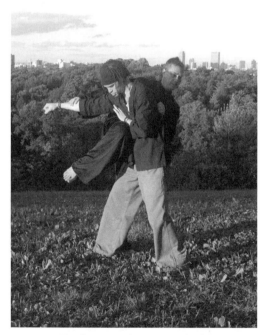

Use knee to strike opponent's rib area while grabbing opponent's head.

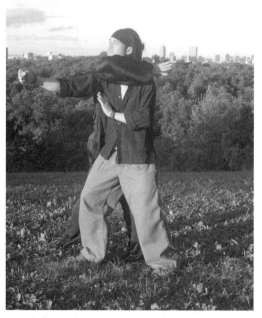

Right foot behind opponent with right arm around opponent's neck, and drop him/her to ground.

To control your opponent, neutralize first.

Then place your left elbow under your opponent's elbow while holding his or her wrist with both your palms.

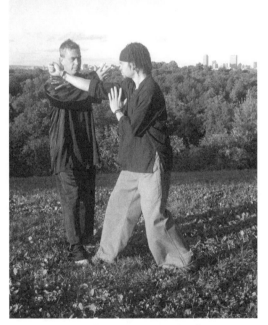

To control opponent, neutralize first.

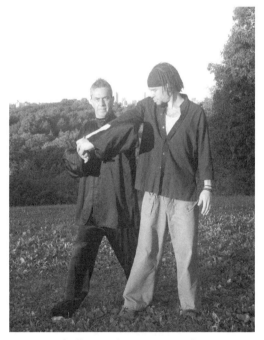

Left elbow under opponent's elbow while holding wrist with both palms.

PICK UP NEEDLE FROM THE SEA BOTTOM
Sunset Tai Chi Form

While turning your waist to the right, inhale and circle both hands and arms clockwise, up across your face with the palms facing forward.

Continue the circle and when you reach 3 o'clock turn the right palm so it faces inward.

Still in horse stance, continue circling the arms down toward the groin area. Now move to left front stance, while pointing with both palms and fingers to the imaginary opponent's groin, left palm facing out, right palm facing in.

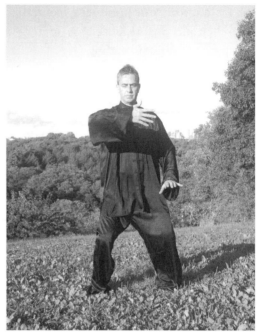

From wave hands, turn waist with arms to left.

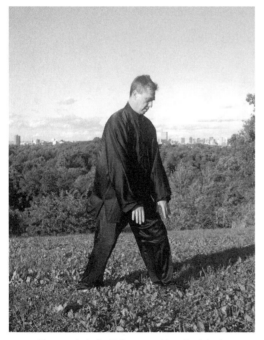

Turn and circle. When reaching 3 o'clock position, turn right palm to face inward.

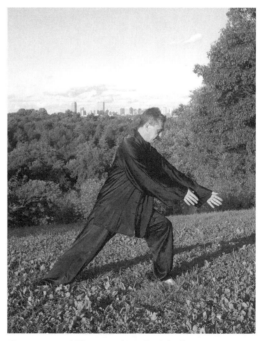

Front stance. When reaching 3 o'clock position, point fingers to imaginary opponent's groin with left palm out and right palm in.

Now move back to empty stance with no weight on the left foot.

At the same time, bring the arms around, still moving clockwise. Cover your face and finish with the arms and palms protecting your face; left arm bent at the elbow with palm facing out, right arm bent at the elbow but the palm faces in.

Exhale and strike forward with the rear, right hand, stinging downward toward an imaginary opponent's lower energy center or groin.

At the same time, the other hand blocks and protects your face.

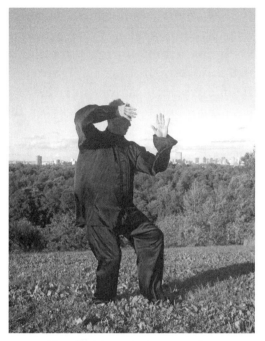

Move back to empty stance, stay low,
arms move clockwise and elbows slightly bent.

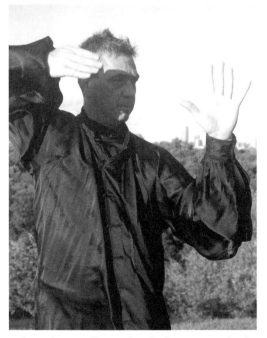

Left arm bent at elbow with palm facing out and right
arm at bent elbow with palm facing in.

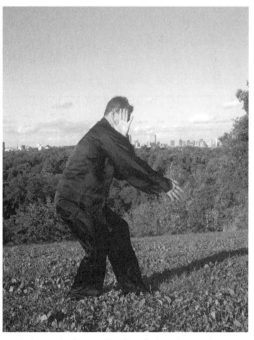

Exhale. Strike forward with right hand toward groin.

Key Points. If you are standing on your right leg and the ball of the left foot is touching the ground, it is your right arm that is by your eyes and ready to attack. Your left arm is in front of you and ready to block. Your mind is actually in all four gates as well as inside your upper and lower energy centers. Your bows are stretched when you are in this posture but when moving to the next one, you release the bows. While the left hand moves toward the right ear, the right one strikes straight to your imaginary opponent's groin area.

If your legs are strong and flexible, you can sink into the standing leg. Make sure the movement is led and directed from the waist and it is not just the arms that are performing the movement.

This move is an excellent opportunity to experience the substantial and insubstantial sensation of energy through the body. First, there is a big difference between the leg that has the weight on it and the one that does not, and second, one arm is attacking, yang, while the other is blocking, yin. As you practice, pay attention to the various sensations from the different positions and intentions of the different limbs. Different muscles are working at different times: tensing and relaxing. Whenever the muscles are tensing (yang), energy flow slows down (yin) in those muscles, and whenever the muscles are relaxing (yin), energy flow is strong (yang), in those muscles.

Pay attention to the various sensations until you can sense the substantial and insubstantial not only in the legs but in the entire body. Practicing this movement near a wall or tree will allow you to experience the energy more strongly and will force you to use the bows. If you do not use the bows, the wall or tree will prevent you from completing the move.

The spirit associated with this move is the sensation of two different winds, the south wind and the north wind. The south wind blocks any negative energy that comes at us while the north wind is the one that attaches to an opponent. The south wind is the left hand that blocks and it also nourishes the right supporting leg. The north

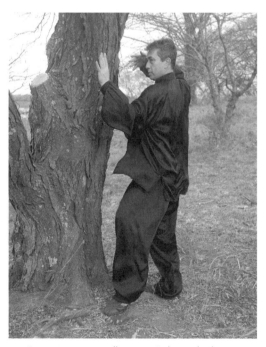

Practicing near wall or tree. Release the bows.

wind, the right hand that attaches, receives energy from the empty left leg. Practicing while sitting on the edge of the chair is also very important. You will find that you can increase the speed of the waist through this practice, and this variation allows you to practice on days that your legs are tired or you are injured.

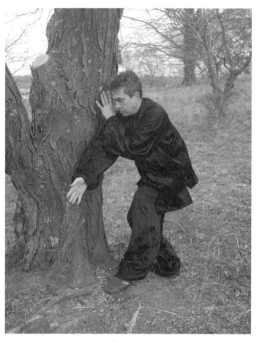

Practicing near wall or tree. Stretch the bows.

Martial Arts Applications of Pick Up Needle from the Sea Bottom

When a punch is coming at you or you are held by a strong grip, one application is to step back or forward with your right leg and use your right arm to block the punch or free yourself from the grip or the punch.

Take your opponent's arm by gripping his or her wrist and lead it up over your head while you are sinking down on one leg. The sinking will make it easier to end up under your opponent's arm rather than trying to lift his or her heavy arm.

Then with your left palm, grab your opponent's elbow.

At this point, you are ready for the application that utilizes all three categories: punch and kick, takedown, and control.

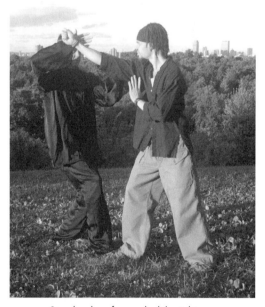

Step back or forward while right arm blocks punch or frees from grip.

If you want to strike and kick, use your right palm fingers to strike the groin area or with your free leg. After you free yourself from the grip, you can kick the patella or the groin.

If you are interested in a control, just pull the arm while you are turning to the right and place your opponent's elbow over your left elbow or shoulder.

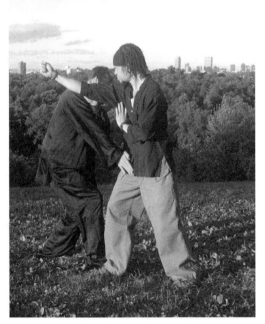

Right palm/fingers strike groin area.

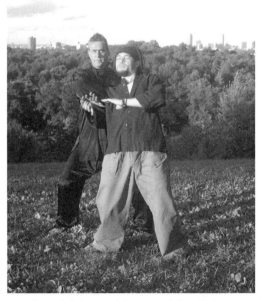

Control. Pull arm while turning left and place opponent's elbow over your left elbow.

For taking down your attacker place your right leg behind your opponent.

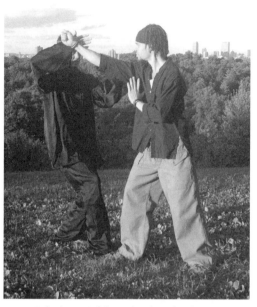

Takedown. Left leg is back and right arm blocks wrist and right leg blocks elbow.

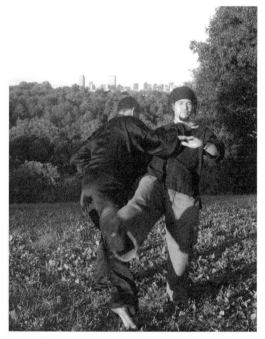

Right arm moves up to opponent's neck.

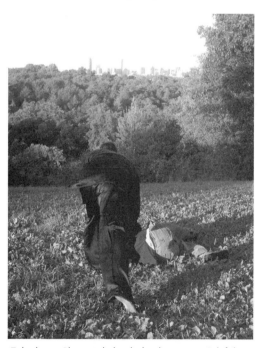

Takedown. Place right leg behind opponent's left leg.

FAN BACK

Sunset Tai Chi Form

Once you finish the pick up needle move, inhale and pull your arms up to your ear area with both palms facing forward. You are still in the empty stance.

As you move forward to front stance, exhale and push both hands at face height.

Key Points. It is interesting that different teachers like to use the long and the cross bows differently with this move. When bringing the palms to ear height, some like to stretch the bows, and then when moving to front stance, release the bows.

Others feel more comfortable releasing the bows when bringing the arms up, and stretching the bows when moving forward to the front stance and pushing your opponent.

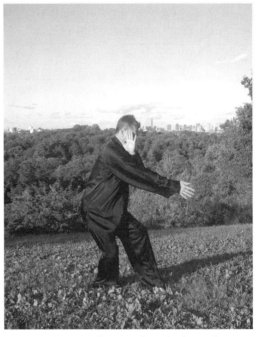

Pick up needle. From the strike forward while in empty stance.

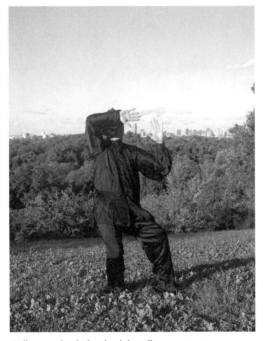

Pull upper body back while still in empty stance, arms are up ear area, and both palms are facing forward.

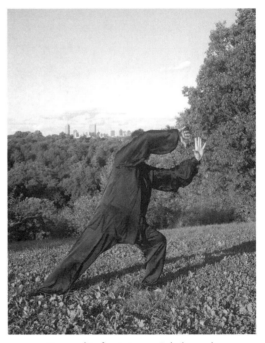

Forward to front stance. Exhale, push both hands shoulder and face height.

You can choose what is best for you. The mind needs to be in all four gates as well as in your energetic baton and bubble.

When you lead your opponent's arm back, an interesting sensation to add to the movement is the sensation of a big wave coming ashore, breaking on the beach. When pushing your opponent, add the sensation of a wave in the middle of the ocean. When pushing your opponent, add a sensation of a lifting wave, which not only pushes your opponent but also lifts him in the same way a big wave will lift a boat. When you are in your empty stance, pretend that you are a giant wave that is forming and as you start to move, move slowly and imagine that you are this great wave moving across the land.

If you are interested in strongly connecting to the spirit of this wave, practice the move fan back from side to side. As you shift backward, inhale and circle both hands down toward your waist, and then raise them on the other side and perform your fan back on the other side. Repeat on both sides.

Remember to eventually integrate all of the internal skills within each tai chi drill and within the tai chi form.

Martial Art Applications of Fan Back

It is not evident in the form how you should use your legs in the applications. This application works well only when using your legs. When a punch is coming at you or you are being gripped at the wrist, chest, or shoulder area, you can do two things at the

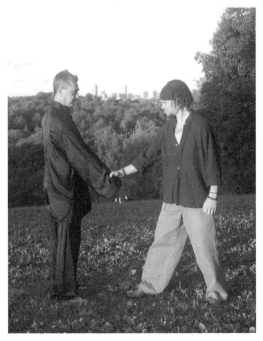

Being gripped at the wrist.

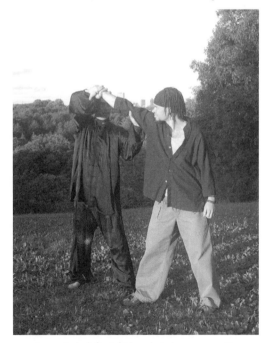

Legs circle left, right hand circles opponent's wrist, and pull up the opponent's arm.

same time: move your right leg behind you to set up an advantageous angle to your opponent, and with your right hand, grip your opponent's right wrist to neutralize the punch or the grip.

Pull toward yourself, like the wave breaking on the beach. Your opponent's natural reaction will be to pull back.

That is when you follow his or her force. Step into him or her, and push and lift, so the crest of the wave creates the power of the force like a wave lifting a boat in the middle of the ocean.

For a takedown, place your right foot behind your opponent.

If you are interested in striking, slide your right hand under your opponent's arm and strike or grab the armpit area.

If you are interested in kicking, a right leg kick to the groin will do the job.

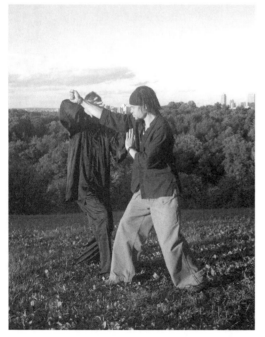

Pull. Wave breaking on beach.

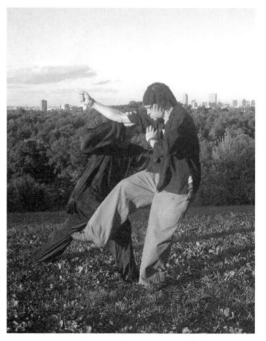

Push and lift. Wave lifting a boat.

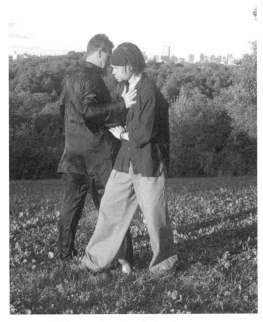

Takedown. Place foot behind opponent.

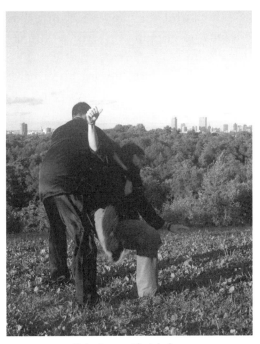

Takedown with right leg.

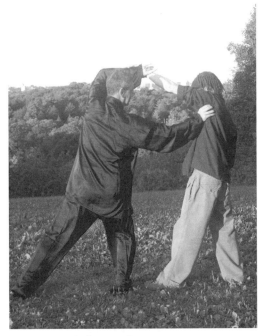

Strike or grab armpit area.

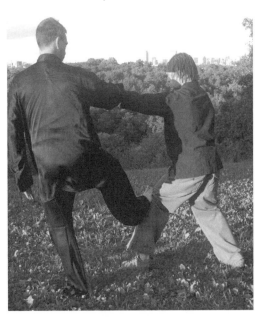

Kicking; right leg kick to groin.

To control your opponent, just slide your right hand under your opponent's arm and end up gripping his wrist with one of your palms and his or her elbow with your other palm.

Fold the forearm toward his or her ear. Grab opponent's wrist and elbow, then lift and squeeze with both of your palms; keep the opponent's arm close to you.

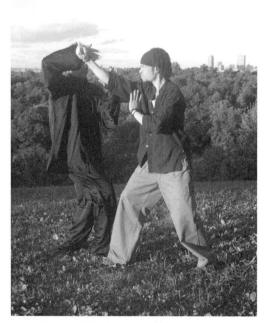

Control. Slide right hand under opponent's arm, gripping his right wrist.

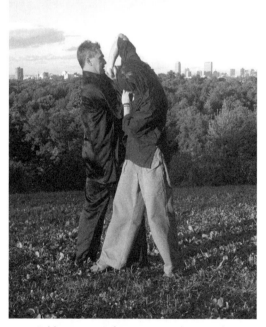

Fold opponent's forearm toward ear, grab opponent's wrist and elbows, and then squeeze.

NOURISH

Sunset Tai Chi Form

From front stance, move to tiger stance with 90% of your weight on your right leg. Drop your arms down and touch palm to palm around the height of your lower energy center.

Continue opening the arms to the sides. Point your fingers to the ground and start pulling earth energy into your core.

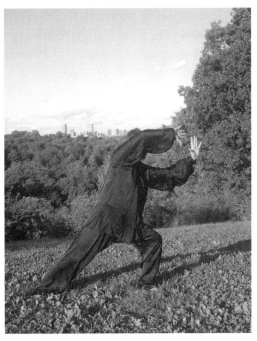

From fan back, shift weight to right leg and bring palms to belly bottom.

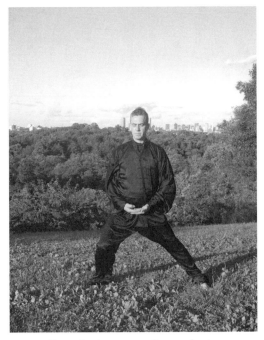

Tame the tiger stance. Drop palms to height of lower energy center.

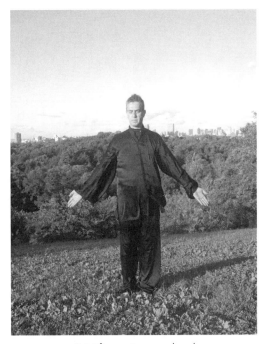

Point fingers to ground and pull earth energy into your core.

Then point to the trees and pull earth energy into your core.

Then point to the oceans and saturate yourself with that energy.

Point to the mountains next and pull in some of that energy.

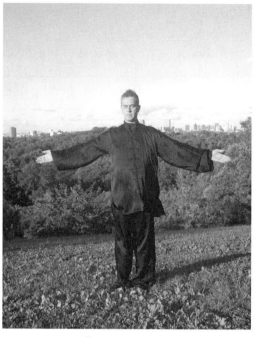

Point fingers to trees and pull earth energy into your core.

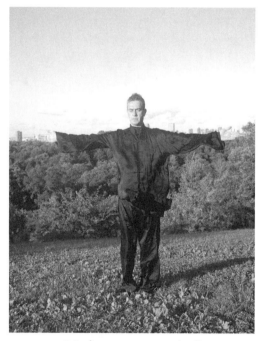

Point fingers to ocean and pull ocean energy into your core.

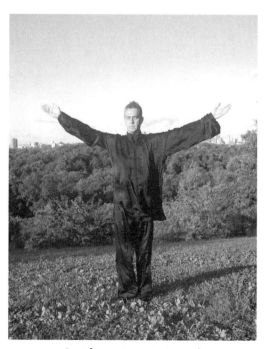

Point fingers to mountains and pull mountain's energy into your core.

The sky is next. Point your fingers and draw sky energy into your core.

Finally point to the heaven and pull and draw heaven energy into your entire being.

Move your left leg and place it beside the right leg.

Bring your arms over your head.

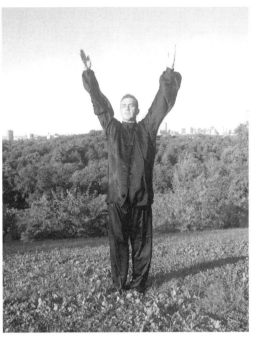

Point fingers to sky and pull sky energy into your core.

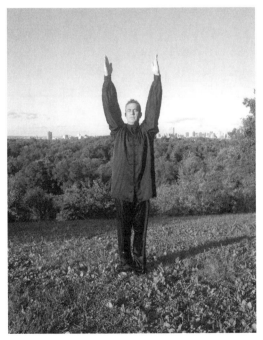

Point fingers to heaven and pull heaven energy into your core.

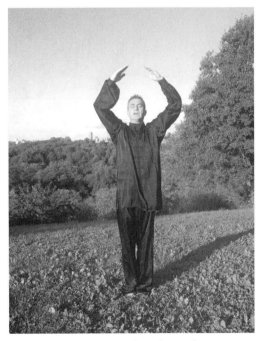

Draw energy through top of head. Nourish entire body.

Draw in energy through the top of the head to nourish the entire body.

Finish with your palms touching gently two inches below the navel connecting to your center of gravity energy center.

Key Points. Inhale and draw clean, healthy energy from your surroundings. Allow the energy to pour in through the top of your head, filling the body from the bottom up, the same way water fills a cup. If you have become comfortable with drawing on the various energies, add four gates breathing and eventually five gates breathing.

Slightly bend your knees. Tuck the tailbone in. Keep your head suspended. Drop your shoulders. Breathe deeply so you can feel the ribs expanding. Visualize your body's energetic circulation. Sense the relationship of your body to the earth. Feel the relationship of your body to the heavens.

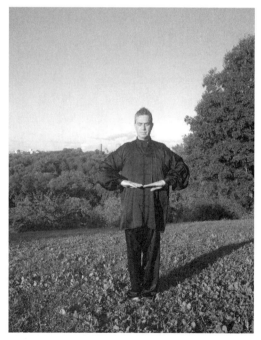

Finish. Palms touching gently two inches below navel.

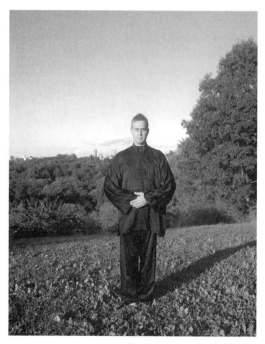

Connecting mentally and physically to your center of gravity energy center.

Move your arms very slowly to allow the mind to strongly experience the various energies that you are going to draw and gather into your body. First, draw earth energy through your fingers as well as your entire body. Then move the arms slightly up and draw in energy from the trees. Move the arms slightly higher and draw in ocean energy. Then move your arms higher and draw in mountain energy. Finish with drawing heaven energy, and then lead all this energy that you have gathered inward through the top of the head (heavenly gate) to nourish your entire body.

Fill your body, plateau by plateau, from the bottom up. Nourish is an excellent way to end your practice for the day and lead your energy to the lower energy center to cool down as well as to conserve.

Some days, your nourishing sensation will be stronger when sitting on the edge of a chair. Of course, when doing the nourishing exercise outside, you will experience a stronger energetic exchange. This will help on the days you are practicing inside. It is very important to really connect to the different elements of nature when drawing on their energies. The best way to do this is to remember your sensation when spending time more intensely in each one of the elements. For example, when you are working in your garden and putting your fingers and palms inside the earth, close your eyes and experience the earth energy. Later when you are standing and visualizing drawing earth energy, your sensations will be stronger. Maybe you need to climb a tree or spend some time under one to better connect to the tree energy. When you are hiking, stop and experience the pure sensation of the mountains or when you are in the ocean, pause and learn new sensations of the ocean. Watch the stars and get a strong sensation of the heavens. Before you know it, this powerful mental visualization will become stronger and stronger. Every now and then, you will experience the sensation of being one with the universe.

Nourish is a traditional qigong exercise. If you feel silly, or skeptical, as you connect to nature and draw in energy, remember this: what you believe will affect the outcome of your practice. If you have strong faith that you are drawing in natural energy and healing your body, the results will be different on a physiological level from if you are just going through the motions. Evoke your spirit, remain focused, relaxed, and alert, and enjoy a light and happy feeling during your training. In this way, you will experience the maximum positive benefit of each exercise, and ultimately, in every moment of your life.

CLOSE TAI CHI

As you finish, return the palms to the front of the body, placing the center of the palms over the lower energy center and keeping them there for a few minutes, or as long as you like. Stand in mountain stance and allow the energy created to return to your lower energy center.

After two or three breaths, move your arms to the side of your body, touch gently with your index finger the middle line on the side of your thighs.

You are back in mountain stance and ready to perform the Sunset Tai Chi form to your right.

Key Points. When standing still in your mountain stance, stand as still as a mountain. Even though you are still when you close your eyes, you will sense many things are moving. It is written in the *Tai Chi Classics* that when being still, look for the motion in the stillness, and when moving, look for the stillness in the movement.

Always end with a few minutes of close tai chi with the mind in the lower energy center. Close tai chi is also important to prepare you for performing the form to the other side. It is a time in which to gather your thoughts and your energy at the lower energy center. You need the energy to become focused and strong before you start the form to the other side or when you want to start any other action throughout your life.

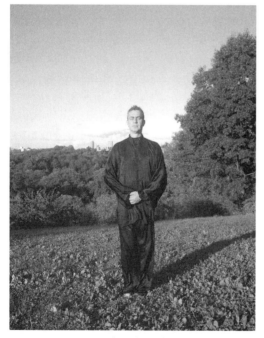

Mountain stance. Mind resides in lower energy center.

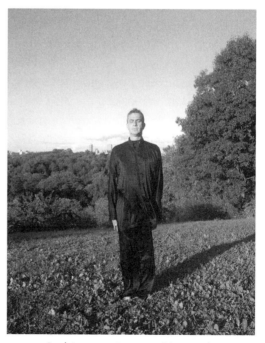

Back in mountain stance. Now ready to perform Sunset Tai Chi form to right.

Practice this skill sitting, standing, as well as moving. The goal is to be able to be in both places, inside as well as outside, at the same time. Usually outside distractions make it hard to be in both places. After years of practice or maybe sooner for you, you will be able to perform this visualization. Of course with your eyes closed, it is much easier to reside in your lower energy center. Try having the eyes half closed, squinting, as an in between stage.

Martial Arts Application of Nourish and Close Tai Chi

You will be surprised that even nourish and close tai chi have applications. If a low punch is coming at you or someone is kicking toward your groin, you can use the right or left arm to block the kick while using the other arm to strike.

Circle your right or left arm the same way you do when performing the beginning of the nourish movement.

Remember to move your feet to angle against your opponent.

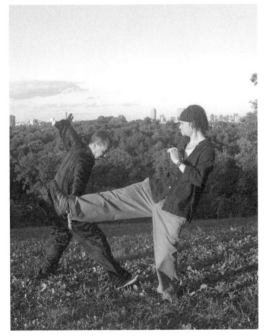

Use right arm to block the kick.

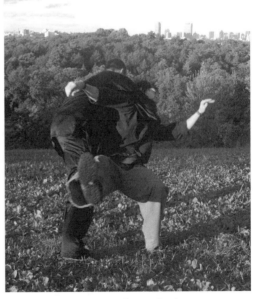

Use arm to strike or take down.

To do a takedown, start with the same neutralization, but this time lift up your opponent's leg and drop him on his back.

You can also place one of your feet behind your opponent and use the striking hand with the leg to take down your opponent.

To control your opponent, neutralize the low punch with your right arm and grab and twist your opponent's wrist as well as his elbow. Move your legs to angle your opponent.

Again, these applications can help you understand the postures more clearly so that your limbs are in the correct place when practicing. But if your intent is to practice tai chi for health, they do not need to be a primary focus of your study.

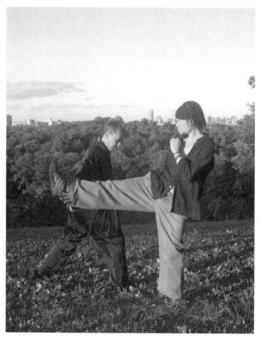

Take down. Lift opponent's leg up.

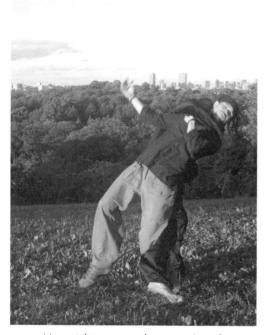

Move right arm around opponent's neck
and drop the opponent on his or her back.

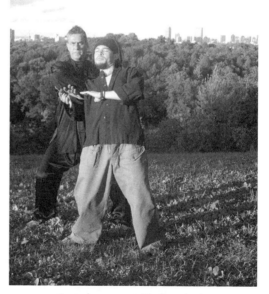

Control opponent. Grab and twist
opponent's wrist and elbow.

FINAL WORDS

As you finish, return the palms to the front of the body, placing them over the lower energy center and keeping them there for a few minutes, or as long as you like. Stand in mountain stance and allow the energy created to return to your lower energy center.

Close tai chi is a fundamentally important part of the practice. Do not skip it. Gathering your energy in your center after your tai chi drills, or form, or any exercise, will help you to build the habit of conserving and settling your energy. Failure to do so may result in scattered energy that can make you hyperactive, anxious, or can keep you up at night.

You may continually practice the Sunset Tai Chi form to the right and left as many times as you like. The key to programming these movements into your body's memory and reflexes is through repetition. Practice, practice, practice. Always end your practice with the close tai chi movement and with your mind in the lower energy center. End the Sunset Tai Chi form to the right. Continue the Sunset Tai Chi form to the left and strive for symmetry.

CHAPTER 6

Epilogue

Training for 25 years under world-renowned masters of the various Eastern arts has given me a unique perspective on the physical body and human behavior. I understand that in order to achieve greater success in the mind and body, I must practice and regulate all five building blocks of my being, not just some. Yes it is true you will still benefit from emphasizing one or two of the blocks, but the benefits and the positive outcome of developing and growing in all five building blocks is a totally different experience that will lead you to greater accomplishment. It is the difference between surviving cancer or not. It is the difference between getting a martial arts gold medal or not. If you investigate different schools, you will see what I mean. Some schools are strongly into the body: lifting weights, emphasizing flexibility. Others are strongly into the mind: relaxation and meditation. There are schools that worship the spirit, with lots of chanting and other Eastern arts and religious elements. Usually the building block that is emphasized is the one that the teacher is interested in or is the stage of the journey he or she is in. It is only the great and rare teachers that know how to lead each student through all five building blocks. And it is also the rare student who seeks balance and desires to reach the levels of understanding, which are essential for mastering any of the Eastern arts.

To make sure you are following this path, always ask yourself in every moment and in any mind/body prescription that you practice: "Am I practicing all five building blocks within this moment?" For example, when standing in mountain stance, your legs are working, but you must also emphasize breathing techniques, tap into the power of the mind and integrate it with the energetic system using various visualizations, and finally, evoke your spirit and experience the three forces: heaven, human, and earth. A simple physical posture then is transformed into being an internal art rather than being only external. This path is the essence of tai chi. When practicing internal arts, your changes and growth will be entirely different than when just exercising. The practice of these internal arts becomes a life-changing, transformative experience.

Your mind/body journey should start with balancing among the five blocks and then harmonizing the blocks with the three forces. You first work on yourself and then you can work on integrating with your surroundings. Remember, there are three kinds of souls, and you can choose which one you want to be. The first soul only wants to take. It is selfish and shallow. The second soul only wants to give. Very quickly this soul will get depleted and empty. The third soul keeps learning in order to give. This one never runs out of knowledge or energy. This soul is available for you if you choose to become it. It is the healthiest soul of the three.

The program in this book and DVD offers you a harmonious approach that will help you to find balance within the body between strength and flexibility. It will teach you breathing techniques that you can mix into your day-to-day living and your tai chi practice. It will teach you ancient techniques to strengthen the horse/wisdom mind and quiet the monkey/emotional mind, using methods and techniques that have been passed down for thousands of years. It will teach you to understand, strengthen, and open your energetic system, and to use the setting sun and your mind to cleanse the physical and energetic body from impurities. And finally, it will challenge you to evoke spirituality in every movement and in every moment throughout your day.

You are encouraged to work with a chair and a wall, both of which are tremendous tools for bringing your practice to higher level. Working with a chair develops your upper body, and working with the wall or a tree will strengthen the sensation of your energetic visualizations. You are taught the tai chi form and drills to both sides, which usually does not happen in most tai chi schools, books, DVDs, or classes, but I feel it is essential for you to strive for symmetry, mentally and physically. This program is about cooling down after a hard day at work, using a powerful cleansing sun meditation and many other mind/body prescriptions. This program is about expecting and adapting to change, and learning how to change from one situation to another in the most effective way.

In the Eastern arts, traumas are believed to be stored in our physical and energetic bodies, and by using this program you can accelerate the natural process of dissolving these stored traumas and assist your recovery and rejuvenation. This program can help you get ready faster for your next task or your next day. It will allow you to enjoy the rest of the time you have before going back to a stressful situation. It is about a smooth transition.

At the same time, Sunset Tai Chi promotes healing. This program is being successfully used at Tufts Medical School in Boston, helping people with fibromyalgia as well as those with osteoarthritis. It is used in the Dana Farber Cancer Institute in Boston, for patients, their families, and its staff, to target the symptoms and stress accompanying the debilitating disease of cancer.

This mind/body program as well as tai chi will increase your muscle mass and increase your bone density. You will increase oxygen intake through deep breathing, which benefits every cell in your body. For those of you who want to evoke the spirit with religious elements, you are more than welcome. I myself like to use the spirit of nature: the earth, mountains, trees, oceans, sky, and heaven, but, for example, when one of my students practices the bubble, instead of visualizing just an energy bubble, she visualizes three angels coming down, holding hands and making a protective and nourishing circle around her. I am just giving you a seed. It is your job to make it grow into whatever kind of flower or tree that best suits your personal needs.

The cool down mind/body program will also prepare you for the stances, tai chi drills, and the tai chi form. This form uses different movements from those found in Sunrise Tai Chi. You will need to learn the stances before you start the tai chi drills and form. The stances will develop your legs and your root, and together with the rest of the program it will give you what I consider leg power rather than just strength. Power is a combination of strength and flexibility.

This book and the *Sunset Tai Chi* DVD is the partner of our first book and DVD, *Sunrise Tai Chi*. Together, they give you a complete mind/body approach for both the morning and the evening. You may choose which movements work best for you, and there is enough variety so that you can have many skills and movements to keep you interested for a long time. When you wake up in the morning, you can use the rising sun to nourish, and when you come home and finish the day, you can use the setting sun to help cleanse and rejuvenate. If you learn and practice these two programs, you will be successful with this goal and your life will change for the better.

This book and its partner are designed for both health and martial arts. For health purposes, do the tai chi drills slowly and in a higher stance. If you are interested in the martial arts aspects of tai chi, perform the drills and form, and over time get into lower stances, and include moving faster. The internal visualizations are from the martial arts world. They are all Taoist and are slightly more aggressive than Buddhist meditations. Because time is of the essence, and I do believe in the concept of awakening the warrior from within, I am a strong believer in the Taoist visualizations. However, over the years, with age and experience, I have learned that emphasizing some of the simpler Buddhist visualizations, when needed, can sometimes bring you further. Balance is the key, and you must determine what best suits your individual needs.

This program will teach you a way to control the fluctuations of your brainwaves. When you are focused, you are in an alpha brainwave state. When you are still thinking, but more scattered, you are in beta brainwaves. When you are in a meditative place, you are in theta brainwaves. When you are between being awake and asleep you are in theta. It is that moment right before you fall asleep when your body is transparent but you can still sense what is around you. It is when you are falling down into that soft place just before you fall asleep. The theta brainwave state is also where healing happens in the body, and that is when your martial arts abilities are at their best. Some people refer to it as being in the zone and some individuals who are partial to running will experience, every now and then, the same meditative sensation when running: the physical transparent sensation with a kind of high mental experience probably due to a surge of positive hormones like endostatin, serotonin, and maybe even endorphins. The phenomenon even has a term: 'high run.'

You will learn through this program to be mindful of your control of your brainwave state. You will learn to adapt more quickly in a situation to the brainwave state that will best suit the situation. You will be able to attain a truly relaxed state more quickly, and be able to stay there much longer than the short time we spend in it right before we fall asleep. This will lead to a better quality of life, a stronger immune system, higher awareness and martial art skills, and greater control and focus in all areas of your life.

Remember to tap into the power of the sun as it rises and sets and you will experience countless benefits for yourself and those around you.

Tai Chi Classics to Ponder

These excerpts from the *Tai Chi Classics* can be applied to each movement in the Sunset Tai Chi form. By seeing how these ancient poems relate to the tai chi movements, you may grasp a deeper understanding of the essence of the internal arts.

Begin Tai Chi

> *Tai Chi, Supreme Ultimate comes from Wu Chi, the Formless Void,*
> *and is the mother of Yin and Yang.*
> *In motion, Tai Chi separates;*
> *in stillness, Yin and Yang fuse and return to Wu Chi.*

When you stand in begin tai chi you are in a posture that has no extreme. The body is relativity relaxed and the effort is distributed evenly through the body. The heart is quiet and the body does not demand extra work from it. Your mind is empty of any thoughts. This stage of stillness is considered a stage of no extremes or in Chinese, wu chi. This energetic place is considered the source or, metaphorically speaking, the mother of the positive/yang and negative/yin energy situation. When you just think of the first move of your tai chi you move away from wu chi. The energy and body begin to differentiate into yin and yang.

Grind

> *Tai Chi is like the water supporting a moving boat.*
> *First sink the chi to the lower energy center,*
> *Then hold the head as if suspended from above.*

In order to create a strong downward energy in the movement of grinding, you need to visualize that you are actually grinding something; this sensation of having an object under your movement of grinding will lead the energy down and will create the sensation you are looking for when performing this motion. Once you create the downward sensation, you need to balance it with a light sensation through your spine up through the top of the head all the way to the heavens. The only way you can have tai chi movements that flow like water is to sink your mind to the ground. The only way you can have tai chi that moves like water and which can support and move the boat is by creating the light upward energy sensation through the spine all the way to the heavens through the top of the head. When you can create both energy sensations, you will begin to understand the meaning of this passage.

Crane Spreads Its Wings

Yield and overcome;
Bend and be straight;
Empty and be full;
Wear out and be New.

As the spirit of the crane, you can take different shapes and forms. The crane's wings when closed are small but once they open they are big and strong. The beak of the crane is sharp and powerful. It can even fight a poisonous snake. Between the wings, the beak, and its speed, the crane is very surprising. One side is attaching while the other wing is blocking. The spirit of the crane is agile and noble. It is a beautiful animal, which stands tall and has great courage. It is used in many paintings because it can be many energies at the same time.

Two Blocks

Have a little and Gain;
Have much and be confused.

The two blocks does not look like much, but if done to its fullest it is a very powerful, simple move, for both health and martial arts. The two blocks, when properly used, can be very effective for blocking and attaching with each block. When done correctly, it pulls your opponent in while breaking and crushing whatever is coming in: a leg or an arm. When utilizing all five building blocks in this movement, the internal organ massage that you are getting is very deep and covers almost every internal organ in our body.

Brush Knee and Step

Sinking to one side allows movement to flow;
Silently treasure knowledge and turn it over in the mind.
Gradually you can do as you like.
A force of four ounces deflects a thousand pounds.

This movement if done correctly is like a stream of water that will lift the boat. Your entire body is setting up to lift the person in front of you the same way a wave in the ocean can lift a boat. Your bows are stretched as you approach your opponent and your mind is ready to release. Some people perform it using the opposite pattern. They approach the opponent with released bows while gripping the opponent. Then to pull the opponent downward, they support the pull with stretched bows. This gives the move extra strength because they are using all the body and not just the hands. As you can see, storing (stretching the bows) is the energy that makes the wave that breaks on the beach, and releasing the bows creates the wave that lifts the boat.

Cloud Hands

> *To adhere means to yield.*
> *To yield means to adhere.*

When performing cloud hands, you want to not only perform this move but you want to be the move: be the clouds that are floating in the blue sky, imitate the slow steady movements and the expanded sensation of a cloud full of rain. The clouds look soft yet they are full of water. They have many shapes and forms and the many shapes and forms give them an unpredictable energy pattern, which cannot be anticipated. A yield can be an attack and an attack could just stick to you like fly paper; once it is on top of you, you cannot shake it off.

Pick Up Needle from the Sea Bottom

> *Within yin, there is yang.*
> *Within yang, there is yin.*
> *Yin and yang mutually aid and change each other.*

When we stand in empty stance, one leg is substantial and the other is insubstantial. When your right hand attaches and stings the groin (yang), the left arm and palm defend the head (yin). When the enemy attacks from the top, punch to the face (yang), and move down to empty stance (yin). All these principles are applied when performing pick up needle from the sea bottom. Yin and the yang are interacting in one move. Yin creates yang and yang leads to yin. One cannot exist without the other.

Fan Back

> *When applied, it is like flowing water.*
> *The substantial is concealed in the insubstantial.*

The movement of fan back can be compared to the flow of a strong river. First, when you stick to your opponent, the movement should be just like a gentle brook, and then it becomes larger and stronger, to make your opponent lose his root. Connect all the way from the floor, then direct with your waist, and finally manifest out the palms. Use the bows and integrate all your internal visualizations, and you will become like the great river, which is a perfect balance of yin and yang in its full strength. This is the goal when performing this movement.

Nourish and Close Tai Chi

When the flow is swift it is difficult to resist.
Coming to a high place, it swells and fills the place up;
Meeting a hollow, it dives downward.
The waves rise and fall,
Finding a hole, they will surely surge in.

The end is divided into two parts. The first is to nourish, tapping into all the higher energy resources until you cannot resist connecting to the natural forces and experiencing each one to its fullest. Can you sense the earth? Can you be a tree? Can you be a great mountain? Can your spirit be one with the oceans? The second part, close tai chi, is about finding peace and quiet on all levels. Can you just let go as the water falls inexorably into a hole? Can you really let go and empty your mind?

Glossary of Sunrise and Sunset Tai Chi Special Terms

The following are special terms used in this book, *Sunset Tai Chi*, and in the companion book, *Sunrise Tai Chi*. We created these unique terms that characterize the special features of our tai chi form and qigong exercises.

baton/bubble breathing. Moving the mind from the energetic bubble to the energetic baton on inhalation and back to the bubble on exhalation,

belt energy vessel breathing. Qigong exercise to strengthen the belt energy vessel around the waist by circling the pelvis.

bone marrow-skin visualization. Moving the mind to the energetic baton while residing a fist away from the skin and then moving the mind to the skin or the bubble while remaining mindful of the energetic baton. (See definition for luo.)

bow breathing. Moving the tailbone and the head inward to stretch the long bow, and rounding the shoulders inward to stretch the cross bow. Do the opposite with both to release the bows.

brain energy. A distracting component in moving energy from the upper energy center to the lower one.

building blocks. The Eastern view of the body sees the human body as being comprised of five building blocks: the body, breath, mind, energy, and spirit.

center of gravity energy center. The lower energy center, two inches below your belly button and three inches inward. An energy ball in the center of your belly.

dissolving the face. A visualization to release stress and tension from the soft tissue of the face.

drain the baton and build the bubble. Leading the energy down from the upper energy center while leading energy out toward the bubble, the energy of which is a fist away from the body.

embrace the tree. Yi Chuan standing meditation

empty moon breathing. Controlled contraction of the abdomen and back muscles during breathing.

energetic baton. The two main energy centers, the upper and lower energy centers with an energetic rod connecting them. The pituitary gland energy center is the top head of the baton and the center of gravity energy center is the lower head of the baton.

energetic block. See building blocks.

energetic bubble. Also known as the guardian energy (wei qi). The bubble surrounds the body.

external energetic baton visualization. An external visualization of the internal energetic baton. You visualize the energetic baton outside your body in front of you. The top of the baton is across your upper energy center and the bottom is across from your lower energy center.

eye energy. A distracting component in moving energy from the upper energy center to the lower one.

fire breath. Inhaling with a sound through your nostrils and exhaling whispering "ha" sound from your mouth. Fire breath breathing helps to move thoughts away from stressful situations and release tension.

five gates. The five gates are 1) The head, especially the face, ears and the center of the top of the head (baihui point), 2) The two palms, especially the center of the palms (laogong point), and 3) The two feet, especially the bottom of the soles (yongquan point).

floating shoulders. Misalignment of shoulders in which a shoulder floats upward.

four gates. Four of the five gates: the palms and feet

full moon breathing. Controlled expansion of the abdomen and back muscles during breathing.

fury eyes. Eyes that resemble the tiger or cat's eyes before it leaps on its prey.

guardian energy. Wei qi, the energetic bubble surrounding the body.

half moon stretch. See rainbow stretch.

happy internal organs. Nourishing the organs with the energy lead from the earth into the internal organs while massaging the internal organs from the outside, using the movements of the trunk muscles. This exercise also enhances the blood and oxygen circulation in the organs.

heavenly gate. A gate at center of the top of the skull, the baihui point (Gv-20).

horse mind. Wisdom mind.

internal energetic baton visualization. Connecting the upper and lower energy centers with a straight line through the center of the body—not the spine but right in front of it—like a baton.

joint pulsing. Meditative pulsing that creates gentle movement in the joints.

latissimus breathing. Also called wing breathing and trapezius breathing. Moving the air into the lungs sideways toward the area from the armpit down a straight line all the way to the hip.

meditative shaking and pulsing. Exercises that starts by charging and igniting the energetic system and then the rest of the body by creating a gentle movement in the joints or in the ligaments.

mind/body prescriptions. Exercises in *Sunset Tai Chi* and *Sunrise Tai Chi* that are part of the mind/body program.

monkey mind. Emotional mind.

multitasking visualizations. Combining several visualizations such as moving the energy from the baton to the bubble and vice versa, while at the same timing move the energy down through the baton.

mushroom breathing. Expanding at the same time the upper front and back of the lungs. Also called umbrella breathing. Breathing deeply toward muscles that go from the bottom of the thoracic spine, between the shoulder blades, out to the middle of each shoulder, and up the neck.

pituitary gland energy center. Upper energy center located uner the two lobes of the brain in the center, i.e., the middle of your head. Where the spinal cord connects to the base of the two brain lobes and the surrounding area that includes the pituitary and pineal glands.

point to heaven. A mind body prescription in which first you point to the heavens with your index fingers when performing a spine stretch while also leading the mind up to the heavens and balancing the movement with moving the mind deep into the earth.

pushing the tablets. Two imaginary tablets, one in front of you touching your front left palm and one behind you touching your back right elbow. At first, the left palm pushes the front tablet and the right elbow pushes the back tablet.

quiet water breathing. The silent and quiet breath with deep, long, and peaceful inhalations and exhalations.

rainbow stretch. Also half moon stretch.

releasing the bows. Straightening up and bringing the top of the head, the tailbone, and shoulders back to the starting position to release both bows.

seesaw breathing. Isolating and moving air into one lung at a time.

side lung breathing. Moving the air into the lungs sideways toward the area from the armpit down a straight line all the way to the hip, isolating air in our imagined wings or leading or pushing air to that area and moving the lungs laterally.

small circulation. Also known as microcosmic orbit. In Chinese, it is xiao zhou tian.

spider climbing. Stretching the sides of the body in opposite directions to release tension around the lungs and to increase lung capacity.

spiritual eye. A tiny spot in the center of the forehead.

spiritual valley. The crack between the two hemispheres of the brain.

stretching the bows. Moving the tailbone and the head inward to stretch the long bow and when rounding the shoulders inward to stretch the crossbow.

surfing the breath. Using the breath to empty the mind from any thoughts.

third eye. A spot right behind the forehead in front of the two brain lobes.

three forces. Heaven, human, and earth.

three spheres. The spheres on top of each other in the torso.

trapezius breathing. Also mushroom breathing.

turtle back. Sinking the chest slightly and arcing the back.

two gates breathing. Moving your mind from the lower energy center to the center of the palms, and back to the lower energy center.

up and down forces. The up and down forces in the body where the bones and some muscles move gently up to lift and hold, while the shoulders and the soft tissue, including the face, melt downward using gravity. The up forces: lower back, thoracic spine, and the top of the head. The down forces: face, shoulders, and abdominal.

vitamin H. Hamstring stretch.

vitamin L. Lower back stretch used in the three musketeers' postures. The first is straight forward and down. The second is left forward and down, and the third is moving forward and down to the right.

wing breath breathing. Another name for latissimus breathing.

zigzag. Working on the up and down forces by lengthening up through the lumbar and dropping down through the abdominal; lengthening through the thoracic spine and then dropping the shoulders, suspending the head, and relaxing the face.

Glossary of Chinese Terms

How to use this glossary: This glossary will serve to help you understand Chinese words and concepts that you will encounter in this book. You will also find words not used in the book that you are likely to encounter in your continued study of tai chi chuan (taijiquan). Some included terms are not commonly-known words in the Chinese language, as they exist only in tai chi society, such as peng, which means 'ward off.'

Common qi cavities are included, with their corresponding acupuncture cavity names, such as huiyin.

This book uses a mixture of both the Wade-Giles and Pinyin methods of Romanizing Chinese words. Usage is based on the mainstream popularity of each term, but the authors also aim to educate the reader by offering both Wade-Giles and Pinyin for many terms. Most terms in this glossary are presented only in Pinyin. Similarly, Chinese names are written in the traditional way of last name first, unless the person is more commonly known by their Westernized name, such as Lao Tzu.

Special thanks to Dr. Yang, Jwing-Ming for his extensive research and knowledge, which comprise much of the contents of this glossary.

an. 'Pressing or stamping.' One of the eight basic moving or jin (jing) patterns of taijiquan. These eight moving patterns are called ba men, which means 'eight doors.' To perform an, first relax the wrist and when the hand has reached the opponent's body, immediately settle down the wrist. This action is called zuo wan in taijiquan practice.

ba men wu bu. Means 'eight doors and five steppings.' The art of taijiquan is built from eight basic moving or jin patterns and five basic steppings. The eight basic moving or jin patterns that can be used to handle the eight directions are called the 'eight doors' (ba men) and the five stepping actions are called the 'five steppings' (wu bu).

bagua (ba kua). Literally, 'eight divinations.' Also called the eight trigrams. In Chinese philosophy, the eight basic variations; shown in the *Yi Jing* (*Book of Changes*) as groups of single and broken lines.

baihui (Gv-20). Hundred meetings. Name of an acupuncture cavity that belongs to the governing vessel. Baihui is located on the crown of the head.

can si jin chan shou lian xi. Silk reeling jin coiling training. One of the important basic trainings in taijiquan.

Chang chuan (changquan). 'long range fist or long sequence.' Chang chuan includes all northern Chinese long-range martial styles. Taijiquan is also called chang chuan simply because its sequence is long.

Cheng, Gin-gsao (A.D. 1911-1976) Ramel Rones' White Crane kung fu grandmaster.

chi (qi). The energy pervading the universe, including the energy circulating in the human body.

chi kung (qigong). The gongfu of qi, which means the study of qi.

chin na (qin na). Literally means 'seize control.' A component of Chinese martial arts that emphasizes grabbing techniques to control your opponent's joints, in conjunction with attacking certain acupuncture cavities.

chong mai. Thrusting vessel. One of the eight extraordinary vessels.

da lu. Large rollback. One of the common taiji techniques.

Da Mo or Bodhidharma. The 28th patriarch of Buddhism, commonly credited for popularizing the practice of Chan (Zen) Buddhism in China in A.D 550. He settled at Shaolin temple to teach Buddhism, and developed qigong exercises during his time there, greatly influencing all Chinese martial arts.

da qiao. To build a bridge. Refers to the qigong practice of touching the roof of the mouth with the tip of the tongue to form a bridge or link between the governing and conception vessels.

da zhou tian. Literally, 'Grand cycle heaven' Usually translated as 'grand circulation.' After a nei dan qigong practitioner completes small circulation, he circulates his qi through the entire body or exchanges the qi with nature.

dai mai. Girdle (or belt) vessel. One of the eight extraordinary vessels.

dan tian. Literally: field of elixir. Locations in the body that are able to store and generate qi (elixir) in the body. The upper, middle, and lower dan tians are located, respectively, between the eyebrows, at the solar plexus, and a few inches below the navel.

Dao De Jing (*Tao Te Ching*). *Morality Classic.* Written by Lao Zi during the Zhou Dynasty (1122-934 B.C.).

Dao. 'The Way.' By implication the 'natural way.'

dazhui (Gv-14). Big vertebra. Name of an acupuncture cavity that belongs to the governing vessel.

deng shan bu. Climbing mountain stance, or forward stance. One of the basic fundamental stances in northern martial arts. Also called bow and arrow stance (gong jian bu).

dian xue. Dian means 'to point and exert pressure' and xue means 'the cavities.' Dian xue refers to those qin na techniques that specialize in attacking acupuncture cavities to immobilize or kill an opponent.

dong jin. Understanding jin. One of the jins that uses the feeling of the skin to sense the opponent's energy.

du mai. Usually translated 'Governing vessel.' One of the eight qi vessels.

fan hu xi (ni hu xi). Reverse breathing. Also commonly called Daoist breathing.

fan tong hu xi. Back to childhood breathing. A breathing training in nei dan qigong through which the practitioner tries to regain control of the muscles in the lower abdomen. Also called abdominal breathing (fu shi hu xi).

fu sui xi. Skin and marrow breathing. Skin breathing is considered as yang. Marrow breathing is classified as yin.

fu xi. Skin breathing. One of the nei dan qigong breathing techniques in which the qi is led to the skin surface.

ha .A yang sound that is used to manifest martial power to its highest efficiency.

han xiong ba bei. To contain or draw in the chest and arc the back.

Han, Ching-tang. A Chinese long fist kung fu great grandmaster.

hen. A yin qigong sound that is the opposite of the yang ha sound. This sound is commonly used to lead the qi inward and to store it in the bone marrow. This sound can also be used for an attack when the manifestation of only partial power is desired.

hou tian. Qi post-birth qi or post-heaven qi. This qi is converted from the essence of food and air and is classified as 'fire qi' because it can make your body too yang.

hua. To neutralize.

huan jing bu nao. Literally, to return the essence to nourish the brain. A Daoist qigong training process wherein qi that has been converted from essence is lead to the brain to nourish it.

huang ting. Yellow yard. 1. A yard or hall in which Daoists, who often wore yellow robes, meditated together. 2. In Daoist qigong, the place in the center of the body where fire qi and water qi are mixed to generate a spiritual embryo, above the lower dan tian.

huiyin. Perineum. An acupuncture cavity belonging to the conception vessel.

hun. The soul. Commonly used with the word 'ling,' which means spirit. Daoists believe that a human being's hun and po originate with his original qi (yuan qi), and separate from the physical body at death.

huo lu. Fire path. One of the paths in small circulation meditation.

ji gong. Spine bow–the long bow. The bow formed from the spine, which is able to store the jin.

ji. Means 'to squeeze' or 'to press.'

jia dan tian. False dan tian. It is called qihai (Co-6) in acupuncture. This place, the front of the belly, is able to produce qi. However, it cannot store qi efficiently.

jia ji Squeeze the spine. The Daoist name of a spot on the spine in small circulation meditation practice. This spot is called lingtai (Gv-10) (i.e., spirit's platform) in acupuncture.

Jin, Shao-feng Ramel Rones' White Crane kung fu great grandmaster.

jing (jin). Chinese martial power. A combination of li (muscular power) and qi.

jing qi. Essence qi. The qi which has been converted from original essence.

jing-shen. Essence-spirit. Often translated as the 'spirit of vitality.' Raised spirit (raised by the qi that is converted from essence), which is restrained by the yi.

kan. One of the eight trigrams meaning 'water.'

Kao, Tao. Ramel Rones' Taijiquan grandmaster.

kao. Means 'to lean or to press against.' In taijiquan, it means to bump someone off balance.

kua. The area on the external hip joint is called 'external kua' (wai kua). The area on the inner side of the hip joints (i.e., groin area) is called 'internal kua' (nei kua).

kung fu (gongfu). 'Energy-time.' Anything which will take time and energy to learn or to accomplish is called kung fu.

kung. (gong) 'energy' or 'hard work.'

Lao Tzu. (or Lao Zi) Considered the creator, or first compiler, of Daoism, also called Li Er. Author of the book, *Dao De Jing*.

laogong (P-8). Labor's palace. A cavity located on the pericardium channel in the center of the palm.

li qi. Li is muscular power, while Qi is inner energy. Li qi means 'to manifest the inner energy into physical power,' which means jin.

Li, Mao-ching. Ramel Rones' Long Fist kung fu grandmaster.

li. The power that is generated from muscular strength.

lian jing hua qi. To refine the essence and convert it into qi.

lian qi hua shen. To refine the qi to nourish the spirit. Leading qi to the head to nourish the brain and spirit.

lian qi sheng hua. To train the qi and sublimate it. A xi sui jing training process by which the qi is led to the huang ting (brain).

Liang, Shou-yu. Ramel Rones' xingyiquan (hsing-yi chuan) and baguazhang (pa kua chang) kung fu master.

lingtai (Gv-10). Spiritual station. In acupuncture, a cavity on the back. In qigong, it refers to the upper dan tian. In Daoist society, the lingtai cavity is called jia ji.

liu yi. The six arts—consisting of writing, music, archery, chariot driving, learning rhetoric, and mathematics—which ancient Chinese scholars were required to master.

lu. Means 'to rollback.'

luo. The small qi channels that branch out from the primary qi channels and are connected to the skin and to the bone marrow.

mingmen (Gv-4). Life's door. Name of an acupuncture cavity that belongs to the governing vessel.

na jin. Controlling jins. The jins that are able to control the opponent through his joints or tendons.

nei shen. Literally, internal kidneys. In Chinese medicine and qigong, the real kidneys.

nei shi gongfu. Nei shi means 'to look internally,' so nei shi gongfu refers to the art of looking inside yourself to read the state of your health and the condition of your qi.

nei shi. Literally, internal vision. It implies feeling to the inner body. It also means 'internal inspection through inner feeling.'

ni wan or ni wan gong. Mud pill, or mud pill palace. Daoist qigong terminology for an area in the brain; the pituitary gland area.

peng. Means 'to ward off.'

po. Vigorous life force. The po is considered to be the inferior or animal soul. It is the animal or sentient life that is an innate part of the body, which at death returns to the earth with the rest of the body. When someone is in high spirits and gets vigorously involved in some activity, it is said he has po li, which means he has 'vigorous strength or power.'

qigong (chi kung). The gongfu of qi, which means the study of qi.

ren mai. Usually translated 'conception vessel.'

renzhong (Gv-26). An acupuncture cavity under the nose.

san guan. Three gates. In small circulation training, the three cavities on the governing vessel which are usually obstructed and must be opened.

seiza. A Japanese sitting style, in which one first kneels on the floor, and then rests the buttocks on the heels, with the tops of the feet flat on the floor and toes pointed. This posture represents willful discipline of the mind and development of spirit.

shang dan tian. Upper dan tian. The brain; it is the residence of the shen (spirit).

Shaolin. A Buddhist temple in Henan Province, famous for its martial arts.

shen gu. Spirit valley. Formed by the two lobes of the brain, with the upper dan tian at the exit.

shen. Spirit. According to Chinese qigong, the shen resides at the upper dan tian (the third eye).

shen xi. Spirit breathing. The stage of qigong training where the spirit is coordinated with the breathing.

shi san shi. Thirteen patterns. Taijiquan is also called shi san shi, because it is constructed from these thirteen moving patterns.

shuai jiao. Means 'wrestling.'

shuang xiu. Double cultivation. A qigong training method in which qi is exchanged with a partner in order to balance the qi in both people.

shuang zhong. Means 'double weighting' or 'double layering.' It means when the opponent has placed a weight or pressure on you, you respond by meeting that pressure with equal or greater pressure of your own. The consequence is stagnation. When this happens, mutual resistance will be generated.

shui lu. Water path. One of the meditation paths in which the qi is led upward through the spinal cord (thrusting vessel, chong mai) to nourish the brain.

si liang po qian jin. Means to use four ounces to repel (i.e., neutralize) one thousand pounds.

si liu bu. Four-six stance, or back stance. One of the basic stances in Northern styles of martial arts training, with 60% of the weight on the rear leg.

tai chi chuan (taijiquan). Grand ultimate fist. A Chinese internal martial style that is based on the theory of taiji (grand ultimate).

Taiji Quan Chan Shou Lian Xi. Taiji (Tai Chi) circle sticking hands training. One of the most important trainings in Yang-style taijiquan (tai chi chuan). This training is used to train listening, understanding, sticking, adhering, connecting, and following skills. In Chen style, it is called 'silk reeling jin coiling training' (chan si jin chan shou lian xi).

Taiji. 'grand ultimate.' It is this force that generates two polarities, yin and yang.

Taiwan. An island to the southeast of mainland China. Also known as Formosa.

ti xi. Body breathing or skin breathing. In qigong, the exchanging of qi with the surrounding environment through the skin.

tian ling gai. Literally, 'heaven spiritual cover.' A person's head is considered to be heaven, and the crown is called 'heaven spiritual cover' by Daoist society. This place is called baihui (Gv-20) in acupuncture.

tian ren he yi. Literally, 'Heaven and man unified as one.' A high level of qigong practice in which a qigong practitioner, through meditation, is able to communicate his qi with heaven's qi.

tian yan. Literally, 'heaven eye.' The third eye or upper dan tian.

tiao qi. To regulate the qi.

tiao shen. To regulate the body.

tiao shen. To regulate the spirit.

tiao xi. To regulate the breathing.

tiao xin. To regulate the emotional mind.

ting jin. Listening jin. A special training that uses the skin to feel the opponent's energy and uses this feeling to further understand his intention.

tu na. Qigong was also called 'tu na,' which means to 'utter and admit,' implying uttering and admitting the air through the nose (i.e. respiration).

tui na. Means 'to push and grab.' A category of Chinese massage for healing and injury treatment.

wai shen. (external kidneys) refer to the testicles.

Wang, Zong-yue A well-known Tai Chi master of the late Qing Dynasty who wrote many comprehensive tai chi chuan documents.

wei qi. Protective qi or guardian qi. The Qi at the surface of the body, which generates a shield to protect the body from negative external influences, such as colds.

weilu. Tailbone. A Daoist name. This cavity is called changqiang (Gv-1) in acupuncture.

wen huo. Scholar fire. Through soft and slender breathing, the qi (i.e., fire) can be built up gently at the abdominal area.

wu bu. Five steppings. They include forward, backward, left, right, and center.

wu huo. Martial fire. Through fast and short breathing techniques, the qi (i.e., fire) can be built up to an abundant level for the physical manifestation in a short time. Though the fire can be built up quickly, it is hard to keep it in the body

wu xin xi. Five gates breathing.

wu xin. Five centers or five gates: the head, the laogong cavities in both palms, and the yongquan cavities on the bottoms of both feet.

wu xing. Five phases, including: metal (jin), wood (mu), water (shui), fire (huo), and earth (tu).

Wudang (Wu Tang). Mountain range Located in Hubei Province in China. Center of Taoist studies and culture.

wuji hu xi (wuji xi). Wuji breathing. Keeping the mind at the real dan tian during breathing practice.

wuji. 'No extremity.'

Xi Sui Jing. Literally: *Washing Brain/Marrow Classic*, usually called *Marrow/Brain Washing Classic*. Credited to Bodhidharma (Da Mo) around A.D 550, this work discusses qigong for washing the marrow or cleaning the brain by qi nourishment.

xia dan tian. Lower elixir field. Located in the lower abdomen, it is believed to be the residence of water qi (original qi) (yuan qi). This cavity in acupuncture is called qihai (Co-6) which means 'qi ocean.'

xian tian qi. Pre-birth qi or pre-heaven qi. Also called dan tian qi. The qi, which is converted from original essence and is stored in the lower dan tian. Considered to be 'water qi,' it is able to calm the body.

xiao lu. Small rollback.

xin yuan yi ma. Xin-monkey and yi-horse. Xin (i.e., heart) is related to the emotional mind, is like a monkey, and is hard to keep steady and calm. Yi is wise and logical thinking, which is like a horse that can be calm and keep still.

xin. 'Heart.' Xin means 'the mind generated from emotional disturbance.'

xiong gong. Chest bow. The bow formed from the chest, which is able to store the jin significantly.

xu ling ding jin. An insubstantial energy leads the head upward. A secret taijiquan phrase which helps a taijiquan practitioner keep the head upright and the neck relaxed.

Yang, Ban-hou (A.D. 1837-1892). Yang, Lu-Shan's second son. Also called Yang, Yu. A second generation practitioner of Yang-style Taijiquan.

Yang, Jwing-Ming. Ramel Rones and David Silver's kung fu master.

yang. Too sufficient. One of the two poles. The other is yin.

Yi Jin Jing. Literally: *Changing Muscle/Tendon Classic*, usually called *The Muscle/Tendon Changing Classic*. Credited to Bodhidharma (Da Mo) around A.D. 550, this work discusses wai dan (external elixir) qigong training for strengthening the physical body.

yi. Wisdom mind. The mind generated from wise judgment.

yin shui. Yin water. The qi stored at the real dan tian is called yin shui, because keeping the qi here may keep you calm.

yin. Deficient. One of the two poles. The other is yang.

yongquan (K-1). Bubbling well or gushing spring. Name of an acupuncture cavity belonging to the kidney primary qi channel in center of sole of the feet.

yuan jing. Original essence. The fundamental, original substance inherited from your parents; it is converted into original qi.

yuan qi. Original qi. Created from the original essence inherited from your parents.

Zen (Chan). A school of Mahayana Buddhism that asserts that spiritual enlightenment can be attained through meditation, self-contemplation, and intuition.

Zhang, San-feng. A monk from Wudang commonly credited as the creator of taijiquan during the Song Dynasty in China (A.D. 960-1127).

Recommended Readings

Beliveau, Richard and Denis Ginbras. *Cooking with Foods that Fight Cancer*. Canada: McClellan & Stewart, 2006.

Beliveau, Richard, PhD. and Denis Ginbras, PhD. *Preventing Cancer through Diet*. McClelland & Stewart Canada 2006.

Benson, Herbert and Miriam Z. Clipper. *The Relaxation Response*. New York: Harper Paperbacks, 2000.

Beurdeley, Michael, Fu-Jui, Chang, Pimpaneau, Jacques, and Schipper, Kristofer. *Chinese Erotic Art*. Hong Kong: Chartwell, 1969

Brizendine, Louann. *The Female Brain*. Morgan Road Books NY 2006

Calais-Germain, Blandine. *Anatomy in Movement*. Translated by Nicole Commarmond, edited by Stephen Anderson. Seattle: Eastland Press, 1993.

Diepersloot, Jan. *Warrior of Stillness*, Vol. 1. Walnut Creek, CA: Center for the Healing and the Arts, 1995.

Diepersloot, Jan. *Warrior of Stillness*, Vol. 2. Walnut Creek, CA: Center for the Healing and the Arts, 1999.

Evans, William and Irwin H. Rosenberg. *BioMarkers: The 10 Determinants of Aging You Can Control*. New York: Simon & Schuster, 1991.

Frantzis, Bruce Kumar. *Opening the Energy Gates of Your Body. Chi Gung for Lifelong Helth*. Berkeley, CA: North Atlantic, 1993.

Frantzis, Bruce Kumar. *Relaxing Into Your Being*. Berkeley, CA: North Atlantic Press, 2001.

Frantzis, Bruce Kumar. *The Great Stillness*. Fairfax, CA: Clarity Press, 1999.

Gorman, David. *The Body Moveable*. 5th Edition. Ontario: Learning Methods Publications, 2002.

Iyengar, B.K.S. and Yehudi Menuhin. *Light on Pranayama. The Yogic Art of Breathing*. New York: The Crossroad Publishing Company, 1985.

Kaptchuk, Ted. *The Web That Has No Weaver: Understanding Chinese Medicine*. New York:McGraw-Hill, 2000.

Lao Tsu. *Tao Te Ching*. Translated by Gia-Fu Feng and Jane English. NY: Vintage, 1972.

Lowry, Lois. The Giver. New York: Random House, 1993.

Mehta, Silva, Mira Mehta, and Shyam Mehta. *Yoga the Iyengar Way*. New York: Knopf, 1990.

Muffs, Yochannan, PhD. *Love & Joy. Law, Language, and Religion in Ancient Israel*. New York and Jerusalem: Meisel Publication, 1992.

Muffs, Yochannan, PhD. *The Personhood of God. Biblical Theology, Faith and the Divine Image*. Woodstock: Jewish Light, 2005.

Nelson, Miriam and Sarah Wernick. *Strong Women Stay Young*. NY: Bantam, 2000.

Netter, Frank W., MD. *The Ciba Collection of Medical Illustrations*. Vols 7 & 8. New Jersey: Ciba Novartis Pharmaceuticals Corporation, 1987

Ralston, Pete. *Cheng Hsin Tui Shou: The Art of Effortless Power.* Berkeley, CA: North Atlantic Books, 1991.

Ralston, Pete. *Cheng Hsin: Principles of Effortless Power.* Berkeley, CA: North Atlantic Books, 1989.

Roizen, Michael F. and Mehmet Oz. *YOU Staying Young.* New York: Free Press, 2007.

Roizen, Michael F. and Mehmet Oz, Mehmet. *YOU The Owner's Manual.* New York: Free Press, 2005.

Rones, Ramel. *Sunrise Tai Chi. Simplified Tai Chi for Health and Longevity.* Boston: YMAA Publishers, 2007.

Sparrowe, Linda, Patricia Walden, Judith Hanson Lasater. *The Woman's Book of Yoga and Health.* Boston: Shambhala, 2002

Wilmore, Jack H., Costill, David L., and W. Larry Kenney. Physiology of Sport and Exercise. 4th Edition, Champaign, IL: Human Kinetics Publishers, 2008.

Yang, Jwing-Ming. *Qigong for Health and Martial Arts.* 2nd ed. Boston, MA: YMAA Publication Center, 1998.

Yang, Jwing-Ming. *Qigong Meditation Embryonic Breathing.* Boston, MA: YMAA Publication Center, 2003.

Yang, Jwing-Ming. *Qigong, the Secret of Youth: Da Mo's Muscle/Tendon Changing, Marrow/Brain Washing Classics.* Boston, MA: YMAA Publication Center, 2000.

Yang, Jwing-Ming. *Tai Chi Secrets of Ancient Masters.* Boston, MA: YMAA Publication Center, 1999.

Yang, Jwing-Ming. *Taiji Theory and Martial Power.* Boston, MA: YMAA Publication Center, 2003.

Yang, Jwing-Ming. *The Root of Chinese Qigong.* 2nd ed. Boston, MA: YMAA Publication Center, 1997.

Index

Acknowledgements
by Ramel Rones

This book is published thanks to the people around me who contribute on many different levels; emotionally, sharing knowledge, and with actual work. The first and foremost recognition goes to my family. First, I must thank my father, Arie Rones, and my great mother, Professor Zichria Zakay-Rones, for teaching me and emphasizing that through hard work and balance I will reach the final goal in life, which is to be happy. Next, I must say "Thank you" to my mother and father in-law, Civia Muffs Rosenberg and Irwin Rosenberg; your kind hearts are our blessing. Then, I must thank my awesome brother and sister, Gady Rones and Nurit Rones, as well as their partners, Ariella and Haim. Our times together are sometimes hard, but it is worth every minute.

I would like to thank my various teachers from the bottom of my heart. First to my Zen teacher Tzvi Harold Weisberg for the many words of wisdom that are still with me, especially, "You are time." And thank you, Dr. Yang, Jwing-Ming for the knowledge you have passed down to me. I hope you are happy and that your dream will come true. Next, I must thank Patricia Walden. You are an inspiration to my students and me.

Because a big part of this book and DVD are used in the program that I created for fibromyalgia, arthritis, and osteoarthritis of the knee research at Tufts University, I would like to thank my principle investigator, Dr. Chenchen Wang, for allowing me to design and implement my knowledge of the Eastern arts in both the osteoarthritis and fibromyalgia research we are conducting and for including, as part of the objective testing, my 'Body Markers.' I would like to also thank Dr. Timothy McAlindon, Chief, Division of Rheumatology at tufts, for having an open mind, for being an important part in making critical decisions, and for giving me and my colleagues a free hand in our quest to prove the efficacy of the Eastern philosophies, especially tai chi. Thank you to Dr. Robert Kalish, Director of Rheumatology Education at Tufts Medical Center for being our 'blind' tester and for all your years of support. Thank you to our research assistant, Judith Ramel. Keep up your smile and positive attitude.

Thank you to Dr. Herbert Benson for writing the testimonial for *Sunset Tai Chi* DVD and book. Special thanks to his colleague Dr. Ann Webster for the testimonial and for your kind soul and all your support over the last 15 years

I would like to thank Dr. Irwin Rosenberg and Dr. Ronenn Roubenoff for years of support of my work, as well as critical constructive advice for both the osteoarthritis and fibromyalgia research. Thank you, Dr. Miriam E. Nelson, for years of sharing your wisdom and continued support and a special thank you for writing me a forward for *Sunrise Ta Chi* DVD and book. I would like to thank Dr. Tamara Vesel for her support and huge heart and her profound ability to diagnose and "find the problem." She is one of a kind. Also, thank you for introducing me to our friend and colleague, Dr. Ahmet Z. Uluer. I wish all three of us good luck in our pursuit for research with cystic fibrosis.

Thank you to my colleagues at the Dana Farber Zakim Center who share my interest in researching and promoting the principles and concepts of the Eastern philosophies to complement health. First a special Thanks to Erica and Rick Kaitz on top of their constant support for sponsoring the tai chi/qigong class at Dana Farber. Thank you for promoting and supporting both my Sunrise and Sunset Tai Chi classes; Susan C., Carol K and Joyce Zakim, and Zakim Director, Dr. Carolyn Hayes. Thank you to the Medical Director, Dr. David Rosenthal, of the Zakim Center, for being willing to be my principle investigator for future Cancer research and for trying to get research going. Thank you, Dr. Elizabeth Dean-Clower, for being simple and wise, and to Susan DeCristofaro, and to Cynthia Medeiros. Thank you Dr. Paul Richardson for taking on the position of principal investigator at Dana Farber for the study comparing modified exercise and qigong. Also, thank you Dr. Ursula A. Matulonis for being my principal investigator for the 12-week pilot study with metastatic breast cancer at Dana Farber.

Thank you to Saul Wisnia and Ray Robbin from the Communication Department. Thank you to Roisin Byrne at the Lance Armstrong Foundation Adult Survivorship Clinic at Harvard for letting me and my knowledge be a part of the Survivor's Life Program. Thank you to all the students who passed through the Farber conferences, presentations, and classes, and to my present students, Julian, Howard, Beatrice, Anna, Nyanna, Susan, Judith, and Billy Joe, Ed, Elizabeth, and Michael, for your hard training and strong spirit. You are all an inspiration to me and to many others.

I must give special thanks to my humble student and friend Dr, Edward Barry for his continued patience throughout the training and for sharing his incredible knowledge while staying humble. Your open mind and strong spirit are an inspiration to me and my students. A special thank you to Ann M. Doherty-Gilman, MPH Program Manager at the Zakim center at Dana Farber, Cancer Institute, for always being positive and getting things done. I appreciate your including me in the various publications and thank you for making the Zakim Center what it is. Good luck with little Tyler Joseph Gilman and big Mark Gilman. Dreams do come true.

A special thank you, to Larry Lucchino, President and CEO, Boston Red Sox for your dedication, support and friendship. You are living proof of the success a mind body program can give you. Thank you to Stacey Lucchino for being so supportive and always having a smile and positive energy.

And a special thanks to Larry's friend and now my friend and baseball teacher, Lou Gorman, Executive Consultant to the Red Sox. Your books, *One Pitch from Glory* and *High and Inside* are very informative and eminent bestsellers. It is an honor to know you.

Thank you to Richard Slone, Reuven. You are the real wandering Jewish Taoist. Thank you, Fay Scheer, your dedication and loyalty is admirable. Thank you to Dwight Michael Evans: Dewey, first, for your great smiles, and second, for being genuine and honest, a lesson for us all. Thank you to Mike Barnacle and his wife Anne Finucane and a special thanks to my student Julia Barnacle for her warm heart and endless joy. Thank you to my dedicated students Dr. Berth Kao and Brian Avery for years of training and brainstorming. You both taught me a lot even thou I was the teacher.

Thank you Dr. Charles L. Shapiro, Professor of Medicine and Director of the Breast Medical Oncology at the Survivorship Center in Columbus, Ohio, for years of friendship and support.

Thank you Susan Kenyon and Rick Abrams, your patience and kindness set an example that only a few can achieve. Many thanks for years and years of support to Billy Star, Pan-Massachusetts Challenge (PMC) founder and executive director, and your lovely partner, Meredith Star. I am impressed and inspired by your positive out look on life. Thank you to Dr. Daniela Sever for helping with the TV program "What's the Alternative?" that airs on a channel called Veria on the Dish Network, channel 9575. Your dedication, hard work, and success are an inspiration. I want to thank this inner circle of students who are there for me whenever I need them.

Thank you Clifford Jay Snider, first for being loyal and honest, and second for designing my fabulous website, and thank you to your lovely partner Kim. I want to thank Adison Martin for years of support and for keeping it down to earth. Thank you Brian Muccio., keep up your spirit.

Thank you to my special students in Dedham, Massachusetts: Carol, Dorothy, Thelma, Mary, Janet, Virginia, Carolyn, Gerrie, Mary, Patricia, Madonna, and Doris. Your success is my joy and when hard times are around for you, it is my challenge to make a difference. Thank you for giving me this opportunity.

For all your support, I thank you Dr. Ted Kaptchuk and Dr. Cathy Kerr, Keep up the good work.

A special thank to Orla Callahan for massaging or needling us when Ilana or I needed it, and thank you for getting involved with the research at Tufts, as well as helping with your time and wisdom in other projects. And thank you to your husband and partner, Jim Callahan. Behind every woman there is a special man.

Thank you to my student and friend Stephen Holda and his partner Peg. You are both an examples of the words, practice, dedication, loyalty, and kindness. I hope this never ends. Thank you to my dear friends in France, Marc Gengoux and Brigitte Lauzat, for years of genuine help and support. Ilana and I love you both as well as your beautiful girls, Valentine and Sandrine. Valentine, we make your Raspberry Pie, at least once a month.

Thank you to my Tai Chi and Qigong colleagues. First, to Paul Mahoney, from Great

Bay Tai Chi & Yoga Center, in Amesbury, Massachusetts, for inviting me a couple of times a year for seminars, but especially for your open mind and the high-quality of students. Then, thank you to my tai chi brother and sister, Lewis and Linda Paleias, for 20 years of friendship, for Linda's beautiful and inspiring heart and paintings, and for Lewis's free sharing of his knowledge.

Many people worked numerous hours on this book. Transcribing it took 100 hours of hard work, so special thanks to Brynn Kessler with lots of appreciation for your patience and excellent work. You will make a great acupuncturist one day. And thank you to David and Ocean Silver, especially to David. Thank you for your patience and for the great profound work you do changing my Hebnish (Hebrew+English) to English and making me look good. It is sometimes said that writing a book with someone is like getting married and having a baby. This is our second baby and we are still in a great relationship. Thank you, again, for great editing and lots of patience, Susan Bullowa.

Thank you to both David Ripianzi and Leslie Takao for publishing my books. I know that you are both wearing more than one hat when it comes to my projects. Again, thank you from the bottom of my heart. Thank you to Barbara Langley for her excellent work as the YMAA publicist and for helping me promotes my publications. Thank you, Tim Comrie, for photography and layout. Thank you to Jeff Warmouth and Ellen Wetmore at MediaManic for the great job on all three DVDs. Thank you Axie Breen, first, for your kindness, and second, for your design work. Thank you for helping in so many other ways.

Thank you Stue Sigel for your support and in your belief in me I hope we can get far. Luckily we have your professional skills and not just hope. A special thank you to Rick Abrams for trying to move me to the next level in sharing my knowledge with the rest of the world good luck.

Thank you to both my older boys Stav and Yahm for helping me with spelling. Keep up the path you are taking and embarking, seeking knowledge, helping your community and staying humble, and you will get very far. You make me proud. Stav, you did an excellent job on the picture list. Thank you Gahl and Danielle for making me so soft with your sweetness and thank you for bringing me down to earth with your honesty. My wish is that this will never end.

Last, but not least, thank you to my lover and partner, Ilana Rosenberg Rones. You are living proof that love can grow stronger with time, like red wine. Thank you for the wonderful job you are doing with our four beautiful children, Stav, Yahm, Gahl, and princess Danielle. Thank you for your brainstorming, advice, proofreading, photographs, design and illustrations, and so much more. I love and cherish you.

Ramel Rones (Rami),
September 2010

Acknowledgements
by David Silver

Thanks to my Mother and Father, Charlotte and Dick, for everything, especially for their patience with the endless train of odd persons and loud music, and my extended absence while traveling. I love you both very much. Ocean, my wife and my friend since 1988, you are really real. My circle of mutant friends, artists, and musicians, you give my life meaning and purpose. Thanks to all my qigong students, from whom I have learned so much over the years, and to Paul Anastasio, Linda Preston, Valerie Twomey, Sasa Reljic, Diana Di Gioia, and Michelle Mashoke for hosting my classes. Thanks to my first Goju Ryu Sensei in the early 1980s for his excellent teaching of meditation and relaxation. Thanks to Ramel Rones for the pleasure of working together on this and various other projects. Thanks to David Ripianzi and all my friends at YMAA Publication Center. Special thanks to Master Yang, Jwing-Ming for his continued inspiration.

David Silver,
September 2010

About the Authors

Ramel 'Rami' Rones is a senior student and certified master of tai chi by renowned teacher and author Dr. Yang, Jwing-Ming, Ph.D. Rones is an award winning martial artist. From 1991 through 1993, he earned gold medals for tai chi, pushing hands, and tai chi sword at the International North American Chinese Martial Arts Competitions. He is a three-time gold medalist in Shanghai, China, at the Grand National Championships in 1994, for tai chi, external and internal weapons, and tai chi and kung fu swords.

Rones has witnessed first hand the profound long-term benefits of tai chi and qigong practice. Since 1989, he has been working to improve the lives of cancer and arthritis patients. He is a scientific consultant of mind/body therapies at Dana Farber Cancer Institute, Harvard, and Tufts Medical Schools, and Children's Hospital, all in Boston.

He actively teaches various age groups. Some he teaches how to improve their martial arts skills. Others he helps to improve the quality of their lives while aging or managing difficult health conditions. His expertise includes guidance on coping with some forms of cancers, fibromyalgia, cystic fibrosis, and various kinds of arthritis. These health and martial goals can be achieved through learning, practicing, and applying the principles and techniques taught in his books and DVDs *Sunrise Tai Chi* and *Sunset Tai Chi.*

Rones created the tai chi component of the "Secrets of Aging," a traveling exhibition for the Museums of Science that toured Boston, Columbus, Los Angeles, Fort Worth, Philadelphia, and Minneapolis between 2000 and 2004.

An active writer and an award-winning book author, Rones is also co-author of numerous scientific publications and articles on healing and the internal arts. Recent works include "Body Markers," "Tai Chi for Fibromyalgia," "Tai Chi for Osteoarthritis of the Knee," "12-Week Intervention for Prostate Cancer," "12-Week Intervention for Cystic Fibrosis."

In August of 2010, the *New England Journal of Medicine* published a report titled, "A Randomized Trial of Tai Chi for Fibromyalgia." This report documented the findings of a Tufts Medical School 12-week tai chi intervention program, developed and implemented by Rones. The tai chi forms and the mind/body programs in his published books and DVDs are used as part of other intervention programs.

Ramel Rones lives with his wife Ilana and four children, and teaches in Boston.

David Silver has been a student of the ancient Chinese art of qigong since the 1990s and became certified to carry on the teaching of qigong by Master Yang, Jwing-Ming in Boston. He works as a producer and director of instructional health and martial arts DVDs and teaches group and private qigong classes. David has also worked as editor of Dr. Yang, Jwing-Ming's qigong books and has contributed his research/writing skills to many other published materials. *Sunset Tai Chi* is his second book collaboration with Ramel Rones.

David Silver lives and teaches on Cape Cod, Massachussetts.

Also by Ramel Rones . . .

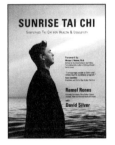

SUNRISE TAI CHI
Simplified Tai Chi for Health & Longevity
Ramel Rones, with David Silver

Based on a modern and unique teaching approach, the simplified, short Tai Chi sequence taught in this book is practiced to help you to develop symmetry and balance in your strength and flexibility. The movements will help loosen and build your muscles, tendons, and ligaments, and will improve your circulation of blood and Qi. Learn to increase the density of your bones, to massage the internal organs through movement, and to generally improve your quality of life and daily physical performance.

216 pages • 320 photos & illus.
Code: B0838 • ISBN: 978-1-886969-083-8

Companion DVD!

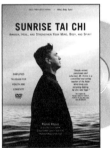

SUNRISE TAI CHI
Ramel Rones

Master-Teacher Ramel Rones gently guides you through the morning with powerful basic exercises and a simple sequence designed to awaken the senses, stimulate the mind, and fill your body and spirit with abundant energy. Created as a comprehensive introduction to a lifetime of practice, the sequence is performed on both the left and right side (for balance) and includes suggestions for intermediate and advanced students to help you grow and improve over time.

300 min. • DVD-NTSC • all regions
Code: D0274 • ISBN: 1-59439-027-4

Also by Ramel Rones . . .

Companion DVD!

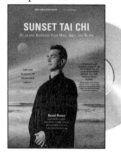

SUNSET TAI CHI
Ramel Rones

This program offers a full mind/body workout, which can be done sitting or standing. The movements in Sunset Tai Chi will help loosen and build your muscles, tendons, and ligaments, which will improve your circulation of blood and Qi energy. You'll learn to find balance between strength and flexibility, counteract the effects of stress and fatigue, and regain conscious control over health and vitality.

This DVD is designed as a companion to the book *Sunset Tai Chi.*

220 minutes • DVD-NTSC • all regions
Code: D0760 • ISBN: 978-1-59439-076-0

SKILL LEVEL
Ⓘ Ⓤ Ⓤ

TAI CHI ENERGY PATTERNS
Ramel Rones

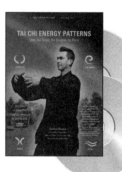

This 2-DVD set teaches essential movements and training exercises, with the focus on four popular Tai Chi Patterns: Ward Off, Rollback, Press, and Push (Peng, Lu, Ji, An). The energy circulation, mental visualizations, extensive breathing techniques, and physical skills can be applied to a deeper understanding of all Tai Chi styles. This DVD set also includes energy exchange exercises for two-person partner training, with comprehensive instruction of health and martial art applications.

385 min. • 2-DVD set • DVD-NTSC • all regions
Code: D0525 • ISBN: 978-1-59439-052-5

SKILL LEVEL
Ⓘ Ⓤ Ⓤ

BOOKS FROM YMAA

more products available from . . .

YMAA Publication Center, Inc. 楊氏東方文化出版中心

1-800-669-8892 • info@ymaa.com • www.ymaa.com

YMAA
PUBLICATION CENTER

BOOKS FROM YMAA (continued)

TAI CHI WALKING	B23X
TAIJI CHIN NA	B378
TAIJI SWORD—CLASSICAL YANG STYLE	B744
TAIJIQUAN THEORY OF DR. YANG, JWING-MING	B432
TENGU—THE MOUNTAIN GOBLIN	B1231
THE WAY OF KATA	B0584
THE WAY OF KENDO AND KENJITSU	B0029
THE WAY OF SANCHIN KATA	B0845
THE WAY TO BLACK BELT	B0852
TRADITIONAL CHINESE HEALTH SECRETS	B892
TRADITIONAL TAEKWONDO	B0665
WESTERN HERBS FOR MARTIAL ARTISTS	B1972
WILD GOOSE QIGONG	B787
WISDOM'S WAY	B361
XINGYIQUAN, 2ND ED.	B416

DVDS FROM YMAA

ADVANCED PRACTICAL CHIN NA IN-DEPTH	D1224
ANALYSIS OF SHAOLIN CHIN NA	D0231
BAGUAZHANG 1, 2, & 3—EMEI BAGUAZHANG	D0649
CHEN STYLE TAIJIQUAN	D0819
CHIN NA IN-DEPTH COURSES 1—4	D602
CHIN NA IN-DEPTH COURSES 5—8	D610
CHIN NA IN-DEPTH COURSES 9—12	D629
EIGHT SIMPLE QIGONG EXERCISES FOR HEALTH	D0037
ESSENCE OF TAIJI QIGONG	D0215
FIVE ANIMAL SPORTS	D1106
KUNG FU BODY CONDITIONING	D2085
KUNG FU FOR KIDS	D1880
NORTHERN SHAOLIN SWORD —SAN CAI JIAN, KUN WU JIAN, QI MEN JIAN	D1194
QIGONG MASSAGE	D0592
QIGONG FOR LONGEVITY	D2092
SABER FUNDAMENTAL TRAINING	D1088
SANCHIN KATA—TRADITIONAL TRAINING FOR KARATE POWER	D1897
SHAOLIN KUNG FU FUNDAMENTAL TRAINING—COURSES 1 & 2	D0436
SHAOLIN LONG FIST KUNG FU—BASIC SEQUENCES	D661
SHAOLIN LONG FIST KUNG FU—INTERMEDIATE SEQUENCES	D1071
SHAOLIN LONG FIST KUNG FU—ADVANCED SEQUENCES	D2061
SHAOLIN SABER—BASIC SEQUENCES	D0616
SHAOLIN STAFF—BASIC SEQUENCES	D0920
SHAOLIN WHITE CRANE GONG FU BASIC TRAINING—COURSES 1 & 2	D599
SHAOLIN WHITE CRANE GONG FU BASIC TRAINING—COURSES 3 & 4	D0784
SHUAI JIAO—KUNG FU WRESTLING	D1149
SIMPLE QIGONG EXERCISES FOR ARTHRITIS RELIEF	D0890
SIMPLE QIGONG EXERCISES FOR BACK PAIN RELIEF	D0883
SIMPLIFIED TAI CHI CHUAN—24 & 48 POSTURES	D0630
SUNRISE TAI CHI	D0274
SUNSET TAI CHI	D0760
SWORD—FUNDAMENTAL TRAINING	D1095
TAI CHI CONNECTIONS	D0444
TAI CHI ENERGY PATTERNS	D0525
TAI CHI FIGHTING SET	D0509
TAIJI BALL QIGONG—COURSES 1 & 2	D0517
TAIJI BALL QIGONG—COURSES 3 & 4	D0777
TAIJI CHIN NA—COURSES 1, 2, 3, & 4	D0463
TAIJI MARTIAL APPLICATIONS—37 POSTURES	D1057
TAIJI PUSHING HANDS—COURSES 1 & 2	D0495
TAIJI PUSHING HANDS—COURSES 3 & 4	D0681
TAIJI WRESTLING	D1064
TAIJI SABER	D1026
TAIJI & SHAOLIN STAFF—FUNDAMENTAL TRAINING	D0906
TAIJI YIN YANG STICKING HANDS	D1040
TAI CHI CHUAN CLASSICAL YANG STYLE	D645
TAIJI SWORD—CLASSICAL YANG STYLE	D0452
UNDERSTANDING QIGONG 1—WHAT IS QI? • HUMAN QI CIRCULATORY SYSTEM	D069X
UNDERSTANDING QIGONG 2—KEY POINTS • QIGONG BREATHING	D0418
UNDERSTANDING QIGONG 3—EMBRYONIC BREATHING	D0555
UNDERSTANDING QIGONG 4—FOUR SEASONS QIGONG	D0562
UNDERSTANDING QIGONG 5—SMALL CIRCULATION	D0753
UNDERSTANDING QIGONG 6—MARTIAL QIGONG BREATHING	D0913
WHITE CRANE HARD & SOFT QIGONG	D637
WUDANG SWORD	D1903
WUDANG KUNG FU—FUNDAMENTAL TRAINING	D1316
WUDANG TAIJIQUAN	D1217
XINGYIQUAN	D1200
YMAA 25 YEAR ANNIVERSARY DVD	D0708

more products available from...

YMAA Publication Center, Inc. 楊氏東方文化出版中心
1-800-669-8892 • info@ymaa.com • www.ymaa.com

PAULINE HAASS PUBLIC LIBRARY
N64 W23820 MAIN STREET
SUSSEX, WISCONSIN 53089
(262) 246-5180

9/11